Theory and History in the Human and Social Sciences

Series Editor

Jaan Valsiner, Department of Communication and Psychology
Aalborg University
Aalborg, Denmark

Theory and History in the Human and Social Sciences fills the gap in the existing coverage of links between new theoretical advancements in the social and human sciences and their historical roots. Making that linkage is crucial for interdisciplinary synthesis across the disciplines of psychology, anthropology, sociology, history, semiotics, and the political sciences. In contemporary human sciences of the 21st century, there exists increasing differentiation between neurosciences and all other sciences that are aimed at making sense of complex social, psychological, and political processes. This series serves the purpose of (1) coordinating such efforts across the borders of existing human and social sciences, (2) providing an arena for possible inter-disciplinary theoretical synthesis, (3) bringing to the attention of our contemporary scientific community innovative ideas that have been lost in the dustbin of history for no good reason, and (4) providing an arena for international communication between social and human scientists across the world.

Gerhart Zeller • Eric J. Engstrom
German E. Berrios

A History of Unitary Psychosis

A Contribution to the Historical Epistemology of Nineteenth Century Psychiatry

Springer

Gerhart Zeller (Deceased)
Berlin, Germany

German E. Berrios
Emeritus Professor for the Epistemology of Psychiatry
Robinson College, University of Cambridge
Cambridge, UK

Eric J. Engstrom
Department of History
Humboldt University
Berlin, Germany

ISSN 2523-8663 ISSN 2523-8671 (electronic)
Theory and History in the Human and Social Sciences
ISBN 978-3-031-90181-2 ISBN 978-3-031-90182-9 (eBook)
https://doi.org/10.1007/978-3-031-90182-9

This Springer imprint is published by the registered company Springer Nature Switzerland AG
The registered company address is: Gewerbestrasse 11, 6330 Cham, Switzerland

Acknowledgments

Support in saving this manuscript from oblivion has been forthcoming from numerous quarters.

Several individuals assisted in finding copies of the typescript. At the Institute for Ethics and History of Medicine in Tübingen, Libuše Rammerstorfer kindly located and reproduced one copy. In Paris, Luigi Grosso generously placed his copy of the manuscript at the disposal of the editors. Dr. Günther Bittel (Duisburg) and Alexander Zahoransky (Freiburg) were also involved in the search.

From the project's inception, Thomas Müller (Ulm), head of the Research Unit for the History of Medicine at the University Clinic of Psychiatry and Psychotherapy and director of the Württemberg Museum of Psychiatry, advised the project, helped garner support for it, and assisted in the final stages of editing. Albrecht Hirschmüller (Tübingen) and Alexander Ananyev (Tübingen) assisted in clarifying the evolution of psychiatric associations in Württemberg. Julia Lieth (Berlin) and Anja Laukötter (Jena) helped locate secondary literature on Friedrich Schleiermacher. Drs. Thomas Götz and Möllhoff-Mylius from Berlin's municipal Department of Science, Health, and Welfare, were engaging interlocutors on Swabian culture.

The project profited especially from the interest and encouragement of numerous members of the Die Brücke e.V. in Berlin, a non-profit organization devoted to extramural care and support for former psychiatric patients: Rüdiger Pfarr, Kurt Tautenhahn, Dagmar Giesen, and Karl Kreutzberg all helped sustain the work at critical junctures. Members of the Zeller family in Berlin, Prof. Ulrich Zeller and Frau Prof. Brigitte Zeller, were likewise consistently supportive.

Archivists and special collection librarians also provided assistance. Wiebke Gröbel-Uhlig and her colleagues at the Handschriften-Abteilung at the Staatsbibliothek in Berlin helped comb through the cryptic finding aids of the Georg Andreas Reimer papers. At the University Archives in Tübingen Dr. Regina Keyler helped navigate the no less labyrinthine papers of Ernst Kretschmer. Drs. Carla Lessing and Matthias Klein of the Archiv des Landschaftsverbandes Rheinland (Pulheim-Brauwieler) assisted with the Jacobi-Zeller correspondence.

At Springer, the patience and support of Catherine Thoms helped guide the manuscript into production.

Generous financial and editorial assistance for the project was forthcoming from Die Brücke e.V. and the Gerhart Zeller Foundation (Berlin), Arkade e.V. (Ravensburg), the Werner-Zeller-Foundation (Leonberg), and the Württemberg Museum of Psychiatry (Ulm).

DIE BRÜCKE
DIE BRÜCKE – Dr. Gerhart Zeller Stiftung

arkade

arkade

Württembergisches
Psychiatriemuseum

EXTINCTA REVIVISCO.

Werner-Zeller-Stiftung
Stiftung für gesellschaftsbezogene Familienforschung
Seedammstraße 1 71229 Leonberg

Declaration of Competing Interests The editors have no conflicts of interest to declare that are relevant to the content of this book.

Contents

About the Authors

Gerhart Zeller (1922–2006) was a German psychiatrist who trained under Ernst Kretschmer at the University of Tübingen in the 1950s. After 1962 he worked as chief physician at the Landesnervenklinik in Spandau near Berlin. He was responsible for establishing the neuropsychiatric ward in the nearby Havelhöhe, Hospital, which he then headed until his retirement. In 1975 he established the patient-aid association *Die Brücke*, which to this day works to bridge the gap between hospitals and local communities by providing extramural housing and psychosocial services to chronically ill patients. During the 1980s, Zeller was intimately involved in the implementation of reforms to the psychiatric infrastructure in Berlin and was a member of the federal Ministry of Health's Advisory Board on Psychiatric Reforms.

Eric J. Engstrom is an historian of psychiatry and a research associate in the Department of History at the Humboldt University in Berlin. He received his BA from Lewis and Clark College in Portland, OR, his MA from the Ludwig-Maximilians-Universität in Munich, and his Ph.D. (in History) from the University of North Carolina at Chapel Hill. He has published widely in the history of psychiatry, including a monograph on *Clinical Psychiatry in Imperial Germany* with Cornell University Press. He has been a member of the working group on the "History of Psychiatry" at the Max-Planck-Institute for Psychiatry in Munich, co-editor of the 9 volume edition of Emil Kraepelin's correspondence, and a lead member of the German Research Foundation (DFG) research group "Cultures of Madness (1870–1930)". He is editor of the journal *History of Psychiatry* and currently researching and writing a book on the history of psychiatric governance in Imperial Berlin, 1880–1914. His full CV can be found online at www.engstrom.de

German E. Berrios is emeritus professor of the epistemology of psychiatry at the University of Cambridge and a Life-Fellow of Robinson College. He has published widely on neuropsychiatry and on conceptual and historical aspects of psychopathology. He is the author of numerous books, including *A History of Clinical Psychiatry* (with Roy Porter) and *The History of Mental Symptoms: Descriptive Psychopathology since the 19th Century*. He has been chairman of the History of Psychiatry Section of the World Psychiatric Association, and was founding editor of the journal *History of Psychiatry*.

Chapter 1
A History of Unitary Psychosis: A Contribution to the Historical Epistemology of Nineteenth-Century Psychiatry

Eric J. Engstrom and German E. Berrios

Editors' Introduction: Threefold Temporality

This monograph is the publication of a book-length typescript (and an abridged English translation of it) written by the German psychiatrist Gerhart Zeller (1922–2006) in 1959/1960. The typescript was awarded a prize by the Association of Southwest German Neurologists and Psychiatrists for the best contribution on the theme "History of Unitary Psychosis." However, until now it had never found its way into print. The book is in part an intellectual biography of the author's great grandfather and first director of the Winnenthal asylum in the southwest German Dutchy of Württemberg, Albert Zeller (1804–1877). It examines the personal experiences as well as the cultural and scientific influences that shaped Albert Zeller, who is commonly described as having been the first author to articulate the doctrine of unitary psychosis. At the same time, however, the book is more than just a biography: it is also the only existing synthetic narrative of the early history of unitary psychosis.

Publishing such a dated historical monograph is beyond unusual and begs explanation. Certainly, readers accustomed to today's research standards will find plenty to criticize about Zeller's rendering of the nineteenth-century history of unitary psychosis. Nevertheless, there are real merits to be had from its publication. Like newly discovered source material, newly discovered historical monographs can also contribute unexpected insights. For one, the author's *intermediate perspective* from the late 1950s, at once distant from our own contemporary research priorities but also more proximate to the events and themes that informed nineteenth-century alienist culture, forces us to think more critically about the evolution of psychiatric concepts and how they are incorporated into historical narratives. In this vein, it is precisely *also* the text's obscure references and putative non-sequiturs that make the document valuable and have the potential to challenge higher-order historiographic conventions and stock narratives.

G. Zeller et al., *A History of Unitary Psychosis*, Theory and History in the Human and Social Sciences, https://doi.org/10.1007/978-3-031-90182-9_1

As this observation suggests, interacting with this historical document involves an engagement with its threefold temporality. The text is first and foremost a study about nineteenth-century psychiatric nosology, specifically about the notion of unitary psychosis which came to dominate alienist theorizing and practice from the 1830s onward. But it is also a work of historical scholarship written in the late 1950s, shortly after the catastrophe of World War II and the Holocaust, just as German psychiatry was beginning to reassess its fraught historical legacy. And finally, it is simultaneously also a text to be read and evaluated in the third decade of the twenty-first century, toward the end of a Neo-Kraepelinian era, at a moment when the assumptions and promises of biological psychiatry are no longer able to command and organize professional loyalties to the degree they once did.

This document is being published in hopes that it can contribute to research in each of these temporal frames. Consider therefore the respective significance of each of the overlain temporalities.

Nineteenth-Century Unitary Psychosis and Its Historiography

In his 1887 inaugural lecture at the University of Dorpat, the renowned German clinical psychiatrist Emil Kraepelin (1856–1926) delivered a cutting critique of mid-nineteenth-century psychiatric nosology:

> [T]here is one doctrine that deserves special mention as a fruit of clinical speculation—a doctrine in which [Albert] Zeller first consolidated his views on disease course. As is well known, Zeller argued that all the different forms of mental illness that had previously been distinguished from one another were really only different phases of one and the same pathological process. That process could lead to recovery from various different phases of its course. The necessary consequence of this dogmatic viewpoint, which Griesinger still used as the basis for the last edition of his textbook, was the adulteration and distortion [*Verkünstelung*] of actual observations and hence the stagnation of clinical research. The initial phase of melancholy and the subsequent phase of excitation were, because Zeller's theory demanded it, read into the casuistic accounts, even where there was absolutely no evidence to support them. Consequently, a great number of well-defined forms of illness that did not fit into the adopted system remained invisible to this biased view.[1]

The doctrine that Kraepelin pejoratively associated with Albert Zeller soon came to be labeled as "unitary psychosis" [*Einheitspsychose*].[2] To Kraepelin and many of

[1] Emil Kraepelin, *Die Richtungen der psychiatrischen Forschung: Vortrag, gehalten bei der Übernahme des Lehramtes an der kaiserlichen Universität Dorpat* (Leipzig: Vogel, 1887), 16–17, reprinted in Eric J. Engstrom and Matthias M. Weber, "The Directions of Psychiatric Research by Emil Kraepelin 1887," *History of Psychiatry* 16.3 (2005): 357–358. Cf. also [Heinrich] Kreuser, "Zu Albert Zellers Gedächtnis," *Medicinisches Correspondenz-Blatt des Würtembergischen Ärztlichen Vereins* 74.45 (1904): 938.

[2] Karl Jaspers (1883–1969) appears to have coined the term in 1913. See Karl Jaspers, *Allgemeine Psychopathologie: Ein Leitfaden für Studierende, Ärzte und Psychologen* (Berlin: Springer, 1913), 257.

his acolytes, the doctrine stood for an outdated and empirically debunked alienist tradition that was antithetical to the new science of clinical psychiatry. As such, it has ever since served as a useful foil in historical narratives of psychiatry's progressive medicalization and modernization. In 1928 the Berlin-based psychiatrist Karl Birnbaum (1878–1950) lamented that the "dogma of unitary psychosis … had long dominated psychiatry, and not always to its advantage." And in 1954 Wolfgang de Boor (1917–2014) associated it with a "preclinical era" of taxonomic "stagnation."[3] And yet at the same time, as Birnbaum conceded, it was out of this very doctrine that Kraepelin's own "clinical approach" evolved.[4] Several subsequent studies have adopted Kraepelin's perfunctory dismissal of unitary psychosis, devoting scant attention to it. The wellsprings of the doctrine and its enormous impact have, until now, never been the object of sustained historical analysis.[5]

A good part of Gerhart Zeller's own research agenda involved reassessing the conventional narrative that Kraepelin had established and correcting what he considered to be its distortions. He sought to recover historical contexts that had been nearly forgotten, even including the importance of Pietism with its emphasis on the spiritual underpinnings of mental anguish. Furthermore, he cautioned that most historical accounts had overstated the influence of the famous Belgian alienist Joseph

[3] Wolfgang de Boor, *Psychiatrische Systematik: Ihre Entwicklung in Deutschland seit Kahlbaum* (Berlin: Springer, 1954), 4.

[4] Karl Birnbaum, "Geschichte der psychiatrischen Wissenschaft," in *Handbuch der Geisteskrankheiten*, edited by Oswald Bumke, vol. 1 (Berlin: Springer, 1928), 11–49. Awareness of Zeller's significance remained palpable in the early twentieth century. By one account, his clinical views had for decades influenced alienists, who modeled their practice on his and Griesinger's work in Winnenthal in the 1840s. See Heinrich Kreuser, "Geschichtlicher Überblick über die Entwicklung des Irrenwesens in Württemberg," *Medicinisches Correspondenz-Blatt des Würtembergischen Ärztlichen Vereins* 72 (1902): 752. In the Dutchy of Württemburg, Zeller's influence was especially pronounced. See Ioannis Pilavas, *Psychiatrie im Widerstreit der Konzepte: Zur Entstehungsgeschichte der Tübinger Nervenklinik* (Sigmaringen: Jan Thorbecke, 1994), 11, 57 footnote 158.

[5] Werner Leibbrand and Annemarie Wettley, *Der Wahnsinn: Geschichte der abendländischen Psychopathologie* (Munich: Karl Albers, 1961; reprint, 2005), are largely silent about unitary psychosis, as are Burkhart Brückner, *Delirium und Wahn: Geschichte, Selbstzeugnisse und Theorien von der Antike bis 1900*, 2 vols. (Hürtgenwald: Pressler, 2007) and Heinz Schott and Rainer Tölle, *Geschichte der Psychiatrie: Krankheitslehren, Irrwege, Behandlungsformen* (Munich: Beck, 2006), 332, 571. Even Bernd Wengler, *Das Menschenbild bei Alfred Adler, Wilhelm Griesinger und Rudolf Virchow: Ursprünge eines ganzheitlichen Paradigmas in der Medizin* (Frankfurt/M: Campus, 1989), 63–64, mentions Zeller and unitary psychosis only in passing. An exception to the rule is Bernhard Pauleikhoff, *Das Menschenbild im Wandel der Zeit: Ideengeschichte der Psychiatrie und der klinischen Psychologie*, vol. 2 (Hürtgenwald: Guido Pressler, 1983), 271–278, who argues that the notion of a unitary psychosis could be traced back to antiquity and had lost none of its contemporary relevance by the end of the twentieth century. In explaining its persistence as a psychiatric conundrum (a "Sphinx," a "Riddle" (277)), he maintained that it was fundamentally about the "essence of the soul" (276) or more specifically the soul's indivisibility. But since Griesinger, efforts to redefine psychiatry as an empirical, natural science had driven the discipline ever deeper into the arms of "speculative materialism" (277). This had "blinded" psychiatry and "blocked" understanding of the unique questions and problems that unitary psychosis sought to address.

Guislain (1797–1860). While these accounts tended to chart a direct lineage from Guislain to Zeller to Wilhelm Griesinger (1817–1868), Gerhart Zeller pointed especially to Guislain's emphasis on psychogenetic etiology and his Gallist focus on the brain as points of stark divergence. Instead of reinforcing this cerebral Belgian lineage, Zeller sought to define a distinctively "Swabian" school of psychiatry centered around scholars working at the university in Tübingen. Specifically, that school traced its roots back from Griesinger through Albert Zeller to J. H. F. Autenrieth (1772–1835). Its basic tenets were that all forms of mental illness were related, often like links in a chain; that *both* mental and somatic causes were prerequisites of psychiatric illness; and that a strict institutional distinction needed to be drawn between therapeutic and nursing care.[6] Zeller cited the influence of Autenrieth and his school as evidence that psychiatry's evolution could not be reduced to scientific discoveries or technical innovations but instead also had to incorporate the influence of Swabian—and more generally German—intellectual contexts.[7]

Beyond Zeller's own aims, as a work of historical scholarship the monograph can still complement and contribute substantively to more recent studies on the history of unitary psychosis. Earlier researchers, although relying in part on Gerhart Zeller's unpublished typescript, radically purged most of the specific historical and

[6] See Gerhart Zeller, "Welcher psychiatrischen Schule hat Wilhelm Griesinger angehört?" *Deutsches Medizinisches Journal* 19 (1968): 331; idem, "Bonhoeffers wissenschaftliches Werk. Entwicklung und Bedeutung," in *Karl Bonhoeffer: Zum hundertsten Geburtstag am 31. März 1968*, edited by Jürg Zutt, Erwin Straus, and H. Scheller (Berlin: Springer, 1969), 121–122; idem, "Die Tübinger Psychiater-Schule," in *Wahn*, edited by Walter Schulte and Rainer Tölle (Stuttgart: Georg Thieme, 1972), 101. Zeller interpreted Ernst Siemerling (1857–1931) and Robert Wollenburg (1862–1942) as neuropsychiatric deviations from this tradition. See ibid., 96.

[7] See Zeller, "Bonhoeffers wissenschaftliches Werk," 122. Zeller touches on this point again in his later publications. On what constituted a specifically Swabian school of psychiatry, he cited Pietist influences on Romanticism and an approach that "places greater emphasis on emotions than on intellect, on transitions than on divisive boundaries, and one that never doubts the unity of body and soul." Zeller, "Die Tübinger Psychiater-Schule," 103. Zeller's account of a culturally inflected psychiatric tradition sits awkwardly alongside the generally neuropsychiatric picture painted in Hanns Ruffin's history of the Association of Southwest German Neurologists and Psychiatrists. See Hanns Ruffin, "Rückblick auf die Geschichte der Wanderversammlung Südwestdeutscher Neurologen und Psychiater," *Deutsche Zeitschrift für Nervenheilkunde* 172.2 (1954): 111–27. However it confirms conclusions drawn from more recent historical analysis, which has underscored the enduring influence of "regional and local communities" prior to German unification in 1870/71. Jürgen Kocka, *Kampf um die Moderne: Das lange 19. Jahrhundert in Deutschland* (Bonn: Bundeszentrale für politische Bildung, 2022), 69. And it also aligns with Anne Harrington's argument that, in the twentieth century, "German holistic science" became so influential because scientists "found ways to craft their most certain truths out of words and images rich with cultural resonances, thus enabling those truths to function in culturally meaningful ways." Anne Harrington, *Reenchanted Science: Holism in German Culture from Wilhelm II to Hitler* (Princeton: Princeton University Press, 1996), 208. This argument has also been made in relation to Kretschmer. See Steffen Dörre, *Zwischen NS- 'Euthanasie' und Reformaufbruch: die psychiatrischen Fachgesellschaften im geteilten Deutschland* (Berlin: Springer, 2021), 69.

personal contexts in which the concept of unitary psychosis evolved.[8] Existing studies also tended to focus narrowly on Wilhelm Griesinger's easily accessible textbook *The Pathology and Therapy of Mental Illnesses*, paying scant or no attention to the impact of significant, albeit more obscure contemporary figures like Autenrieth, Maximilian Jacobi (1775–1858), Albert Zeller, or Joseph Guislain.[9] An otherwise exemplary study of nineteenth-century anthropological psychiatry is written from a philosophical perspective that downplays the impact of Romanticism and religion on early psychiatric nosology.[10] Gerhart Zeller's narrative corrects these deficits, engaging a wider *dramatis personae* and reintroducing important historical contexts and contingencies. It furthermore situates itself in relation to the larger historical transition from Romanticism to Naturalism (i.e., in relation to the era of so-called *Biedermeiermedizin*) that comprised an essential backdrop to the rise of Kraepelinian psychiatry.[11] Along a threshold extending from about 1830 to 1850, this era's practitioners were enthusiastically empirical and descriptive, they showed an aversion to heroic therapies, and they were decidedly wary of the speculative flights of natural philosophy and Romanticism. Elucidating these historical contexts and trajectories must be an important prerequisite for any more comprehensive study of the epistemology of nineteenth-century psychiatry.

More generally, while historical biographies may have gone out of fashion, they remain important portals that open onto personal experiences and subjectivities. For example, one of the striking claims advanced in this monograph disputes the conventional explanations used to differentiate psychological and somatic schools of thought (so-called *Psychiker* vs. *Somatiker*), for it insists that the difference was in good part a consequence of alienists' own *personal experiences*. This self-reflexive, experiential dimension has often been elided from historical analyses. Just as the history of psychiatry has too often lost sight of the personal experiences of patients, so too has it tended to discount or underestimate the personal experiences and emotions of psychiatrists themselves. Zeller's text enables us to reflect more meaningfully about cross-currents in various domains of subjectivity (biographic, nosologic, historiographic). As such, and throughout these domains, it can also contribute to greater awareness of the importance of emotions in biomedical and psychiatric historiography.[12]

[8] See Josef Vliegen, *Die Einheitspsychose: Geschichte und Problem* (Stuttgart: Enke, 1980).

[9] See Maurício Viotti Daker, *The Continuum of Mental Disorders and Unitary Psychosis: History and Perspectives* (Newcastle on Tyne: Cambridge Scholars Publishing, 2021).

[10] See Gerlof Verwey, *Psychiatry in an Anthropological and Biomedical Context: Philosophical Presuppositions and Implications of German Psychiatry, 1820–1870* (Dordrecht: Reidel, 1985). For another study that omits Albert Zeller, see Udo Benzenhöfer, *Psychiatrie und Anthropologie in der ersten Hälfte des 19. Jahrhunderts* (Hürtgenwald: Pressler, 1993).

[11] See Johanna Bleker, "Biedermeiermedizin: Medizin der Biedermeier? Tendenzen, Probleme, Widersprüche," *Medizinhistorisches Journal* 23.1/2 (1988): 5–22.

[12] See Otniel E. Dror, Bettina Hitzer, Anja Laukötter, and Pilar León-Sanz, eds. *History of Science and the Emotions* (Chicago: University of Chicago Press, 2016).

Finally, the text also helps counter a tradition that has often indulged in the casual expunging of religious sentiments from nineteenth-century psychiatric historiography. Certainly, many older asylum histories have dealt extensively with religious themes. But in recent decades it has become apparent that historians of science have tended to downplay the broader religious and humanistic agendas that frequently informed the work of nineteenth-century alienists. Largely elided post hoc, in the wake of psychiatry's evolution toward medical science, there remains an inadequately charted realm of religious experience that suffused alienist culture. Paying greater attention to this realm, as Zeller's account does, can enrich our understanding of the early history of unitary psychosis and help rectify some of the "epistemic injustices" that have come with the blithe adoption of latter nineteenth-century scientistic narratives.[13]

Twentieth-Century Contexts of Unitary Psychosis

To fully understand Gerhart Zeller's own discontents, and to unpack the wider historiographic potential of the manuscript, it is worth examining more closely the context in which the manuscript was written. As a historical document crafted in post-World War II Germany, Zeller's account helps us examine efforts by psychiatrists to revamp the historical legitimacy of their profession in the wake of the Holocaust and the complicity of medical professionals in implementing the biopolitical policies of the National Socialist regime.

The author, Gerhart Zeller, was born in Stuttgart on July 4, 1922. Straight out of high school, he entered German military service in the summer of 1940. He served as junior noncommissioned officer in the reserve medical corps and began studying medicine in Giessen before he was eventually captured and held in British custody.[14] Upon release and after briefly working as an orthopedic nurse in Stuttgart, he resumed his medical studies in Tübingen.[15] Drawing on evaluations of the records of nearly 2600 schizophrenic patients treated at the Württemberg Asylum in Winnenthal, Zeller completing his dissertation on "Birth-Month and Age at Onset

[13] Gordana Jovanović, "How Psychology Repressed Its Founding Father Wilhelm Wundt," *Human Arenas* 4 (2021): 36. On efforts to recover Wilhelm Griesinger's fuller scientific persona, see also Gerlof Verwey, *Wilhelm Griesinger: Psychiatrie als ärztlicher Humanismus* (Nijmegen: Arts & Boeve, 2004).

[14] Zeller had been a member of the *Deutsche Jungvolk* and the *Hitlerjugend*. He was released from British custody under an amnesty order in August of 1946. See "Antrag auf ein Studienplatz," February 22, 1947, and "Personalbogen Georg Andreas Gerhart Zeller," April 22, 1954, 695/39197 and 155/6069, respectively, University Archive Tübingen.

[15] On the medical faculty in Tübingen under French occupation after World War II, see Bernd Grün, "Schuld und Sichtweise: Versuch einer Kategorisierung der 'Entnazifizierung' am Beispiel der Tübinger medizinischen Fakultät," in *Vergangenheitspolitik in der universitären Medizin nach 1945: institutionelle und individuelle Strategien im Umgang mit dem Nationalsozialismus*, edited by Sigrid Oehler-Klein and Volker Roelcke (Stuttgart: Steiner, 2007), 277–304.

of Schizophrenics and their Biological Meaning" in 1951.[16] In October of 1952, on the strength of his dissertation, he began working under the influential postwar psychiatrist Ernst Kretschmer (1888–1964) at the university hospital in Tübingen, where he remained through April 1959.[17] Thereafter he worked briefly on a ward for internal medicine at the municipal hospital in Esslingen and an asylum in Landau before moving to Berlin, where the remainder of his career unfolded, first as senior physician at the State Psychiatric Hospital in Spandau and from 1974 until his retirement as head of the neuropsychiatric section of the general hospital in Havelhöhe.

Shortly after Gerhart Zeller's tenure in Tübingen had ended, the regional Association of Southwest German Neurologists and Psychiatrists issued a call for manuscript submissions on the theme "History of Unitary Psychosis." The call was associated with a prize of 1000 marks, to be awarded by a jury comprised of the directors of the university psychiatric hospitals in Tübingen, Freiburg, and Heidelberg, respectively, Ernst Kretschmer, Hanns Ruffin (1902–1979), and Walter Ritter von Baeyer (1904–1987). Zeller was announced as the winner of the prize in July of 1961.

The impetus behind the choice of topic is unclear. It may well have been tailored to suit Gerhart Zeller, supporting the early career of a young psychiatrist from southwest Germany and one of Kretschmer's own students. Or perhaps it was the postwar inadequacies of existing diagnostic categories that "forced" the Association to embark on a historical reevaluation of psychiatric nosologies.[18] Indeed, according to one assessment of the diagnostic quandaries facing German psychiatrists in the 1950s, psychiatric diagnosis was bereft of the analytical tools needed to verify its results and could in no way be described as scientific.[19]

Whatever the reason, the Association and the jurors seem to have had an interest in engaging with the historical legacy of their profession, albeit not its deeply fraught immediate past but instead its nineteenth-century roots. For example, in a

---

[16] See Kretschmer and Mall to Medizinische Fakultät der Universität Tübingen, July 27, 1951, 125/254,223, University Archive Tübingen. The issues examined in Zeller's dissertation echo throughout Kretschmer's earlier work on marriage hygiene. See Ernst Kretschmer, *Mensch und Lebensgrund: Gesammelte Aufsätze* (Tübingen: Rainer Wunderlich Verlag, 1966), 117–144, and Esther Krähwinkel, "Formen der Umsetzung des 'Gesetzes zur Verhütung erbkranken Nachwuchses' an der Marburger Medizinischen Fakultät." *Medizinhistorisches Journal* 34.2 (1999): 159–209.

[17] See the recommendation of Kretschmer to Akademische Rektoramt, March 14, 1958, 155/6069, University Archive Tübingen.

[18] Günther Bittel, "Entwicklung und Wirkung der Heilanstalt Winnental: Zur Anwendung der historischen Methode in der Psychiatrie," Medical Dissertation, Albert-Ludwigs-Universität Freiburg, 1980, 101–102. Cf. also Werner Janzarik, "Nosographie und Einheitspsychose," in *Schizophrenie und Zyklothymie: Ergebnisse und Probleme*, edited by Gerd Huber (Stuttgart: Thieme Verlag, 1969), 30.

[19] See K[laus] Conrad, "Das Problem der 'nosologischen Einheit' in der Psychiatrie," *Der Nervenarzt* 30.11 (1959): 494. Cf. also Nicolas Henckes and Lara Rzesnitzek, "Performing Doubt and Negociating Uncertainty: Diagnosing Schizophrenia at its Onset in Post-War German Psychiatry," *History of the Human Sciences* 31.2 (2018): 65–87.

review of the Association's history published in 1954, Hanns Ruffin had underscored the importance of historical research. Ruffin made only oblique reference to the Nazi era, conceding merely that the Association's purportedly "liberal spirit" had encountered real limits.[20] He believed, however, that historical retrospectives could help provide the Association with a "new sense of purpose."[21] He also hoped to build on the work of earlier, nineteenth-century neuropsychiatric "paragons" like Wilhelm Griesinger, Carl Ludwig (1816–1895), and Wilhelm Erb (1840–1921) and now help reinforce "awareness of larger biological and anthropological relationships."[22]

Ruffin's reference to "larger biological and anthropological" relationships is worth special note for what it suggests about the contemporary context in which Zeller produced his manuscript. From its inception in 1876, the Association had represented a platform for academic neuropsychiatrists working to distance themselves from the supposedly more mundane concerns of alienist practitioners. However, under the Nazi regime, such professional rivalries had been mostly papered over by the policy of *Gleichschaltung*.[23] In the postwar era, Ruffin and his colleagues now sought to reconcile these two long-standing biological and anthropological traditions with the aid of historical research. Gerhart Zeller's manuscript, it would seem, served these ends.

The manuscript also resonated with a larger turn toward medical anthropology after World War II. The founder of the so-called Heidelberg School, Viktor von Weizsäcker (1886-1957), sought to reorient medical science around patients' subjective experiences and biographies.[24] The members of the Association's jury shared many of von Weizsäcker's views, advocating holistic, anthropological, and psychotherapeutic approaches to psychiatric practice. Ruffin had been a student of von Weizsäcker in Heidelberg and later came to head the General Medical Society for Psychotherapy. Walter Ritter von Baeyer was instrumental during his tenure as

---

[20] For an overview of how medical professionals sought to come to terms (or not) with their complicity in the genocidal policies of the Nazi regime, see Sigrid Oehler-Klein and Volker Roelcke, *Vergangenheitspolitik in der universitären Medizin nach 1945: institutionelle und individuelle Strategien im Umgang mit dem Nationalsozialismus* (Stuttgart: Steiner, 2007). On the specific situation in Tübingen, see therein Grün.

[21] Ruffin, 127.

[22] Ibid.

[23] On these efforts more generally, see Hans-Walter Schmuhl, *Die Gesellschaft Deutscher Neurologen und Psychiater im Nationalsozialismus* (Berlin: Springer, 2016), and Aaron Pfaff, *Geschichte der verfassten Ärzteschaft auf dem Gebiet des heutigen Bundeslandes Baden-Württemberg von 1920 bis 1960* (Stuttgart: Franz Steiner Verlag, 2024). On the Nazi's "euthanasia" practices in southwest Germany, see Hermann J. Pretsch, *'Euthanasie': Krankenmord in Südwestdeutschland* (Zwiefalten: Verlag Psychiatrie und Geschichte, 1996). On the history of psychiatric professional organizations in Germany after World War II, see Dörre.

[24] See Viktor Freiherr von Weizsäcker, *Grundfragen medizinischer Anthropologie* (Tübingen: Furche Verlag, 1948). On Weizsäcker's ambiguous legacy, see Harrington, 200–206, and Alexa Geisthövel, "Viktor von Weizsäcker oder die 'monumentale Unruhe' einer subjektiven Medizin," in *Auf der Suche nach einer anderen Medizin: Psychosomatik im 20. Jahrhundert*, edited by Alexa Geisthövel and Bettina Hitzer (Berlin: Suhrkamp, 2018), 144–53.

professor of psychiatry in Heidelberg in promoting psychosomatic and psychosocial practices and pioneering anthropologically oriented research on the traumatic impact of political persecution under the Nazis.[25] And two of von Baeyer's students, Heinz Häfner (1926–1922) and Karl-Peter Kisker (1926–1997), became key architects of major reforms of psychiatric care during the 1960s and 1970s.

But it was undoubtedly Ernst Kretschmer who had the greatest impact on Zeller's early career. A fellow Swabian, Kretschmer too had cut his teeth in clinical psychiatry working at the Winnenthal asylum.[26] His affinity with the doctrine of unitary psychosis dated back to his research on constitutional body types and their association with psychiatric disorders in the 1920s.[27] Kretschmer's enormously influential *Physique and Character* and his textbook on *Medical Psychology* found avid readers throughout the mid-twentieth century and not just in Germany.[28] In the 1930s, Kretschmer had supported the Nazi's sterilization and eugenic marriage-hygiene laws with enough fervor to impress his academic colleagues, albeit not enough to

---

[25] See Walter Baeyer, Heinz Häfner, and Karl-Peter Kisker, *Psychiatrie der Verfolgten: Psychopathologische und gutachtliche Erfahrungen an Opfern der nationalsozialistischen Verfolgung und vergleichbarer Extrembelastungen* (Berlin: Springer, 1964); Volker Roelcke, "Psychosomatic Medicine in Post-War Germany: The Domestication of Psychoanalysis by Public Institutions. The Case of the Psychosomatic Hospital at the University of Heidelberg," in *Proceedings of the 1st European Congress on the History of Psychiatry and Mental Health Care*, edited by Leonie de Goei and Joost Vijselaar (Rotterdam: Erasmus, 1993), 51–58; and Maike Rotzoll, "Die Entstehung der 'Sozialpsychiatrischen Klinik Heidelberg' in den 1960er Jahren: Sozialpsychiatrie in Heidelberg," *Jahrbuch des Heidelberger Geschichtsvereins* 17 (2012): 133–48.

[26] See Ernst Kretschmer, *Gestalten und Gedanken* (Stuttgart: Thieme, 1963), 82–83, 107–108; F[riedrich] Mauz, "Ernst Kretschmer - von innen gesehen," *Zeitschrift für Psychotherapie und medizinische Psychologie* 15.2 (1965): 61; and W. Schulte, "Ernst Kretschmer: Werk und Persönlichkeit in ihren Auswirkungen auf die Klinik," *Zeitschrift für Psychotherapie und medizinische Psychologie* 15.2 (1965): 65. Kretschmer shared with Zeller a deep-seated affiliation with Swabian culture. In his autobiography, he made much of his own southwest German lineage. This predilection spurred not only Kretschmer's own research on geniality but also inspired other collaborators, like Hans-Jörg Weitbrecht (1909–1975), who studied specifically Swabian forms of psychosis, especially within pietist religious communities. See Kretschmer, *Gestalten*, 12–48; Ernst Kretschmer, *Geniale Menschen*, 3rd ed. (Berlin: Springer, 1942); Hansjörg Weitbrecht, "Zum Problem der Rassen- und Stammespsychopathologie," *Der Nervenarzt* 15 (1942): 145ff; and idem, *Beiträge zur Religionspsychopathologie: Insbes. zur Psychopathologie d. Bekehrung* (Heidelberg: Scherer, 1948).

[27] On Kretschmer's oeuvre and "holistic biologism," see the excellent summary by Heinz Häfner, "Ernst Kretschmer: Beständiges und Vergangenes," *Fundamenta Psychiatrica* 3 (1989): 56–64, here 64. See also Bernhard Matz, "Die Konstitutionstypologie von Ernst Kretschmer: Ein Beitrag zur Geschichte von Psychiatrie und Psychologie des Zwanzigsten Jahrhunderts," Medical Dissertation, Free University of Berlin, 2000; Michael Hau, "The Holistic Gaze in German Medicine (1890–1930)," *Bulletin of the History of Medicine* 74 (2000): 495–524; and Martin Priwitzer, *Ernst Kretschmer und das Wahnproblem* (Stuttgart: Franz Steiner, 2007).

[28] Ernst Kretschmer, *Körperbau und Charakter: Untersuchungen zum Konstitutionsproblem und zur Lehre von den Temperamenten*, 1st ed. (25th edition, 1967) (Berlin: Julius Springer, 1921), and idem, *Medizinische Psychologie: Ein Leitfaden für Studium und Praxis*, 1st ed. (14th edition, 1975) (Leipzig: Thieme, 1922). On the popularity of these works, see also Ludwig J. Pongratz, ed., *Psychiatrie in Selbstdarstellungen* (Bern: Hans Huber, 1977), 61.

satiate hard-line racial hygienists, who denounced his "vacillations" [*Bedenkenmeierei*].[29] After the war, Kretschmer became one of the most influential and decorated psychiatrists in Germany.[30] Endorsed by the occupying powers, he published a survey of psychiatric research undertaken in Germany between 1939 and 1946.[31] He was at the heart of controversial efforts to rehabilitate psychiatric colleagues and to reconstitute biomedical professional organizations, himself founding the Society for Constitutional Research in 1948.[32] In the eyes of many, Kretschmer became a postwar symbol for the reemergence of psychiatric science guided by Christian values.[33] For his accomplishments, he was awarded the prestigious "Kraepelin Medallion" in 1956 and the German government's Order of Merit (*Bundesverdienstkreuz*) in 1958.

In good part, these attempts to reorient psychiatry targeted the profession's scientific ethos, specifically whether it properly belonged to either the natural sciences or the humanities, especially to anthropology.[34] But these reassessments also involved a reevaluation of psychiatry's historical lineages. Framed as a critique of the materialistic and positivistic convictions of latter nineteenth- and early twentieth-century medical science, anthropologically minded reformers looked back to the Romantic era for inspiration.[35] For example, Weizsäcker was fond of citing Wolfgang Goethe's holistic understanding of the sciences in his efforts to restore a purportedly lost unity of not just body and mind but of the sciences in general.[36] And

[29] Thus Gisela Bock as cited in Peter Weingart, Jürgen Kroll, and Kurt Bayertz, *Rasse, Blut, und Gene: Geschichte der Eugenik und Rassenhygiene in Deutschland* (Frankfurt/M: Suhrkamp, 1992), 474. On Kretschmer's ambiguous conduct under the Nazi regime, see Dörre, 64–74; Schmuhl, 132, 156, 193; Ernst Klee, *Das Personenlexikon zum Dritten Reich: Wer war was vor und nach 1945*, 2nd ed. (Frankfurt/M: Fischer, 2016), 339; Krähwinkel, 166–171, 183–186, 192–194, 207–208; and Regine Lockot, *Erinnern und Durcharbeiten: Zur Geschichte der Psychoanalyse und Psychotherapie im Nationalsozialismus* (Frankfurt/M: Fischer-Taschenbuch-Verl., 1985), 74–79. Kretschmer's promotion of eugenic marriage counseling dated back at least to his 1925 article "Spousal Fitting in Marriage" [*Die Zusammenstimmung in der Ehe*] and drew substantially on traditional, patriarchal norms of interventionist social welfare. See Ernst Kretschmer, *Mensch und Lebensgrund: Gesammelte Aufsätze* (Tübingen: Rainer Wunderlich Verlag, 1966), 117–144.

[30] See H. C. Rümke, "Ernst Kretschmer und die Psychiatrie gestern, heute und morgen," *Zeitschrift für Psychotherapie und medizinische Psychologie* 15.2 (1965): 53–60.

[31] Ernst Kretschmer, ed. *Psychiatrie*, Naturforschung und Medizin in Deutschland 1939–1946 [Field Information Agency, Technical (FIAT) Review of German Science] (Wiesbaden: Dieterich, 1948). The book was entirely silent about the entanglement of psychiatric research with the biopolitical agendas of the National Socialist regime.

[32] See Lockot, 79; Weingart, 587, 623–24; and Dörre, 91–99. Gerhart Zeller was a member of the society. See "Gesellschaft f. Konstit.foschg.," 749–S42, Kretschmer Papers, University Archive Tübingen.

[33] See Dörre, 67.

[34] Thus Hubertus Tellenbach as cited in Klaus Dörner, *Bürger und Irre: Zur Sozialgeschichte und Wissenschaftssoziologie der Psychiatrie* (Frankfurt/M: EVA, 1984 [1969]), 333–334.

[35] Dörner described developments as a "backlash against the Age of Reason." Ibid., 333.

[36] See Sophie Witt, "Einleitung: Ganzheitswissen?" *Body Politics* 10.14 (2022): 8.

immediately after the war in 1947, Kretschmer was already singing the praises of "Romantic physicians."[37]

One example of these efforts to reframe psychiatry's past looked explicitly to the work of Albert Zeller. In his examination of the rise of psychiatry as a science in the nineteenth century, the psychiatrist Joachim Bodamer (1910–1985) cast Albert Zeller in prophetic terms. In light of the surging interest in "physiological subjectivity" and the "anthropological turn," Albert Zeller could now rightly "claim some credit for these modern views, given his resistance against the rising tide of materialism in medical science."[38] Hoping to spawn greater interest in these historical origins, Bodamer even had that most iconic account of Romantic medical interventions—Justinus Kerner's treatment of the Seeress of Prevorst—republished in 1958.[39]

Needless to say, such efforts at historical revisionism elicited forceful ripostes from more somatically minded psychiatrists. Wolfgang de Boor worried that recourse to any notion of an earlier "romantic psychiatry" would open gates to "metaphysical" and "transcendental" definitions of insanity that lay outside the laws of organic nature. Others mocked the growing use of terms like "holistic" and "dynamic" as fashionable fads.[40] Indeed, the very concept of unitary psychosis soon exuded a kind of "magical aura" bound to elicit contrarian reactions.[41]

Well aware of these tensions within the psychiatric profession, Gerhart Zeller himself reflected on the prospects for his manuscript in a letter to a colleague in 1963. Zeller had just arrived in Berlin to take up a position as senior physician and medical director of the state asylum in the suburb of Spandau. In Berlin he was burdened by his new responsibilities and also encountered a starkly divided professional landscape:

> As you know, psychiatrists in Berlin are very analytical, i.e. they're either extreme somaticists like [Helmut] Selbach[42] or Freudians. Whoever can't associate with one of the factions must be able to synthesize. But where else could one learn this if not under [Ernst] Kretschmer? I think you can now understand why I've not yet published my award-winning

[37] Ernst Kretschmer, "Romantische Ärzte," in *Mensch und Lebensgrund: Gesammelte Aufsätze* (Tübingen: Rainer Wunderlich Verlag, 1966 [1947]), 40–60.

[38] Joachim Bodamer, "Zur Entstehung der Psychiatrie als Wissenschaft im 19. Jahrhundert," *Fortschritte der Neurologie, Psychiatrie und ihrer Grenzgebiete* 21 (1953): 523.

[39] Joachim Bodamer, *Die Seherin von Prevorst* (Stuttgart: J. F. Steinkopf, 1958). Furthermore, a decade earlier in the immediate aftermath of the war, Bodamer had published an intellectual history of psychiatric science that took as its point of departure the pietist physician Georg Ernst Stahl (1659–1734), arguably the inspiration for many subsequent unitarian interpretations of madness. See Joachim Bodamer, "Zur Phänomenologie des geschichtlichen Geistes in der Psychiatrie," *Der Nervenarzt* 19 (1948): 299–310.

[40] See Johannes Hirschmann, "Medizinische Psychologie," in *Psychiatrie*, edited by Ernst Kretschmer, Naturforschung und Medizin in Deutschland 1939–1946 (Wiesbaden: Dieterich, 1948), 184, and Vliegen, 52.

[41] Bittel, 102.

[42] Selbach was a neuropsychiatrist who in 1950 had become head of the psychiatric clinic of the Free University in Berlin.

> manuscript, even though I've circulated it among colleagues. Indeed, I've reached an agreement with the publisher Gustav Fischer in Stuttgart, specifically with professors Herrlinger and Rothschuh.[43] They are the editors of a new and—with the exception of *Sudhoffs Classics*[44]—only German book series in the history of medicine entitled *Medicine in History and Culture*[45] […]. Unfortunately, I need to shorten the text, substantially. I'm only too aware of the text's weaknesses. Revisions are necessary and for that I'm now reading.[46]

This professional situation of an early-career psychiatrist helps to explain why Zeller may have been reluctant to pursue publication of his manuscript, for it was unlikely to find favor among either his somatic or his psychoanalytic colleagues. But that Zeller had found a publisher in a series edited by Karl Eduard Rothschuh (1908–1984) is indicative of his intentions. For in the history of medicine, the physiologist Rothschuh would soon become Germany's foremost advocate of historical anthropology. Echoing the views of Ruffin, Rothschuh envisioned historical inquiry as having a vital integrative function within medicine, helping to guide the research and practice of medical professionals.[47] Concerned that scientific progress toward understanding the nature of organic life was being harmed by disciplinary divides, Rothschuh had just published a new attempt at synthesizing biology, psychology, and pathology into a single complex of scientific problems.[48]

Within German psychiatry, similar synthetic agendas informed the research of other psychopathologists. One of them was another representative of the Heidelberg School and successor to Walter Ritter von Baeyer, Werner Janzarik (1920–2019). With the publication his *Basic Dynamic Constellations in Endogenous Psychoses* in 1959, Janzarik outlined a program that used unitary psychosis as a "regulative idea," as a "hypothesis" of a holistic psychopathology."[49] Janzarik's so-called structural-dynamic method drew on Albert Zeller's dynamic understanding of unitary psychosis and applied the notion of a "dynamic disruption" [*dynamische Entgleisung*] as a heuristic principle for investigating potentially common origins among idiopathic

[43] Robert Herrlinger (1914–1968) was an anatomist who from 1951 taught the history of medicine at the University of Würzburg. Karl Eduard Rothschuh (1908–1984) was a physiologist who in 1960 had become director of the Institute for the History of Medicine in Munich.

[44] *[Sudhoffs] Klassiker der Medizin* (Leipzig: Barth, 1910–1942, 1960–1990).

[45] *Medizin in Geschichte und Kultur* (Stuttgart: Fischer, 1961–1998).

[46] Gerhart Zeller to Herrn Dr. Langen [May 1963], 749/T4, Kretschmer Papers, University Archive Tübingen. On Dietrich Langen, a fellow student of Kretschmer's, a clinical psychologist, and a proponent of group psychotherapy and so-called active hypnosis, see B. Peter, "Langen, Dietrich," in *Personenlexikon der Psychotherapie*, edited by G. Stumm, et al. (Vienna: Springer, 2005), 269–70.

[47] See Volker Roelcke, "Die Entwicklung der Medizingeschichte seit 1945," *NTM* n.s. 2 (1994): 204–205.

[48] K[arl] E[duard] Rothschuh, *Theorie des Organismus: Bios, Psyche, Pathos* (Munich: Urban & Schwarzenberg, 1959).

[49] Werner Janzarik, *Dynamische Grundkonstellationen in endogenen Psychosen* (Berlin: Springer, 1959), 67.

syndromes.[50] In East Germany, the doctrine of unitary psychosis found its most vocal advocate in Helmut Rennert (1920–1994), whose work on mixed states or schizoaffective psychoses in the 1950s led him to develop a model of the universal genesis of psychoses.[51] The work of Janzarik, Rennert, and others helped to fuel ambitions of combining psychopathological and biological strategies in ways that would culminate in a "post-nosological, integrative psychiatry."[52]

Not just in Germany but, more generally, observers have discerned a renaissance of interest in unitary psychosis in the postwar era.[53] In his introduction, Gerhart Zeller himself noted this surge of interest and used it to justify his investigation, citing especially the work of the Spanish psychiatrist Bartolomé Llopis (1905–1966).[54] Pointing to the late work of the American psychiatrist Adolf Meyer (1866–1950), as well as Karl Menninger (1893–1990), Henri Ellenberger (1905–1993), and several others, German Berrios has written of a "reactivation" of unitarian views after World War II.[55] This introduction cannot do justice to the convoluted debates, competing interests, and global networks that accompanied this mid-twentieth-century renaissance. Further historical research is needed to explain its continuities and disjunctions, and Gerhart Zeller's manuscript represents a contribution to these efforts.

---

[50] J. Klosterkötter, "Die Idee der Einheitspsychose im Zeitalter der biologischen Psychiatrie," in *Für und wider die Einheitspsychose*, edited by Christoph Mundt and Henning Saß (Stuttgart: Thieme, 1992), 95.

[51] See Ekkehardt Kumbier and Sabine C. Herpertz, "Helmut Rennert's Universal Genesis of Endogenous Psychoses: The Historical Concept and Its Significance for Today's Discussion on Unitary Psychosis," *Psychopathology* 43 (2010): 335–44.

[52] Klosterkötter, 97.

[53] See Werner Janzarik, "Nosographie und Einheitspsychose," in *Schizophrenie und Zyklothymie: Ergebnisse und Probleme*, edited by Gerd Huber (Stuttgart: Thieme Verlag, 1969), 30; L[uis] Valenciano, "La Tesis de la Psicosis única en la Actualidad," in *Introducción Dialéctica a la Psicopatologia*, edited by Bartolomé Llopis (Madrid: Morata, 1970), 113–59; and Vliegen, 28–33, 53–55.

[54] Bartolomé Llopis, "Single Psychosis," in *Anthology of Spanish Psychiatric Texts*, edited by Juan José López-Ibor, Carlos Carbonell, and Jean Garrabé (Paris: World Psychiatric Association, 2001 [1954]), 344–401, and Bartolomé Llopis, "Das allen Psychosen gemeinsame Achsensyndrom," *Fortschritte der Neurologie und Psychiatrie* 28.2 (1960): 106–29.

[55] G. E. Berrios and D. Beer, "Unitary Psychosis in English Speaking Psychiatry: A Conceptual History," in *Für und wider die Einheitspsychose*, edited by Christoph Mundt and Henning Saß (Stuttgart: Thieme, 1992), 18–19; see also idem, "Unitary Psychosis Concept," in *A History of Clinical Psychiatry: The Origin and History of Psychiatric Disorders*, edited by German E. Berrios and Roy Porter (London: Athlone, 1994), 311–35.

Contemporary Twenty-First-Century Resonances

Gerhart Zeller's text was a near contemporary of several other major German-language contributions to the history of psychiatry. Werner Leibbrand's and Annemarie Wettley's *Insanity* (1961) and Klaus Dörner's *Madmen and the Bourgeoisie* (1969), which Dörner began researching in 1962, became dominant pillars of latter twentieth-century West German psychiatric historiography. The enormous heft of these magna opera may well also have been a factor in dissuading Zeller from publishing his manuscript. Taking these works into consideration, combined with Erwin Ackerknecht's lighter and far more accessible *Short History of Psychiatry*,[56] it is unclear what kind of reception Zeller's work could have received. In the shadow of these studies, Zeller's text represents an undeveloped strand of psychiatric historiography. But recent research trends in both psychiatry and history suggest that recovering and expanding upon this strand have the potential to yield unanticipated gains. A few examples can help illustrate this point.

Among the most important findings of recent work in psychiatric genetics is that genetic influences transcend traditional diagnostic categories and that at the level of DNA sequence, there is "substantial overlap among disorders."[57] Researchers interested in assessing genetic risks have found them to be pleiotropic, that is to say, "associated not only with schizophrenia and psychotic disorders but also with other psychiatric and medical disorders."[58] This fact that genetic influences do not generally correlate directly with specific psychiatric diagnoses has spurred interest in transdiagnostic frameworks, like the American Psychiatric Association's Research Domain Criteria (RDoc),[59] and reinforced calls for a denosologization of psychiatry. In one recent provocative intervention published in the *American Journal of Psychiatry*, Caspi and Moffitt put these diagnostic concerns bluntly:

> Diagnostic systems that are currently used in research and practice regard psychiatric disorders as categorical, independent, and distinct. But these systems are being questioned on multiple fronts. On scientific and clinical grounds, there is evidence that symptoms are continuous rather than categorical and that overlap between disorders is the rule rather than the exception (1). On social and cultural grounds, there is concern that diagnostic expansiveness is pathologizing everyday life (2). On philosophical grounds, there are ontological

[56] Erwin Heinz Ackerknecht, *Kurze Geschichte der Psychiatrie* (Stuttgart: Enke, 1957).

[57] Jordan W. Smoller, "Psychiatric Genetics Begins to Find Its Footing," *American Journal of Psychiatry* 176.8 (2019): 610.

[58] Elisabeth B. Binder, "Polygenic Risk Scores in Schizophrenia: Ready for the Real World," *American Journal of Psychiatry* 176.10 (2019): 783.

[59] See Thomas Insel, et al., "Research Domain Criteria (RDOC): Toward a New Classification Framework for Research on Mental Disorders," *American Journal of Psychiatry* 167 (2013): 748–51, and William T. Carpenter, "The RDoC Controversy: Alternate Paradigm or Dominant Paradigm," *American Journal of Psychiatry* 173.6 (2016): 562–63. For more on RDoc and the "epistemological and ontological politics" of contemporary (US) psychiatry, see Martyn Pickersgill, "Psychiatry and Sociology of Novelty: Negotiating the US National Institute of Mental Health 'Research Domain Criteria' (RDoc)," *Science, Technology, & Human Values* 44.4 (2019): 612–33.

reservations about whether psychiatric disorders are "natural kinds" whose causes can be discovered (3).[60]

In response to these challenges to the causal specificity of psychiatric disorders, Caspi and Moffitt argue that genetic and neuroscientific research must turn its attention toward nonspecific shared pathogenesis or what they call the "p-factor." And for them, the p-factor is nosological "lumping with a vengeance."[61] In view of such developments, revisiting the early history of unitary psychosis appears timely.

These nosological debates have also contributed to a revival of interest in non-cerebrocentric explanations of mental illness. One of the hallmarks of the early history of unitary psychosis was the emphasis placed on the vegetative nervous system. This perspective still resonates in contemporary psychiatric theorizing. For example, vagus nerve stimulation is being actively used in the treatment of depression as an alternative to more conventional forms of treatment like psychotherapy and psychopharmacology.[62] Furthermore, as part of a wider explosion of research on microbiomes, recent work on the gut microbiome has focused on its pathogenic significance in the development of depression.[63] According to one recent study, gut microbiota modulate brain function and human behavior primarily via a bidirectional communication pathway known as the "brain-gut axis."[64] This has led researchers to conclude that "changes in the intestinal flora and the brain–gut axis constitute important mechanisms by which the pathogenesis of depression can be explained and potential depression treatment regimens be predicted."[65] Although so far the clinical evidence is "equivocal at best,"[66] it too suggests that early nineteenth-century alienists like Albert Zeller who discounted the etiological primacy of the brain were not quite as misguided as sometimes depicted.

It remains to be seen whether or how historical scholarship can engage with this psychiatric research. But recent studies on the history of melancholia and depression suggest some common concerns. For example, in her study of nineteenth-century melancholia, Åsa Jansson has found that while "physicians conceptualized mental pain as a physiological phenomenon, most patients continued to experience

---

[60] Avshalom Caspi and Terrie E. Moffitt, "All for One and One for All: Mental Disorders in One Dimension," *American Journal of Psychiatry* 175.9 (2018): 831.

[61] Ibid., 836.

[62] J. Douglas Bremmer and Mark Hyman Rapaport, "Vagus Nerve Stimulation: Back to the Future," *American Journal of Psychiatry* 174.7 (2017): 609–10.

[63] Akash Kumar, et al., "Gut Microbiota in Anxiety and Depression: Unveiling the Relationship and Management Options," *Pharmaceuticals* 16.4 (2023): 565.

[64] Lijia Chang, Yan Wei, and Kenji Hashimoto, "Brain-Gut-Microbiota Axis in Depression: A Historical Overview and Future Directions," *Brain Research Bulletin* 182 (2022): 44–56.

[65] Wen-Zhi Hao, Xiao-Juan Li, Pei-Wen Zhang, and Jia-Xu Chen, "A Review of Antibiotics, Depression, and the Gut Microbiome," *Psychiatry Research* 284 (2020).

[66] Nitin K. Ahuja, "Gut Instincts," *The New York Review of Books*, 70.19 (2023): 16.

their pain in spiritual terms."[67] Bridging this gap between biological explanations and life-world experiences has been an abiding aim of unitarian endeavors.[68] And in his recent monograph on the history of depression, Jonathan Sadowsky has poignantly observed that the "medical ideas under-pinning the idea of melancholia were never just mental or just physical. They assumed mind and body constantly influence one another. How did we lose that?"[69] Studying the early history of unitary psychosis reminds us of a time when this assumption had not yet been lost.

If nothing else, unitary psychosis has exhibited remarkable historical staying power. It has certainly already outlasted many specific psychiatric diagnoses and is arguably likely to outlast many more. Explaining this persistence can, in and of itself, well justify further historical inquiry. But obviously, exactly what its various advocates and detractors have meant by the term has shifted radically over time. Untangling the fluctuating and layered meanings of the concept is the challenge—and opportunity!—facing any historical epistemology of nineteenth-century psychiatry.[70]

It has been argued that unitary psychosis can plausibly be understood as a product of nosological skepticism. By this reasoning, unitary psychosis is a necessarily speculative artifact of any and all nosologies, an inherent "other" embedded in those nosologies that contests their very structures and logics.[71] Understanding unitary psychosis in this way harbors significant analytic potential, both for psychiatrists seeking to stress test the validity of their categories and for historians tracking the continuities and shifts in psychiatric nosology over time. May the publication of this monograph help exploit this potential.

The Typescript and Its Translation

At least three copies of the typescript are known to have survived. One is held by the library of the Institute for Ethics and History of Medicine in Tübingen. Of the two other copies, one is held by the Zeller family (Berlin) and the other by Luigi Grosso

[67] Åsa Jansson, "From Melancholia to Depression: Disordered Mood in Nineteenth-Century Psychiatry," *History of Psychiatry* 33.1 (2022): 56. Cf. likewise the recent findings of Owen Davies, *Troubled by Faith: Insanity and the Supernatural in the Age of the Asylum* (Oxford: Oxford University Press, 2023).

[68] See Christoph Mundt, "Einheit und Vielfalt von Endogenität der Psychosen?" in *Für und wider die Einheitspsychose*, edited by Christoph Mundt and Henning Saß (Stuttgart: Thieme, 1992), 81–90.

[69] Jonathan Sadowsky, *The Empire of Depression: A New History* (Cambridge: Polity, 2020), 22.

[70] For an analytic model to aid in the study of the historical epistemology of the concept of unitary psychosis, see German E. Berrios and Ivana S. Marková, "Historical Epistemology of the 'Unitary Psychosis'," in *Psychotic Disorders: Comprehensive Conceptualizations and Treatments*, edited by Carol A. Tamminga et al. (Oxford: Oxford University Press, 2021), 12–20.

[71] See Michael Schmidt-Degenhard, "Einheitspsychose - Begriff und Idee," in *Für und Wider der Einheitspsychose*, edited by C[hristoph] Mundt and H[ans-Martin] Saß (Stuttgart: Thieme, 1992).

(Paris). The three versions are essentially identical, except for an appended bibliography in the Berlin and Paris versions and a "concluding summary" and handwritten revisions in the Paris version. For the purposes of this publication, the Paris version has been taken to be the full and authoritative original. At some point prior to his death in 2006, Gerhart Zeller began revising the typescript, deleting substantial amounts of material related to the Zeller family's early history. Almost all of this editing targeted the first 60 pages of the typescript; thereafter, he undertook only light editing. These edits are preserved in the Paris version and have been incorporated into this published version without annotation.

The editorial aim has been to produce a faithful rendering of the original typescript. For the most part, the editors have refrained from appending scholarly commentary to the text. All editorial additions or deletions have been placed in square brackets ([]). Wherever possible, incomplete or missing references have been added. References to secondary sources in the original text body have been rendered as footnotes. Where appropriate, cross-references to the 2007 publication of Albert Zeller's *Travel Diary* have been added.[72] Insofar as quotations from the diary deviate from the 2007 publication, this later publication has been used. References to Albert Zeller's as yet unpublished diaries have not been subjected to editorial scrutiny. Simple misspellings and typographical errors have been corrected.

The English translation is an abridgement of the original typescript. The primary aim of the abridgement is to eliminate digressions that distracted from the narrative account of the history of unitary psychosis. All abridgements have been referenced in the footnotes, including their approximate length and subject matter.

References

Ackerknecht, Erwin Heinz. 1957. *Kurze Geschichte der Psychiatrie*. Stuttgart: Enke.

Ahuja, Nitin K. 2023. Gut instincts. *The New York Review of Books* 70 (19): 16–17.

Benzenhöfer, Udo. 1993. *Psychiatrie und Anthropologie in der ersten Hälfte des 19. Jahrhunderts*. Hürtgenwald: Pressler.

Berrios, G. E., and D. Beer. 1992. Unitary psychosis in English speaking psychiatry: A conceptual history. In *Für und wider die Einheitspsychose*, ed. Christoph Mundt and Henning Saß, 12–21. Stuttgart: Thieme.

Berrios, G. E., and D. Beer. 1994. Unitary psychosis concept. In *A history of clinical psychiatry: The origin and history of psychiatric disorders*, ed. German E. Berrios and Roy Porter, 311–335. London: Athlone.

Berrios, German E., and Ivana S. Marková. 2021. Historical epistemology of the 'unitary psychosis'. In *Psychotic disorders: Comprehensive conceptualizations and treatments*, ed. Carol A. Tamminga et al., 12–20. Oxford: Oxford University Press.

Binder, Elisabeth B. 2019. Polygenic risk scores in schizophrenia: Ready for the real world. *American Journal of Psychiatry* 176 (10): 783–784.

[72] Albert Zeller and Gerhart Zeller, *Albert Zellers medizinisches Tagebuch der psychiatrischen Reise durch Deutschland, England, Frankreich und nach Prag von 1832 bis 1833*, 2 vols. (Zwiefalten: Psychiatrie und Geschichte, 2007).

Birnbaum, Karl. 1928. Geschichte der psychiatrischen Wissenschaft. In *Handbuch der Geisteskrankheiten*, ed. Oswald Bumke, vol. 1, 11–49. Berlin: Springer.

Bittel, Günther. 1980. *Entwicklung und Wirkung der Heilanstalt Winnental: Zur Anwendung der historischen Methode in der Psychiatrie*. Medical Dissertation, Albert-Ludwigs-Universität Freiburg.

Bleker, Johanna. 1988. Biedermeiermedizin: Medizin der Biedermeier? Tendenzen, Probleme, Widersprüche. *Medizinhistorisches Journal* 23 (1/2): 5–22.

Bodamer, Joachim. 1948. Zur Phänomenologie des geschichtlichen Geistes in der Psychiatrie. *Der Nervenarzt* 19:299–310.

Bodamer, Joachim. 1953. Zur Entstehung der Psychiatrie als Wissenschaft im 19. Jahrhundert. *Fortschritte der Neurologie, Psychiatrie und ihrer Grenzgebiete* 21:511–535.

Bodamer, Joachim. 1958. *Die Seherin von Prevorst*. Stuttgart: J. F. Steinkopf.

Bremmer, J. Douglas, and Mark Hyman Rapaport. 2017. Vagus nerve stimulation: Back to the future. *American Journal of Psychiatry* 174 (7): 609–610.

Brückner, Burkhart. 2007. *Delirium und Wahn: Geschichte, Selbstzeugnisse und Theorien von der Antike bis 1900*. 2 vols. Hürtgenwald: Pressler.

Carpenter, William T. 2016. The RDoC controversy: Alternate paradigm or dominant paradigm. *American Journal of Psychiatry* 173 (6): 562–563.

Caspi, Avshalom, and Terrie E. Moffitt. 2018. All for one and one for all: Mental disorders in one dimension. *American Journal of Psychiatry* 175 (9): 831–844.

Chang, Lijia, Yan Wei, and Kenji Hashimoto. 2022. Brain-gut-microbiota axis in depression: A historical overview and future directions. *Brain Research Bulletin* 182:44–56.

Conrad, K. 1959. Das Problem der 'nosologischen Einheit' in der Psychiatrie. *Der Nervenarzt* 30 (11): 488–494.

Daker, Maurício Viotti. 2021. *The continuum of mental disorders and unitary psychosis: History and perspectives*. Newcastle upon Tyne: Cambridge Scholars Publishing.

Davies, Owen. 2023. *Troubled by faith: Insanity and the supernatural in the age of the asylum*. Oxford: Oxford University Press.

de Boor, Wolfgang. 1954. *Psychiatrische Systematik: Ihre Entwicklung in Deutschland seit Kahlbaum*. Berlin: Springer.

Dörner, Klaus. 1984 [1969]. *Bürger und Irre: Zur Sozialgeschichte und Wissenschaftssoziologie der Psychiatrie*. Frankfurt: EVA.

Dörre, Steffen. 2021. *Zwischen NS-'Euthanasie' und Reformaufbruch: die psychiatrischen Fachgesellschaften im geteilten Deutschland*. Berlin: Springer.

Dror, Otniel E., Bettina Hitzer, Anja Laukötter, and Pilar León-Sanz, eds. 2016. *History of science and the emotions*. Chicago: University of Chicago Press.

Engstrom, Eric J., and Matthias M. Weber. 2005. The directions of psychiatric research by Emil Kraepelin 1887. *History of Psychiatry* 16 (3): 345–364.

Geisthövel, Alexa. 2018. Viktor von Weizsäcker oder die 'monumentale Unruhe' einer subjektiven Medizin. In *Auf der Suche nach einer anderen Medizin: Psychosomatik im 20. Jahrhundert*, ed. Alexa Geisthövel and Bettina Hitzer, 144–153. Berlin: Suhrkamp.

Grün, Bernd. 2007. Schuld und Sichtweise: Versuch einer Kategorisierung der 'Entnazifizierung' am Beispiel der Tübinger medizinischen Fakultät. In *Vergangenheitspolitik in der universitären Medizin nach 1945: institutionelle und individuelle Strategien im Umgang mit dem Nationalsozialismus*, ed. Sigrid Oehler-Klein and Volker Roelcke, 277–304. Stuttgart: Steiner.

Häfner, Heinz. 1989. Ernst Kretschmer: Beständiges und Vergangenes. *Fundamenta Psychiatrica* 3:56–64.

Hao, Wen-Zhi, Xiao-Juan Li, Pei-Wen Zhang, and Jia-Xu Chen. 2020. A review of antibiotics, depression, and the gut microbiome. *Psychiatry Research* 284:112691.

Harrington, Anne. 1996. *Reenchanted science: Holism in German culture from Wilhelm II to Hitler*. Princeton: Princeton University Press.

Hau, Michael. 2000. The holistic gaze in German medicine (1890-1930). *Bulletin of the History of Medicine* 74:495–524.

Henckes, Nicolas, and Lara Rzesnitzek. 2018. Performing doubt and negociating uncertainty: Diagnosing schizophrenia at its onset in post-war German psychiatry. *History of the Human Sciences* 31 (2): 65–87.

Hirschmann, Johannes. 1948. Medizinische Psychologie. In *Psychiatrie*, ed. Ernst Kretschmer, 168–193. Wiesbaden: Dieterich.

Insel, Thomas, et al. 2013. Research domain criteria (RDOC): Toward a new classification framework for research on mental disorders. *American Journal of Psychiatry* 167:748–751.

Jansson, Åsa. 2022. From melancholia to depression: Disordered mood in nineteenth-century psychiatry. *History of Psychiatry* 33 (1): 47–64.

Janzarik, Werner. 1959. *Dynamische Grundkonstellationen in endogenen Psychosen*. Berlin: Springer.

Janzarik, Werner. 1969. Nosographie und Einheitspsychose. In *Schizophrenie und Zyklothymie: Ergebnisse und Probleme*, ed. Gerd Huber, 29–38. Stuttgart: Thieme Verlag.

Jaspers, Karl. 1913. *Allgemeine Psychopathologie: Ein Leitfaden für Studierende, Ärzte und Psychologen*. Berlin: Springer.

Jovanović, Gordana. 2021. How psychology repressed its founding father Wilhelm Wundt. *Human Arenas* 4:32–47.

Klee, Ernst. 2016. *Das Personenlexikon zum Dritten Reich: Wer war was vor und nach 1945*. 2nd ed. Frankfurt: Fischer.

Klosterkötter, J. 1992. Die Idee der Einheitspsychose im Zeitalter der biologischen Psychiatrie. In *Für und wider die Einheitspsychose*, ed. Christoph Mundt and Henning Saß, 91–98. Stuttgart: Thieme.

Kocka, Jürgen. 2022. *Kampf um die Moderne: Das lange 19. Jahrhundert in Deutschland*. Bonn: Bundeszentrale für politische Bildung.

Kraepelin, Emil. 1887. *Die Richtungen der psychiatrischen Forschung: Vortrag, gehalten bei der Übernahme des Lehramtes an der kaiserlichen Universität Dorpat*. Leipzig: Vogel.

Krähwinkel, Esther. 1999. Formen der Umsetzung des 'Gesetzes zur Verhütung erbkranken Nachwuchses' an der Marburger Medizinischen Fakultät. *Medizinhistorisches Journal* 34 (2): 159–209.

Kretschmer, Ernst. 1921. *Körperbau und Charakter: Untersuchungen zum Konstitutionsproblem und zur Lehre von den Temperamenten*. 1st ed. (25th edition, 1967). Berlin: Julius Springer.

Kretschmer, Ernst. 1922. *Medizinische Psychologie: Ein Leitfaden für Studium und Praxis*. 1st ed. (14th edition, 1975). Leipzig: Thieme.

Kretschmer, Ernst. 1942. *Geniale Menschen*. 3rd ed. Berlin: Springer.

Kretschmer, Ernst, ed. 1948. *Psychiatrie, Naturforschung und Medizin in Deutschland 1939-1946 [Field information agency, technical (FIAT) review of German science]*. Wiesbaden: Dieterich.

Kretschmer, Ernst. 1963. *Gestalten und Gedanken*. Stuttgart: Thieme.

Kretschmer, Ernst. 1966a. *Mensch und Lebensgrund: Gesammelte Aufsätze*. Tübingen: Rainer Wunderlich Verlag.

Kretschmer, Ernst. 1966b [1947]. Romantische Ärzte. In *Mensch und Lebensgrund: Gesammelte Aufsätze*, 40–60. Tübingen: Rainer Wunderlich Verlag.

Kreuser, Heinrich. 1902. Geschichtlicher Überblick über die Entwicklung des Irrenwesens in Württemberg. *Medicinisches Correspondenz-Blatt des Würtembergischen Ärztlichen Vereins* 72:749–757.

Kreuser, Heinrich. 1904. Zu Albert Zellers Gedächtnis. *Medicinisches Correspondenz-Blatt des Würtembergischen Ärztlichen Vereins* 74 (45): 935–939.

Kumar, Akash, et al. 2023. Gut microbiota in anxiety and depression: Unveiling the relationship and management options. *Pharmaceuticals* 16 (4): 565.

Kumbier, Ekkehardt, and Sabine C. Herpertz. 2010. Helmut Rennert's universal genesis of endogenous psychoses: The historical concept and its significance for today's discussion on unitary psychosis. *Psychopathology* 43:335–344.

Leibbrand, Werner, and Annemarie Wettley. 1961. *Der Wahnsinn: Geschichte der abendländischen Psychopathologie*. Munich: Karl Albers. Reprint, 2005.

Llopis, Bartolomé. 2001 [1954]. Single psychosis. In *Anthology of Spanish psychiatric texts*, ed. Juan José López-Ibor, Carlos Carbonell, and Jean Garrabé, 344–401. Paris: World Psychiatric Association.

Llopis, Bartolomé. 1960. Das allen Psychosen gemeinsame Achsensyndrom. *Fortschritte der Neurologie und Psychiatrie* 28 (2): 106–129.

Lockot, Regine. 1985. *Erinnern und Durcharbeiten: Zur Geschichte der Psychoanalyse und Psychotherapie im Nationalsozialismus*. Frankfurt: Fischer-Taschenbuch-Verl.

Matz, Bernhard. 2000. *Die Konstitutionstypologie von Ernst Kretschmer: Ein Beitrag zur Geschichte von Psychiatrie und Psychologie des Zwanzigsten Jahrhunderts*. Diss. med., Free University of Berlin,

Mauz, F. 1965. Ernst Kretschmer - von innen gesehen. *Zeitschrift für Psychotherapie und Medizinische Psychologie* 15 (2): 60–64.

Medizin in Geschichte und Kultur. Stuttgart: Fischer, 1961–1998.

Mundt, Christoph. 1992. Einheit und Vielfalt von Endogenität der Psychosen? In *Für und wider die Einheitspsychose*, ed. Christoph Mundt and Henning Saß, 81–90. Stuttgart: Thieme.

Oehler-Klein, Sigrid, and Volker Roelcke. 2007. *Vergangenheitspolitik in der universitären Medizin nach 1945: institutionelle und individuelle Strategien im Umgang mit dem Nationalsozialismus*. Stuttgart: Steiner.

Pauleikhoff, Bernhard. 1983. *Das Menschenbild im Wandel der Zeit: Ideengeschichte der Psychiatrie und der klinischen Psychologie*. Vol. 2. Hürtgenwald: Guido Pressler.

Peter, B. 2005. Langen, Dietrich. In *Personenlexikon der Psychotherapie*, ed. G. Stumm et al., 269–270. Vienna: Springer.

Pfaff, Aaron. 2024. *Geschichte der verfassten Ärzteschaft auf dem Gebiet des heutigen Bundeslandes Baden-Württemberg von 1920 bis 1960*. Stuttgart: Franz Steiner Verlag.

Pickersgill, Martyn. 2019. Psychiatry and sociology of novelty: Negotiating the US National Institute of Mental Health 'Research Domain Criteria' (RDoc). *Science, Technology, & Human Values* 44 (4): 612–633.

Pilavas, Ioannis. 1994. *Psychiatrie im Widerstreit der Konzepte: Zur Entstehungsgeschichte der Tübinger Nervenklinik*. Sigmaringen: Jan Thorbecke.

Pongratz, Ludwig J., ed. 1977. *Psychiatrie in Selbstdarstellungen*. Bern: Hans Huber.

Pretsch, Hermann J. 1996. *'Euthanasie': Krankenmord in Südwestdeutschland*. Zwiefalten: Verlag Psychiatrie und Geschichte.

Priwitzer, Martin. 2007. *Ernst Kretschmer und das Wahnproblem*. Stuttgart: Franz Steiner.

Roelcke, Volker. 1993. Psychosomatic medicine in post-war Germany: The domestication of psychoanalysis by public institutions. The case of the Psychosomatic Hospital at the University of Heidelberg. In *Proceedings of the 1st European congress on the history of psychiatry and mental health care*, ed. Leonie de Goei and Joost Vijselaar, 51–58. Rotterdam: Erasmus.

Roelcke, Volker. 1994. Die Entwicklung der Medizingeschichte seit 1945. *NTM* 2:193–216.

Rothschuh, K. E. 1959. *Theorie des Organismus: Bios, psyche, pathos*. Munich: Urban & Schwarzenberg.

Rotzoll, Maike. 2012. Die Entstehung der 'Sozialpsychiatrischen Klinik Heidelberg' in den 1960er Jahren: Sozialpsychiatrie in Heidelberg. *Jahrbuch des Heidelberger Geschichtsvereins* 17:133–148.

Ruffin, Hanns. 1954. Rückblick auf die Geschichte der Wanderversammlung Südwestdeutscher Neurologen und Psychiater. *Deutsche Zeitschrift für Nervenheilkunde* 172 (2): 111–127.

Rümke, H. C. 1965. Ernst Kretschmer und die Psychiatrie gestern, heute und morgen. *Zeitschrift für Psychotherapie und Medizinische Psychologie* 15 (2): 53–60.

Sadowsky, Jonathan. 2020. *The empire of depression: A new history*. Cambridge: Polity.

Schmidt-Degenhard, Michael. 1992. Einheitspsychose - Begriff und Idee. In *Für und Wider der Einheitspsychose*, ed. Christoph Mundt and Henning Saß, 1–11. Stuttgart: Thieme.

Schmuhl, Hans-Walter. 2016. *Die Gesellschaft Deutscher Neurologen und Psychiater im Nationalsozialismus*. Berlin: Springer.

Schott, Heinz, and Rainer Tölle. 2006. *Geschichte der Psychiatrie: Krankheitslehren, Irrwege, Behandlungsformen*. Munich: Beck.

Schulte, W. 1965. Ernst Kretschmer: Werk und Persönlichkeit in ihren Auswirkungen auf die Klinik. *Zeitschrift für Psychotherapie und Medizinische Psychologie* 15 (2): 65–72.

Smoller, Jordan W. 2019. Psychiatric genetics begins to find its footing. *American Journal of Psychiatry* 176 (8): 609–614.

Sudhoff, K., ed. 1910–1942, 1960–1990. *Klassiker der Medizin*. Leipzig: Barth.

Valenciano, L. 1970. La Tesis de la Psicosis única en la Actualidad. In *Introducción Dialéctica a la Psicopatologia*, ed. Bartolomé Llopis, 113–159. Madrid: Morata.

Verwey, Gerlof. 1985. *Psychiatry in an anthropological and biomedical context: Philosophical presuppositions and implications of German psychiatry, 1820-1870*. Dordrecht: Reidel.

Verwey, Gerlof. 2004. *Wilhelm Griesinger: Psychiatrie als ärztlicher Humanismus*. Nijmegen: Arts & Boeve.

Vliegen, Josef. 1980. *Die Einheitspsychose: Geschichte und Problem*. Stuttgart: Enke.

von Baeyer, Walter, Heinz Häfner, and Karl-Peter Kisker. 1964. *Psychiatrie der Verfolgten: Psychopathologische und gutachtliche Erfahrungen an Opfern der nationalsozialistischen Verfolgung und vergleichbarer Extrembelastungen*. Berlin: Springer.

von Weizsäcker, Viktor Freiherr. 1948. *Grundfragen medizinischer Anthropologie*. Tübingen: Furche Verlag.

Weingart, Peter, Jürgen Kroll, and Kurt Bayertz. 1992. *Rasse, Blut, und Gene: Geschichte der Eugenik und Rassenhygiene in Deutschland*. Frankfurt: Suhrkamp.

Weitbrecht, Hansjörg. 1942. Zum Problem der Rassen- und Stammespsychopathologie. *Der Nervenarzt* 15:145ff.

Weitbrecht, Hansjörg. 1948. *Beiträge zur Religionspsychopathologie: Insbes. zur Psychopathologie d. Bekehrung*. Heidelberg: Scherer.

Wengler, Bernd. 1989. *Das Menschenbild bei Alfred Adler, Wilhelm Griesinger und Rudolf Virchow: Ursprünge eines ganzheitlichen Paradigmas in der Medizin*. Frankfurt: Campus.

Witt, Sophie. 2022. Einleitung: Ganzheitswissen? *Body Politics* 10 (14): 6–14.

Zeller, Gerhart. 1968. Welcher psychiatrischen Schule hat Wilhelm Griesinger angehört? *Deutsches Medizinisches Journal* 19:328–334.

Zeller, Gerhart. 1969. Bonhoeffers wissenschaftliches Werk. Entwicklung und Bedeutung. In *Karl Bonhoeffer: Zum hundertsten Geburtstag am 31. März 1968*, ed. Jürg Zutt, Erwin Straus, and H. Scheller, 115–143. Berlin: Springer.

Zeller, Gerhart. 1972. Die Tübinger Psychiater-Schule. In *Wahn*, ed. Walter Schulte and Rainer Tölle, 95–104. Stuttgart: Georg Thieme.

Zeller, Albert, and Gerhart Zeller. 2007. *Albert Zellers medizinisches Tagebuch der psychiatrischen Reise durch Deutschland, England, Frankreich und nach Prag von 1832 bis 1833*. Vol. 2. Zwiefalten: Psychiatrie und Geschichte.

Chapter 2
The History of Unitary Psychosis Before Kraepelin

Gerhart Zeller and Eric J. Engstrom

Section 2.1

Introduction

"All perceptions of the past are enlightened and colored by the present."[1] This self-evident assertion by the eminent historian from Tübingen, Johannes Haller, justifies our asking at the outset of this historical study, why recently so much interest has been shown in an aspect of the history of our science that was heretofore seen as hopelessly outdated and hence uninteresting: the concept of "unitary psychosis."

Our task is not to examine the scientific guise in which this turn to ancient history today appears. To illustrate the seriousness and intensity of this retrospection, and its impact on current debate about psychosis, one can simply point to an article by the Madrilenian clinician Bartolomé Llopis on "The Axial Syndrome Common to All Psychoses."[2] There Llopis explicitly uses the old term "unitary psychosis" in the way Griesinger defined it in the first edition of his *Pathology and Therapy of Mental Illnesses* in 1845. Instead of an elusive, abstract definition of the term, which would do little to advance the study of its shifting historical meanings, one can cite Griesinger himself:

> Clinical analysis reveals that two large fundamental groups of abnormal mental conditions comprise the two most significant distinctions within insanity. On the one hand, insanity involves the morbid emergence, predominance, and fixation of affects and affect-like states. Under their influence, all mental life [*psychisches Leben*] suffers from the affects' characteristic modifications. On the other hand, insanity involves cognitive and volitional distur-

Author "Gerhart Zeller" is deceased at the time of publication.

[1] Johannes Haller, *Die Epochen der deutschen Geschichte* (Stuttgart: Port Verlag, 1950), 15. [Haller's monograph was first published in 1923 and was a popular success.]

[2] Bartolomé Llopis, "Das allen Psychosen gemeinsame Achsensyndrom, *Fortschritte der Neurologie und Psychiatrie* 28.2 (1960): 106–129.

G. Zeller et al., *A History of Unitary Psychosis*, Theory and History in the Human and Social Sciences, https://doi.org/10.1007/978-3-031-90182-9_2

> bances that don't (or no longer) originate from the predominance of an affective state, but instead represent independent and calm, albeit false cognition and volition (usually predominated by mental debility), without deeper emotional agitation [*Gemütserregtheit*]. Observation further reveals that, in the vast majority of cases, states in the first group precede those in the second; and those in the second, which are generally only a consequence and outcome of the first, arise when the brain disease remains uncured. Furthermore, within the first group, one again observes on average a certain sequence of the specific kinds of affective states. This view recognizes, in the different forms of insanity, different stages of one disease process. Although this process can be modified, interrupted, and altered by countless different intervening pathological events, overall it runs a constant course that can end in the total disintegration of mental life.[3]

In what medical discipline or branch of science could such a Renaissance of a century-old and long-dismissed theory be possible? To answer this question, we must examine the causes of such a turn of events.

The term "unitary psychosis" is of rather recent vintage and was used by none of the founders examined in this study. And yet for us, the term has a unique meaning that helps animate our historical interest. It appeals to us because today many psychiatrists have grown weary of symptomatology and its sharp delineation of specific diseases. By 1919, in his ground-breaking study on the psychogenesis of psychoses in cases of traumatic brain debility, Ernst Kretschmer had already given voice to this discontent: "What we gain in nosology [*Systematik*], we lose in understanding."[4] We are also weary of never-ending individualization that, under the flag of "no diagnosis at all," has led in some quarters to an abandonment of science, which is necessarily systemic and based on rules.

It is the yearning for a generally satisfactory, unified view of mental diseases—a view that might correspond to a long-sought, unified concept of the soul—that enlightens and colors our psychiatric past. Unity, as opposed to the diversity we encounter in both the scientifically organized life's work of Emil Kraepelin and in an approach that discerns only individual life stories and dispenses of all systemic order.

German Literature on Unitary Psychosis

Although it is therefore mostly psychiatry's current situation that elicits interest in the concept of unitary psychosis, we can hardly hope to learn much from older studies in the history of medicine. Hence, our overview of the existing literature can be brief.

The most extensive and richest treatment of the topic is Sigmund Kornfeld's *History of Psychiatry*, where we find this clue: "Albert Zeller (1804–1877) (Reports on the Mental Asylum Winnenthal, especially the second report 1840) distinguishes

[3] Wilhelm Griesinger, *Die Pathologie und Therapie der psychischen Krankheiten* (Stuttgart: A. Krabbe, 1845), 151.

[4] Ernst Kretschmer, "Über psychogene Wahnbildungen bei traumatischer Hirnschwäche," *Zeitschrift für die gesamte Neurologie und Psychiatrie - Originalien* 45.3/4 (1919): 298.

two large groups of abnormal mental conditions. On the one hand, insanity involves the morbid emergence, predominance, and fixation of affects and affect-like states …"[5] Here Kornfeld quotes, as cited above, directly from Griesinger's *Pathology and Therapy of Mental Illnesses*; he is neither paraphrasing nor quoting the five reports that [Albert] Zeller published between the inauguration of the Winnenthal asylum on March 1, 1834, and February 28, 1854.[6] We will later examine those reports, especially how Griesinger appropriated them. The differences between Griesinger and his mentor Zeller are not so trivial that one can assume, as Kornfeld does, that Griesinger simply adopted Zeller's terminology. Based on Kornfeld's rendering, one must assume that he never examined the reports.

We are little better served by Emil Kraepelin's study *One Hundred Years of Psychiatry*,[7] although he was likely the first to sketch a fuller history of unitary psychosis. Kraepelin proceeds from Guislain, whose views he incisively grasps. Guislain believed that diverse clinical pictures represented the expressions of evermore afflicted regions attempting to compensate in the face of invasive mental injury. Consequently, in response to direct stimulus, an initial feeling of sadness and depression [*Schwermut*] arises, provoking a "survival instinct" that produces fits of anger and rage, i.e., "craziness" [*Tollheit*]. Further attempts to compensate for the strain then involve "strange deviations in reasoning," hypochondria vaga [*Grillen*] manifesting "lunacy" [*Narrheit*], "nervous tension" in the form of "ecstasy," convulsions, and finally false ideas as presented to us in "derangement" [*Verrücktheit*], as either "distressing" or "comforting" delusions, as delusions of persecution or grandeur. Differences in the clinical picture are due to differences in personal disposition. Kraepelin then writes:

> It seems that Zeller drew on Guislain's ideas in later developing his views, which were adopted by Hagen and which formed the basis of Griesinger's account of mental medicine [*Seelenheilkunde*]. According to Zeller, the clinical forms of insanity represent, for the most part, stages in the course of an illness. The first stages of the affliction, characterized by depression, frenzy, and delusions, manifest acute emotional distress [*lebhafter Gemütsbewegung*] and are considered curable. Cognitive and volitional disturbances, such as

[5] S[igmund] Kornfeld, "Geschichte der Psychiatrie," in *Handbuch der Geschichte der Medizin*, ed. Max Neuburger and Julius Pagel (Jena: Fischer, 1905), 688.

[6] [[Albert v.] Zeller, "[Erster] Bericht über die Wirksamkeit der Heilanstalt Winnenthal von ihrer Eröffnung den 1. März 1834 bis zum 28. Februar 1837," *Medicinisches Correspondenz-Blatt des Würtembergischen Ärztlichen Vereins* (*MCblWÄV*) 7.30 (Beilage #11) (1837): 321–335; idem, "Zweiter Bericht über die Wirksamkeit der Heilanstalt Winnenthal vom 1. März 1837 bis zum 29. Februar 1840," *MCblWÄV* 10.17–19 (1840): 129–147; idem, "[Dritter] Dreijähriger Bericht über die Wirksamkeit der Heilanstalt Winnenthal vom 1. März 1840 bis zum 28. Februar 1843," *MCblWÄV* 13.38–39 (1843): 297–310; idem, "[Vierter] Dreijähriger Bericht über die Wirksamkeit der Heilanstalt Winnenthal vom 1. März 1843 bis 28. Februar 1846," *MCblWÄV* 18.2–3 (1848): 9–20; idem, "[Fünfter] Bericht über die Wirksamkeit der Heilanstalt Winnenthal vom 1. März 1846 bis 28. Februar 1854," *MCblWÄV* 24.38 (1854): 297–318.]

[7] Emil Kraepelin, "Hundert Jahre Psychiatrie: Ein Beitrag zur Geschichte menschlicher Gesittung," *Zeitschrift für die gesamte Neurologie und Psychiatrie* 38 (1918): 161–275.

> derangement and dementia [*Blödsinn*], tend to emerge independently and reflect the transition to conditions of incurable mental debility.[8]

But this Zeller-Griesinger concept became untenable, according to Kraepelin, once Snell and Westphal found that derangement was by no means always the result of an affective mental disturbance but could instead also emerge independently as a "primary" condition.

Ever since Kraepelin's account, Guislain has been viewed as an immediate predecessor to Zeller and Griesinger. However, it must be noted that this connection has been overstated. Kraepelin failed to see that Zeller responded to Guislain with his own critical perspective.[9] As a result, one can conclude that Guislain was not simply Zeller's predecessor. And one suspects Kraepelin was unaware of Zeller's introduction and addenda to the translation of Guislain's book on phrenopathy. Otherwise he would not have described Zeller as Guislain's translator.[10]

Another interpretation of the historical development of unitary psychosis has been put forth by Theodor Kirchhoff, best known for his 1921 biographic collection *Deutsche Irrenärzte*.[11] Kirchhoff writes about Griesinger:

> His seminal textbook on mental illnesses was based on Reil's concept of the general sense of condition [*Gemeingefühl*] (Zeller's unitary psychosis) and joined Herbart's psychology with Griesinger's own clinical and anatomic experiences. Especially noteworthy is Griesinger's unitary interpretation of the origins of mental disturbances which seeks to recognize in a certain, specific sequence of different forms simply different stages of *one* morbid process. This viewpoint, which dates back to antiquity, proved to be impractical, although it exerted great influence over the development of psychiatric classification.[12]

Notably, Heinrich Haeser pays no attention to the concept of unitary psychosis.[13] One is inclined to think that he stood a bit too far from psychiatry to take more than casual interest in the historical development of its problems. Haeser is content with this elegant, oft-cited summary:

> Since its reestablishment in the eighteenth century, psychiatry has traversed the same general developmental phases as pathology has: the strictly theoretical phase represented by

---

[8] Ibid., 240.

[9] Joseph Guislain, *Abhandlung ueber die Phrenopathien oder neues System der Seelenstörungen, gegründet auf praktische und statistische Beobachtungen und Untersuchung der Ursachen, der Natur, der Symptome, der Prognose, der Diagnose und der Behandlung dieser Krankheiten. Mit einem Vorwort und Zusätzen von Dr. Zeller* (Stuttgart: Rieger, 1838), 1–28, 440–518.

[10] [See Kraepelin, "Hundert Jahre Psychiatrie," 197.]

[11] Theodor Kirchhoff, *Deutsche Irrenärzte: Einzelbilder ihres Lebens und Wirkens*, 2 vols. (Berlin: J. Springer, 1921/24).

[12] Idem, *Geschichte der Psychiatrie*, in *Handbuch der Psychiatrie*, edited by Gustav Aschaffenburg (Leipzig and Vienna: Deuticke, 1912), 46.

[13] See Heinrich Haeser, *Geschichte der Medicin in der neueren Zeit*, 3rd ed., vol. 2 (Jena: Fischer, 1881). [Heinrich Haeser was a nineteenth-century historian of medicine who published a textbook in 1881.]

> Stahl's animism, the descriptive phase founded by Pinel and Esquirol, the patho-anatomic phase led by Spurzheim, and the physiological phase represented by Griesinger.[14]

Having expected little from the older publications, more recent literature also lacks in-depth examination of the topic. Diepgen's *History of Medicine* does not mention the term "unitary psychosis."[15] On Griesinger, Diepgen remarks: "He came from internal medicine and neurology and was entirely committed to physiological medicine, which one associated with a natural science mindset. In his younger years, he was briefly an assistant to the eminent psychiatrist Albert Zeller (1804–1877) at the Winnenthal asylum. He had never headed a psychiatric clinic, not even later in Berlin. But his experiences in Winnenthal joined with those from internal medicine and neurology."[16]

In the most comprehensive study since Kraepelin and Kornfeld, Erwin H. Ackerknecht's *Short History of Psychiatry* remarks on the teacher-student relationship between Zeller and Griesinger: "Although Griesinger followed his mentor Zeller in assuming only one kind of psychosis that evolves in two stages, he provided detailed descriptions of hypochondria, melancholia, mania, monomania, and dementia."[17] But Ackerknecht fails to examine the deeper interconnections and touches on the problem only once: "A large number of tedious classifications emerged in response to the Zeller-Griesinger unitary psychosis (Schüle, v. Krafft-Ebing, Meynert, Skae, Maudsley, Tuke, Blandford)."[18]

In his study on "The Development of Psychiatric Classification in Germany Since Kahlbaum,"[19] Wolfgang de Boor briefly touches on the issue. Notably, de Boor is the first author to discuss the heretofore ignored relationship between Heinrich Neumann and Zeller/Griesinger.

In a lecture on Griesinger's concept of psychiatric illnesses and his importance for subsequent developments, Roland Kuhn summarized what is known about Griesinger:

> Griesinger adopted Guislain's and Zeller's 'unitary psychosis', specifically the view that there was only one kind of mental illness, and that its different clinical manifestations were simply different stages of one and the same process. This process could cease at any moment; it first afflicted the affective side and could be reversed; but later it evolved through cognitive disturbances to dementia [*Verblödung*]. In most cases, the first stage was supposed to be melancholic, followed by mania, which according to Griesinger took two different forms of 'exaltation', namely 'frenzy' [*Tobsucht*] and 'delusional states' [*Wahnsinn*]. 'Mental debility' follows, accompanied by 'partial derangement', 'confusion or general

---

[14] Ibid., 1028.

[15] Paul Diepgen, *Geschichte der Medizin: die historische Entwicklung der Heilkunde und des ärztlichen Lebens*, 2nd ed., vol. 2/1: Von der Medizin der Aufklärung bis zur Begründung der Zellularpathologie (etwa 1740 - etwa 1858) (Berlin: Walter de Gruyter, 1959).

[16] Ibid., 180.

[17] Erwin Heinz Ackerknecht, *Kurze Geschichte der Psychiatrie* (Stuttgart: Enke, 1957), 66.

[18] Ibid., 70.

[19] Wolfgang de Boor, *Psychiatrische Systematik: Ihre Entwicklung in Deutschland seit Kahlbaum* (Berlin: Springer, 1954).

> derangement', 'apathic dementia'. In his textbook's second addition Griesinger then added a chapter on 'idiocy and cretinism'. 'Progressive Paralysis' and 'Epilepsy' are then described as 'complications of insanity'. In his study of Griesinger, which unfortunately is available only in manuscript form, Bodamer has shown how this interpretation of mental illness necessarily follows from Herbart's psychology.[20]

In this brief survey of secondary literature in the history of medicine, there is no need to examine the views of Heinrich Damerow[21] and C. A. Wunderlich[22] because neither dealt with our topic. But the historical chapter in Jaspers' *General Psychopathology*[23] is worth brief consideration. Famously, Jaspers distinguished two kinds of nineteenth-century psychiatric authors: analytical writers and descriptive ones. Among the analysts, he counted Heinrich Neumann, Johann Spielmann, and Carl Wernicke. However, most were descriptive writers, like Griesinger. However, this distinction does not really hold, as Bodamer had already demonstrated in the case of Griesinger,[24] who was both an analytic and a descriptive writer. Jaspers' account of the dispute between somaticists and psychists is likewise unfortunate. He failed to recognize that the positions adopted by somaticists were just as bound to their worldview as those adopted by psychists. This is especially evident in the case of M[aximilian] Jacobi. Jacobi believed that the immortal soul could not possibly fall ill and hence, because of his Christian beliefs, he had to search for the cause of insanity in the body.

Foreign Language Literature on Unitary Psychosis

Having found the German language literature on the history of unitary psychosis mostly unsatisfactory, we can hardly expect foreign language literature to have dealt thoroughly with an issue of concern mostly to German researchers. Gregory Zilboorg's *History of Medical Psychology*[25] is doubtless a commendable and substantive work, the only history of psychiatry to have been published in English. But

[20] Roland Kuhn, "Griesingers Auffassung der psychischen Krankheiten und seine Bedeutung für die weitere Entwicklung der Psychiatrie," in *Beiträge zur Geschichte der Psychiatrie und Hirnanatomie*, edited by Alfred Glaus (Basel: Karger, 1957), 49. [See Joachim Bodamer, "Wilhelm Griesinger und die Entwicklung der Psychiatrie im 19. Jahrhundert" (Medical Dissertation, University of Heidelberg, 1944).]

[21] Heinrich Philipp August Damerow, *Die Elemente der nächsten Zukunft der Medizin, entwickelt aus der Vergangenheit und Gegenwart* (Berlin: Reimer, 1829). [On Damerow, see also Gerhart Zeller, ed., *Albert Zellers medizinisches Tagebuch der psychiatrischen Reise durch Deutschland, England, Frankreich und nach Prag von 1832 bis 1833*, Bd. 2 (Zwiefalten: Psychiatrie und Geschichte, 2007), 13–14.]

[22] Carl August Wunderlich, *Geschichte der Medizin: Vorlesungen gehalten im Sommersemester 1858* (Stuttgart: Ebner & Seubert, 1859).

[23] Karl Jaspers, *Allgemeine Psychopathologie*, 5th ed. (Berlin: Springer, 1948), 703–716.

[24] See Bodamer, "Wilhelm Griesinger".

[25] Gregory Zilboorg, *A History of Medical Psychology* (New York: Norton, 1941).

unfortunately, the author stands conceptually and geographically so far afield of the problems confronting Europe in the early nineteenth century that one cannot expect more than general pronouncements about this historical era—pronouncements that are also often distorted by a rigid schema. For example, he views somaticists as materialists and psychists as Romantics. He views Griesinger as having arbitrated the dispute between both parties. Over the course of our study, we will see that this claim is completely untenable.

In the French literature we note only the book *Les Malades de l'Esprit et leurs Médecins du XVIe au XIXe siècle* by M. Laignel-Lavastine and Jean Vinchon, although it contains nothing relevant to our topic.[26]

Surveying this literature, one finds that the concept of unitary psychosis is usually associated with the Winnenthal psychiatrist Albert Zeller, Griesinger's mentor. It is commonplace to speak of the Zeller-Griesinger unitary psychosis. Griesinger himself remarked that "thanks to this idea, most clearly expressed by Zeller, it is possible to move a bit further along the path of symptomatology toward the preeminent tasks of explaining and diagnosing mental illness pathoanatomically."[27] In subsequent editions of his textbook, the quote remained unchanged, as a memorial to his mentor. The first edition of the textbook is dedicated to Zeller:

> It has been very satisfying to eventually complete this work, although I am well aware of its many flaws. Writing it has been the more pleasurable for reminding me of my earlier work as a practicing alienist at one of the best German asylums. There, my initial psychiatric research profited under the direction of a distinguished friend, privy councilor Dr. Zeller in Winnenthal. May this publication give him too occasion to recall pleasant memories.[28]

However, to this day no one has bothered to study Albert Zeller's predecessors. Authors usually mention Joseph Guislain, claiming that Zeller either followed or even adopted his theories. Kirchhoff then links to Reil, Gruhle to Knight, Bodamer, and later Kuhn to Herbart. None of these linkages have been conclusively demonstrated. It remains entirely unclear how Zeller's unitary psychosis relates to Neumann's and which of them then influenced Arndt and Kahlbaum.

Given so many unresolved questions, one must ask what methods will be used to answer them. Two approaches are available: intellectual history and biography. The former approach would need to draw on existing literature to pursue the questions in all their variations. The sources would have to be examined as to whether they have a common intellectual origin or whether they are associated to one another by tradition. However, this approach cannot produce definitive answers to the unresolved questions, especially regarding the relationship between Guislain and Zeller. The other approach seems to be more viable. However, a scientific biography of

---

[26] M. Laignel and Jean Vinchon, *Les malades de l'esprit et leur médecins du 16e au 19e siècle* (Paris: Maloine, 1930).

[27] Griesinger, *Die Pathologie und Therapie*, 151.

[28] Ibid., vi.

Albert Zeller detailed enough to clarify his concept of unitary psychosis faces nearly insurmountable difficulties, given that he published very little.[29]

Unpublished Sources

This study must therefore also rely on Zeller's unpublished papers if the analysis of his ideas is to succeed. However, to date those papers have been all but unreadable, and all attempts to decipher them have failed, such that so far only fragments could be evaluated. Among the unpublished sources are the diaries. The most important of these is a 344-page "Medical Diary of the Psychiatric Trip Through Germany, England, and France from February 1832 to May 1833."[30] This diary, which Robert Gaupp had hoped to have medical students decipher, has rebuffed all such attempts, not just because of the handwriting but also because in France it is written in French, in England English, and otherwise occasionally in Latin. Only recently has the manuscript been translated and transcribed. A second diary is much shorter, exists as a typescript,[31] and was used by Gaupp for his biographic research.[32] It was written when Albert Zeller was a student. A third, yet to be transcribed, diary recounts his impressions of Berlin when he studied there in 1827.[33]

Almost no relevant letters have survived. During World War II the entire Zeller-Jacobi correspondence was destroyed.[34] It comprised 162 letters from Jacobi and 151 from Zeller, beginning in 1832 until Jacobi's last letter on May 8, 1858, 10 days before his death. Unfortunately, the correspondence was never fully investigated, although for a time it was on loan to the Research Institute for Psychiatry in Munich.[35] However, both Johannes Herting and Hermann Zeller used part of the correspondence for their publications.[36] There remains also a small, handwritten,

---

[29] [Abridgement (ca. 570 words): Annotated bibliography of Albert Zeller's publications. See the titles in the bibliography marked with an asterisk (*).]

[30] [Shortly after his death in 2006, Gerhart Zeller's full transcription and commentary of the medical diary was published in two volumes. See Gerhart Zeller, ed., *Albert Zellers medizinisches Tagebuch*.]

[31] Albert Zeller, Studientagebücher, 1824–1827, Albert Zeller Papers, Berlin.

[32] [Robert Gaupp, "Ein zyklothymer Psychiater über seine seelischen Krankheitszeiten," *Zeitschrift für die gesamte Neurologie und Psychiatrie* 166 (1939): 705–710; idem, "Albert Zeller," *Schwäbische Lebensbilder* 1 (1940): 574–582.]

[33] Albert Zeller, Studientagebücher.

[34] [Only copies of Jacobi's letters to Zeller have survived. See Archiv des Landschaftsverband Rheinland (Pulheim-Brauweiler), Nos. 31557 and 31656.]

[35] [Gerhart Zeller is referring here to the Max-Planck-Institute of Psychiatry.]

[36] Johannes Herting, *Carl Wigand Maximilian Jacobi: Ein deutsche Arzt (1775-1858)* (Görlitz: C. A. Starke, 1930); Hermann Zeller, "Ernst Albert Zeller," in *Deutsche Irrenärzte*, edited by Theodor Kirchhoff (Berlin: J. Springer, 1921), 208–218.

and incomplete paper "On the Consensus of Internal Organs and Systems" written in the summer of 1824.[37]

The following study will reveal whether this heretofore unexamined source material will promote new insights about the history of unitary psychosis.

Section 2.2

Albert Zeller's Family, Culture, and Intellectual Background

To understand someone's intellectual development, one should first ask where they come from. There are two aspects to this question: genealogy and cultural heritage, including that heritage's unique tribal aspects. One must carefully examine the person's schooling, teachers, and independent development, given their circumstances. Considering Albert Zeller's personality, the first question is easily answered.[38]

The roots of the Zeller family can be traced back to the year 1521. His great-grandfather was a Catholic prelate and his grandfather a physician and medical officer in the town of Laufen on the Neckar river. His father (1769–1846) Johann Friedrich married Johanna Regine Andreae, whose father Jakob Eberhard was a royal physician in Stuttgart. Albert Zeller's father Johann Friedrich was a jurist closely involved in the incorporation of territorial acquisitions of the state of Württemberg: he became the chief administrator of the free Imperial City of Heilbronn and was named commissioner in charge of river traffic on the Neckar. He was well-known at the time, a cosmopolitan, no-nonsense politician, upright and energetic. He is rendered in a portrait by Johann Baptist Seele (1774–1814), a member of the elite Carlsschule and otherwise known for his character portraits and genre scenes.

Zeller's mother was a deeply spiritual woman. In a letter that survives, she recounts to her grown son Albert "How I raised my children."[39] The letter exudes an attitude to life that we recognize as sentimentalism, which evolved from—and in constant interaction with—Pietism. In Pietism we have the foundation of Albert Zeller's personality and perhaps even of modern psychiatry and psychology.[40] This historical context has been all but forgotten. The nineteenth-century historian

---

[37] Albert Zeller, "Versuch über den Consens der inneren Organe und Systeme, 1824," Albert Zeller Papers, Berlin.

[38] [In Gerhart Zeller's revised manuscript, treatment of the Zeller family history has been radically shortened. On the history of the Zeller family, see Gerhart Zeller, ed., *Albert Zellers medizinisches Tagebuch*, vol. 1, 10–14.]

[39] [The letter was lost during World War II. In the original manuscript, extended excerpts are cited. However, in revising the manuscript, Gerhart Zeller deleted most of these passages. But see Gerhart Zeller, ed., *Albert Zellers medizinisches Tagebuch*, vol. 1, 14.]

[40] [Gerhart Zeller would later emphasize the decisive impact of Pietism on the development of alienism in Germany. See Gerhart Zeller, "Bonhoeffers wissenschaftliches Werk. Entwicklung und

Haeser still recognized this in his treatment of [the founder of a prominent eighteenth-century branch of Pietism] August Hermann Francke (1663–1772), a minister, professor of theology, and founder of an orphanage in the city of Halle. Although the importance of Pietism has been noted by some authors,[41] in more recent literature the term Pietism is rarely mentioned. This is mainly because Pietism as we know it today in Württemberg suggests the narrow-mindedness, resentment, and moralizing of cabalists. But to properly assess the significance of Pietism, one must recognize it as part of an enormously influential intellectual movement stretching from medieval German mysticism to Romanticism. Pietism's emphasis on the mind and the will, as opposed to perception, feeling, and imagination, initially allied it, albeit unintentionally, with the Enlightenment. One sees this in the fact that the otherwise enlightened founder of Pietism, Jakob Spener (1635–1705), still engaged in the practice of "thumbing," i.e., consulting the bible for personal instruction. However, Pietism increasingly became a reaction against the stale superficiality and intolerance of a religious and philosophical orthodoxy that had disparaged the importance of the imaginative and mysterious in religious belief. Francke's brand of Pietism recalled the moral content of Christianity and the inner revelation in conscience. From this emerged the doctrine that everyone born again in Christ should be constantly preoccupied with God and their own unworthiness and ignore everything preventing one's immersion into oneself. And from this doctrine there evolved in turn a movement that was indifferent to the sciences, the church, and even different religions, believing that salvation and contentment could be found only in the pleasure derived from one's inner light. The consequences of this evolution of popular religious consciousness were threefold.[42]

First, an emphasis on inner experience and a preference for subjective mental facts [*subjektivistischen seelischen Tatsachen*]. There emerged an intimate sense of the inner life. [The pietist revivalist Gerhard] Tersteegen (1697–1769) wrote to a friend: "Everything in me tends to seclusion, silence, imagelessness, and unity with God."[43] "To be able to live like that means truly to live."[44]

Second, a revived appreciation for human involuntariness. [The Lutheran pietist theologian Johann Albrecht] Bengel reminded his readers: "The divine force of the simplest truths, which enter the heart apart from one's own effort, proceeds to spread on its own in many directions. One seeks not to compel some sensual experience in oneself, but simply to endure in true loyalty."[45]

Bedeutung," in *Karl Bonhoeffer: Zum hundertsten Geburtstag am 31. März 1968*, edited by Jürg Zutt, Erwin Straus and H. Scheller (Berlin: Springer, 1969), 119–121.]

[41] Max Dessoir, *Geschichte der neueren deutschen Psychologie*, vol. 1, 2nd ed. (Berlin: Duncker, 1902).

[42] Dessoir.

[43] [The original source of this quotation could not be identified.]

[44] [The original source of this quotation could not be identified.]

[45] [The original source of this quotation could not be identified.]

Third, an interest in understanding the psychological life of pious individuals, regardless of their social standing.

Just as Francke's Halle-based Pietism was stagnating, it was revived in Württemberg, which in the eighteenth century was something of a backwater of intellectual life in Germany. There, because the aristocracy played no role outside the royal court, clergy and government officials assumed the traditional roles of the nobility. As Schelling once mocked, there evolved a "preacher and scribe state." This arrangement proved especially durable because of an extensive meritocratic system that funneled nearly all of the country's intelligentsia into Christian ministry. Instead of enriching himself at the church's expense like other aristocrats, Duke Christoph, son of the controversial reformation Duke Ulrich, established an office to administer church property, pay clerical salaries, and fund convent schools and the seminary in Tübingen. These educational resources were accessible to gifted children who passed a state exam.

As a result of this arrangement, Württemberg's bourgeois nobility sustained itself, shunning both Enlightenment ideals and aristocratic norms. However, Pietism was widely championed and became so powerful as to require measures curbing it in 1773. Communal life in Württemberg was thus lived within the bosom of the Lutheran state church.

Albrecht Bengel (1687–1752) and Christoph Friedrich Oetinger (1702–1782) invigorated this movement. Oetinger drew on the teachings of Jakob Böhme and influenced Schelling. He combined Pietist sensibilities and a sober, Swabian sense of reality. His affinity with nature and life aligns him with the artistic tradition of *Sturm und Drang*. Pietism's outlook shifted toward originalism, the believer becoming the visionary, religion becoming a divinely inspired art form. At the same time, the apolitical aversion to life evolved into a sober-minded embrace of life.

Returning to Zeller, we know that his father sent him, together with his brothers, to be schooled by a minister in Horkheim near Heilbronn. When his father returned to Stuttgart, he attended the local gymnasium. After completing his schooling, he enrolled at the university in Tübingen, fulfilling his long-standing wish to study medicine.

Records documenting this period include a 54-page copy of his diary and the 19-page manuscript "On the Consensus of Internal Organs and Systems." Both were written in the mid-1820s and provide important insight into his mental development, as well as the sources of his scientific views. We begin with a verse that Zeller committed to his diary in 1825 and that could serve as the diary's motto:

Go ahead and descend into yourself!
Forces that have long slumbered
Are held by your unfathomable self
Deep in its inner depths.[46]

[46] Albert Zeller, Studientagebücher.

Throughout his diary, we encounter the 20-year-old student as an "analyst of the subjective" [*subjektivistischer Analytiker*],[47] i.e., an individual striving to know themselves, searching not for general scientific knowledge but instead struggling to analyze internal evidence of the self. This tendency to self-observation was hardly a youthful fad. Well into old age, and long after their popularity had waned, Zeller was reading introspective accounts of the self, such as the writings of Adam Bernd, whom Dessoir described as the first decadent psychologist. In Zeller's copy of Bernd's classic, but long forgotten monument to psychological introspection,[48] he highlighted this passage:

> The beast of irascibility continued to rage in me, until God drove out one affect with another, using awful anxiety and melancholy to put an end to the fury, or to at least much weaken it; and until I found the roots of the immoderate affects in the flesh and with the help of medication resisted the hot and fiery feelings [*Gemüte*] of the body.[49]

We will later see how strongly Zeller inevitably found himself validated by these words.

The young self-analyzing student remarks about himself:

> It is strange that, from the outset, I lagged behind my fellow pupils in everything, from my A-B-Cs to the logic of chess, in arithmetic to this day, in drawing and languages, especially in everything demanding reasoning. And yet, I was not dumb and soon surpassed the others, at least in some areas. I think about it to this day and still don't know where the mistake in my cognitive abilities lies. I more easily comprehended the beautiful and the good, but not rational forms and formulae.[50]

This passage reminds one of Goethe's remark "Division and numbers were not part of my nature"[51] or Bengel's critique of mathematics: "In some things, mathematics can be helpful, but applied to truths that lie outside its forum, it saps our understanding. In wanting nothing but definitive concepts, one loses the vital ones."[52] We see that Albert Zeller's reasoning was better suited to grasping a totality than to analyzing details. He readily participated in the holistic impetus of Romanticism, which Werner Leibbrand has rightfully identified as being "addicted to unity" [*einheitssüchtig*].[53] But he also brought with him considerable talents of Romantic absorption that for him, whom Bodamer called an "anima naturaliter christiana," necessarily

---

[47] Dessoir, 301–302.

[48] Adam Bernd, *Eigene Lebens-Beschreibung Samt einer aufrichtigen Entdeckung, und deutlichen Beschreibung einer der grösten, obwohl großen Theils noch unbekannten Leibes- und Gemüths-Plagen, Welche Gott zuweilen über die Welt-Kinder, und auch wohl über seine eigene Kinder verhänget: Den Unwissenden zum Unterricht, Den Gelehrten zu weiterem Nachdencken, Den Sündern zum Schrecken, und Den Betrübten, und Angefochtenen zum Troste* (Leipzig: Johann Samuel Heinsius, 1738).

[49] Ibid., 103.

[50] Albert Zeller, Studientagebücher.

[51] Johann Wolfgang Goethe, "Der Verfasser teilt die Geschichte seiner botanischen Studien mit," in *Sämtliche Werke* (Leipzig: Insel, 1917 [1817]), 259.

[52] [The original source of this quotation could not be identified.]

[53] [The original source of this quotation could not be identified.]

found expression in religious channels.[54] In his diary he writes: "If I wouldn't find God in nature, nature would not attract my interest."[55] Zeller experienced the mysteries of the soul with God in a truly mystical fashion, hence his devotion to John the Evangelist. But he also clearly recognizes the hazards this poses for him as a physician. In his diary he admonishes himself: "I must very much beware of mysticism."[56] Throughout his diary, a Romantic search for unity is coupled with a Christian mindset: "A person can wrestle and strive for as long as he wants, but as long as he is not Christian, he will find no harmony."[57]

One of Zeller's own observations demonstrates just how emotionally subtle his empathy—likely the strongest source of his effectiveness as a mental doctor—was:

> I have often found that I can guess, for no obvious reason, the thoughts of others. I lit upon the strangest words that others sought, especially the words that friends of mine sought. The same is true when someone loses the thread of a poem: I can often recite the still unspoken lines. And it seems natural to me. I adopt the feelings and atmosphere and the entire situation of the poet, so that the subsequent course then proceeds in me as it would in the poet.[58]

Given this constant striving toward self-awareness, Zeller necessarily also encountered the depressive predisposition that Robert Gaupp diagnosed.[59] Albert Zeller writes about himself:

> In the moments of greatest pleasure, the image of death hangs over me. As a boy, I lost in rapid succession a brother and two playmates, whom I loved dearly. And so the thought of death very often came to me as a child at play, especially because one of them suddenly fell ill in our midst and was buried within just three days. I saw them in the coffin, I can still see them, the lovely pale boys, and my early death seemed certain. And so the foundations of melancholy were already laid in my childhood and grew with me into a young man with lowered torch. I must shake off the melancholy and raise the torch before the flame dies, so that lowering it will have served only to make it burn brighter.[60]

It seems that Albert Zeller's temperament was inclined to very serious waves of depression, something of the utmost importance for the later development of his psychiatric schema. Must not the question of the boundary between morbid and premorbid melancholia have been posed to him more urgently than to his contemporaries? On the other hand, from observing himself he must have derived a sense, through no fault of his own, of constant mental endangerment. This led to his adamant rejection of any overly moralistic interpretation of mental illness and cleared a path to truly humane engagement with patients. One is reminded of Zeller's

---

[54] [Joachim Bodamer, "Zur Entstehung der Psychiatrie als Wissenschaft im 19. Jahrhundert," *Fortschritte der Neurologie, Psychiatrie und ihrer Grenzgebiete* 21 (1953): 523.]

[55] Albert Zeller, Studientagebücher.

[56] Ibid.

[57] Ibid.

[58] Ibid. [Empathy and sympathy are reputed to have comprised the "leitmotif" of Albert Zeller's life. See Gerhart Zeller, ed., *Albert Zellers medizinisches Tagebuch*, vol. 2, 38.]

[59] Gaupp, "Ein Zyklothymer Psychiater" and idem, "Albert Zeller".

[60] Albert Zeller, Studientagebücher.

contemporary Søren Kierkegaard, who wrote in 1844: "The alienist who is dumb enough to believe that he is forever smart and that his portion of reason will never wane, is in some sense smarter than the mad, but at the same time also dumber than them, and unlikely to cure many of them."[61] Thanks to his personal experience, Albert Zeller had always been immune from such "stupidity."

Whereas the diary reveals something of the inner life of the young man, his incomplete 1824 manuscript "On the Consensus of Internal Organs and Systems"[62] sheds light on his studies at the University in Tübingen and especially its foremost scholar, Johann Heinrich Ferdinand v. Autenrieth (1772–1835), since it is nothing other than an excerpt of Autenrieth's *Handbook of Empirical Human Physiology*.[63]

[J. H. F. Autenrieth and Higher Education in Württemberg]

Autenrieth entered the elite Carlsschule in Stuttgart in 1785 at the height of its late eighteenth-century influence, and a decade after it had acquired a medical division.[64] There, like his fellow student Friedrich Schiller, he participated actively in student life, joining the scientific club founded and headed by Georges Cuvier (1769–1832). Medical instruction in Stuttgart distinguished itself pedagogically in that upper division students were given teaching responsibilities and all students, including medical students, were required to take courses and pass a final examination in philosophy. Medical instruction remained mostly theoretical, in spite of Herman Boerhaave's (1668–1738) model of clinical teaching in Leyden. And yet practical instruction appears to have been more pronounced in Stuttgart than at the university in Tübingen. Course catalogs in Stuttgart reveal that the city's surgeon taught classes at the local hospital and that two of the school's professors offered practical instruction in pathology at public hospitals.[65] The publications of Friedrich Schiller clearly show that Thomas Sydenham (1624–1689) and Boerhaave were highly regarded at the school.[66] And the animism of Georg Ernst Stahl (1659–1721)

---

[61] Søren Kierkegaard, *Der Begriff Angst* (Leipzig: Fr. Richter, 1844), 50.

[62] Albert Zeller, "Versuch".

[63] Johann Heinrich Ferdinand v. Autenrieth, *Handbuch der empirischen menschlichen Physiologie*, 3 vols. (Tübingen: Heerbrandt, 1801–02).

[64] See Gustav Schleich, *Ein Stück aus der Geschichte der medizinischen Fakultät der Universität Tübingen* (Tübingen: Schnürlen, 1910); Eberhard Stübler, *Johann Heinrich Ferdinand v. Autenrieth (1772–1835)* (Stuttgart: Schröder, 1948). [On Autenrieth, see also Gerhart Zeller, ed., *Albert Zellers medizinisches Tagebuch*, vol. 1, 14–18 and vol. 2, 14–17. There Autenrieth is described as a "Vitalist and Zeller as an animist". Ibid, vol. 1, 15.]

[65] [Abridgement (ca. 270 words): Details about the Carlsschule, its curriculum and staff.]

[66] See Friedrich Schiller, "De discrimine febrium inflammatoriarum et putridarum," in *Medizinische Schriften* (Miesbach: W. F. Mayr, 1959 [1780]), 63–134; idem, "Versuch über den Zusammenhang der tierischen Natur des Menschen mit seiner geistigen," in *Medizinische Schriften* (Miesbach: W. F. Mayr, 1959 [1780]), 135–180.

was banished into the realm of speculation in favor of the ideas of Friedrich Hoffmann (1660–1721).

Instruction at the Carlsschule was strongly influenced by the views of Thomas Sydenham, especially the idea that different illnesses shared a deep affinity with one another. In his work on infectious diseases, Sydenham maintained that epidemics were variable and that they brought forth illnesses that, although they belonged together, did not share the same symptoms. For example, in a smallpox epidemic, Sydenham tended to diagnose all cases of fever as cases of smallpox. Sydenham also argued that a secondary, derivative illness, for example fever, could elicit symptoms from an entirely different organ system. Evidence of Sydenham's impact on psychiatric thinking can be gleaned from a prominent nineteenth-century publication, where his work on hysteria and hypochondria was cited to illustrate how a case of mania that devolved into dementia could emerge from a case of intermittent fever.[67]

In philosophy, the Carlsschule was a "product of the Protestant Enlightenment and late-absolutist welfare state"[68] and embodied two rather different intellectual standpoints. On one side stood Gottfried Ploucquet (1716–1790), a champion of speculative rationalism, who drew on the ideas of Reformed Calvinism and Swabian Pietism to criticize and debunk the theodicies of Descartes and Leibniz. On the other side stood Jakob Friedrich Abel (1751–1829), who used the writings of John Locke in combination with post-Leibnizian notions of spiritual powers [*Seelenkräfte*] to develop a mechanistic system of forces (*vires*) governing thought, feeling, perception, imagination, memory, etc. Abel also used these forces to describe the soul's influence on the body, and we can assume that students of medicine and philosophy at the Carlsschule engaged these ideas.[69]

In these two figures we clearly see two sources of Autenrieth's thought. In spite of his many speculations, he remained a sober empiricist. Writing in the *Tübinger Blätter*, which he edited alongside the physicist J. G. Bohnenberger, he proclaimed: "Any mind that wishes to recognize the world as it is, rather than as it can be dreamed, and that loves to examine one specific thing in order to gain reliable general knowledge, will have its place in these pages."[70] In these words, one recognizes that Kant's transcendental critique had not yet arrived at the Carlsschule. Autenrieth's naïve rationalism had not yet learned to doubt itself. But he remained committed to philosophical and theoretical questions, publishing articles on "The Soul's Connection to

[67] Heinrich Laehr, *Gedenktage der Psychiatrie und ihre Hilfswissenschaften in allen Ländern*, 4th ed. (Berlin: G. Reimer, 1893).

[68] Müller, "Forschung, Erziehung und Lehre untersucht nach den Druckschriften der Carlsschule," in *Die Hohe Carlsschule [Ausstellungskatalog]* (Stuttgart: Turmhaus, 1960), 41.

[69] According to Müller, Abel's writings on sympathy and character mirrored those of Johann Friedrich Consbruch, who taught internal medicine at the Carlsschule, and that both scholars drew on the works of Haller, Boerhaave, Gaubius, Hume, and de Wytt. Ibid., 45.

[70] [J. H. F. Autenrieth and J. G. v. Bohnenberger, "Vorrede," *Tübinger Blätter für Naturwissenschaften und Arzneykunde* 1.1 (1815), 1.]

Organic Forces," "Man and His Hope for Everlasting Life from a Scientific Perspective," and "On the Book of Job."[71]

Strangely, some historians have claimed that Autenrieth was a student of Johann Peter Frank (1745–1821), the famous pioneer of public hygiene and medical policing.[72] In fact, however, Autenrieth studied only briefly with Frank in Pavia and was highly critical of his views.[73] Indeed, Autenrieth remained a devoted student of the Carlsschule and its values.[74]

In June of 1797 he was appointed professor at the Carlsschule, and in May of 1805 he established and began teaching at an *institutum clinicum* with 15 beds. From the outset, he also treated mentally ill patients; and because they often disturbed other patients and were a danger to themselves, he devised means of keeping them safe and quiet, such as a mask and a pear that prevented patients from screaming and so-called palisade cells. These cells were simply rooms in which the window and oven were encased in wooden fencing. Today, such things belong in museums. And yet they are the only things we know about his psychiatric work, and that Autenrieth resorted to such disagreeable methods in treating the mentally ill in his clinic is testament to his great interest in them. As a theoretician and in practice, he is said to have had little impact on the development of psychiatry.[75] But we have reason to disagree with this view. His legacy in general medicine is likewise all but forgotten: one knows only that he believed many illnesses could be traced to recurrent scabies and that he went on the war path against the use of mercury to treat scabies.

Autenrieth's public stature was confirmed when he became the first non-theologian whom the king appointed vice chancellor of the University of Tübingen in 1819 and chancellor in 1822. During his difficult tenure, he had to dampen the revolutionary fervor of the fraternities and face down opposition to transforming the university into a state institution. His greatest influence was as a teacher, and his "Tübingen School" counted among its most prominent students Albert Zeller, Wilhelm Griesinger, and C. A. Wunderlich.

Autenrieth was a humoral pathologist in the tradition of Sydenham and Franz de le Boë (Sylvius) (1614–1672). From Sydenham he adopted the conviction that different illnesses shared a deep affinity with one another and that it was possible for one to change into the other (*transmutatio morborum*); from Sylvius he adopted the concept of acrimony whereby acrid humors arose in certain organs and took hold metastastically in others. Autenrieth distinguished between acute and chronic acrimony, counting among the later scabious, hemorrhoidal, and arthritic acrimony. The

[71] Johann Heinrich Ferdinand v. Autenrieth, *Ansichten über Natur- und Seelenleben* (Stuttgart: Cotta, 1836).

[72] Diepgen.

[73] Stübler, 24–29.

[74] [Abridgement (ca. 90 words): remarks on Autenrieth's personality drawn from Robert v. Mohl, *Lebens-Erinnerungen von Robert von Mohl (1799-1875)* (Stuttgart: DVA, 1902).]

[75] Robert Gaupp, "Ferdinand Autenrieth (1772-1835)," in *Deutsche Irrenärzte: Einzelbilder ihres Lebens und Wirkens*, edited by Theodor Kirchhoff (Berlin: J. Springer, 1921).

regularity he believed often to have witnessed in metastasis led him to believe that there was a connection or consensus between the organs. The notion of a consensus of inner organs gradually came to dominate his medical thinking and led to remarkable results. Among other things, Autenrieth spoke of organs connected by habit, possibly imagining what Pavlov (1859–1936) would later describe as a conditional reflex.

The essential therapeutic task was to redirect the acrimony outward, preferably through the intestines. This idea was commonplace among humoral pathologists. Applying a setaceum to the neck to produce an artificial boil, reopening an ulcerous wound when its acridity had turned inward, and provoking hemorrhoidal or menstrual flows—all of these were well-accepted measures that somatically inclined psychiatrists and then also put to generous use, not to mention bleedings with the aid of a scarificator or leeches.

Understanding the scientific outlook of physicians around 1800 also entails an assessment of their views about a *vis vitalis* and the relationship between body and soul. Most eighteenth-century physicians followed the Montpellier school in their understanding of the *vis vitalis* as a *force hypermécanique*. Even in France they had distanced themselves from Descartes' view of life processes as a kind of clock or machine: "According to the rules of mechanics which are the same as those of nature."[76] Georg Ernst Stahl[77] then identified the soul with forces that invigorated, developed, and protected the body from decay. Max Dessoir has rightly noted how awkward for us Stahl's view is, because we tend to associate the word "soul" simply with the sum of conscious processes. But originally, in its most common usage, the term "soul" encompassed not just mental but all vital phenomena. Aristotle's *anima vegetativa* later evolved into a vital force. Stahl too writes that the body, lacking this principle, is a machine that is not self-sufficient and soon decays. But he expands the concept of this invigorating and developmental principle by including the animal soul, the site of movement and sensation. He concludes that the vital force is identical to the soul because seemingly unconscious movements can become conscious ones or vice versa voluntary movements involuntary ones. Finally, he even binds life to reason, thereby not only transforming a strictly human condition into a general one but also positing a causal relationship between the two, with the mental soul acting as a necessary condition of that relationship.

Stahl's follower Robert Whytt (1714–1766) then restricted vitality to the "merely perceiving" soul. For him, the soul is the site at which the force of perception is transformed into motor force; because the entire body is sensitive and mobile, the soul must permeate it. He concludes that the spinal cord is more than simply a subordinate conduit. Whytt's argument was adopted by E. Pflüger's early work on the

[76] Oeuvres I, 184.

[77] Georgii Ernesti Stahl, *Theoria Medica Vera* (Hallae: Orphanotropheum, 1708).

"spinal soul" [*Rückenmarksseele*], where he claimed to have proven that "the sensorium is spread throughout the entire cerebro-spinal organ."[78]

These issues are important because Albert Zeller repeatedly cites Stahl and likewise claims that the spinal cord is related to mental life [*Seelenleben*]. August Unzer revamped Stahl's teachings, stripping them of their peculiarities. He did this by introducing a nervous force between the soul, as the seat of consciousness, and bodily functions. As a result, the body's dependence on the soul became indirect. We will see that this concept of an intermediate force [*Mittelkraft*] reappears in the work of Schiller and Autenrieth. However, Autenrieth links it to the ideas of Friedrich Hoffmann, a friend of Schiller's.

[¶] There were two major differences between Stahl's mental vitalism [*psychischer Vitalismus*] and Hoffmann's dynamic vitalism.[79] First, Hoffmann recognized that some life functions (e.g., circulation) were based on strictly mechanical laws. In this he agreed with the so-called iatro-mathematicians, who sought to explain all non-volitional processes using the laws of mechanics and hydraulics. Apart from these mechanical processes, he posited a *vis vitalis solidi*, which comprised a vital force specific to solid tissue, especially the muscles and nerves. Hoffmann argued that this force circulated in minute tubes as a neural ether [*Nervenäther*], like blood in veins and arteries. Second, Hoffman claimed that, as an ether, this force could be found throughout nature and be drawn out of the atmosphere by organic bodies, as Franz Anton Mesmer (1733–1815) maintained. According to Mesmer, the entire universe was saturated with an ethereal fluid finer still than light's ether. The movement or "flood" of this fluid—specifically, oscillations attributable to the laws of polarity—influences not only how celestial bodies interact with one another and with the earth but also how animal bodies interact, as manifested in well-known phenomena. According to Mesmer, the universal fluid can collect in or dissipate from an individual, creating a microcosmic analogy to waxing and waning tides. Just as one can collect electromagnetic force in metal—a force like or even identical to the fluid—so too can, in certain individuals, natural magnetism be increased to the point that it too can produce effects analogous to magnets. Animal magnetism is thus merely a variant of natural magnetism, of the cosmic flux; it is based on the receptivity of all organic bodies to the universal fluid, which initially affects the nerves. After Galvani (1737–1798) then discovered that living animals and nerves produced electricity, Alexander von Humboldt concluded that the yet unknown nerve fluid, muscular stimulation, and indeed the entire life process were galvanic processes. In his handbook, Autenrieth writes: "Even if galvanic fluid is itself not the source of the vital force, among all of the imponderable alternatives, it comes closest to it.[80]

[78] Thus Eduard Friedrich Wilhelm Pflüger, *Die sensorischen Functionen des Rückenmarks der Wirbelthiere: Nebst einer neuen Lehre über die Leitungsgesetze der Reflexionen* (Berlin: Hirschwald, 1853) as cited in Dessoir, 503 footnote 2.

[79] [See] Dessoir, 505 f.

[80] Autenrieth, *Handbuch*, vol. 1, §200, 124.

In his understanding of the connection of the soul to the organic body, Autenrieth like Schiller concurs with Unzer's idea of an intermediate force:

> The connection of the mind [*Geist*] to the body, regardless of its own constant non-spatialty [*Unräumlichkeit*], is possible because the body coexists in connection with an organic vital force. Insofar as that force is incorporated in organic matter and expressed spatially, it becomes spatial. But the mind manifests itself non-spatially insofar as the relationships of every individualized life force are conditional upon a common source of all life that is non-spatial. It can therefore also be related to the essentially non-spatial. It is only by means of the organic life force that the soul enters into a close, but as noted above potentially fluctuating connection to the body. The two-sided vital force binds the soul, in its non-spatial world, to the body.[81]

Remarkably, Friedrich Schiller develops the same ideas, albeit more clearly and elegantly, in his philosophy of physiology:

> Or finally there must exist a force between mind [*Geist*] and matter that connects both. A force that can be changed by matter and that can change the mind. And so this force would be a partly mental, partly material, an essence partly penetrable and partly impenetrable. Is such a force even conceivable? Certainly not! Be that as it may, a force really exists between matter and mind. This force is very different from the world and the mind. If I remove it, all the world's effects on the mind disappear. And yet the mind remains. And yet the object remains. Its loss has torn world and mind apart. Its existence enlightens, awakens, enlivens everything around it. I call it an intermediate force [*Mittelkraft*].[82]

Before turning to Autenrieth's theory of disease, we briefly consider whether he was really a child of his own time and not just a belated one of the Enlightenment. This is not the case because, for one, he often and happily used Romanticism's magic wand of analogy, and furthermore, he worked, much along the lines of Oken, on a theory of anatomy and on morphological laws [*Bildungsgesetzen*]. In his theory of anatomy, the Romantic concept of polarity plays an important role: "all these appearances lead ultimately to a deep, natural polarity that is manifested everywhere, even in humans."[83] Elsewhere he claimed that the structure of the female thorax was attributable to less need for oxygen due to a negative polarity of the female.[84] The positive polarity of the man was due to a stronger oxidation process. These examples suffice to show that Autenrieth was a true Romantic physician. And yet his ideas about polarity prevented him from adopting the Brownianism that was

---

[81] Johann Heinrich Ferdinand v. Autenrieth, "Verbindung der Seele mit dem organischen Körper: Entwicklung des Charakters der Persönlichkeit in der Reihe der Wesen," in *Ansichten über Natur- und Seelenleben*, edited by Hermann Friedrich Autenrieth (Stuttgart: Cotta, 1836), 358.

[82] Friedrich Schiller, "Philosophie der Physiologie," in *Friedrich Schiller: Medizinische Schriften. Eine Buchausgabe der Deutschen Hoffmann-La Roche AG aus Anlaß des 200. Geburtstages des Dichters* (Miesbach: W. F. Mayr, 1959 [1779]), 41.

[83] Autenrieth, *Handbuch*, vol. 3, § 917, 121. [Zeller misquotes Autenrieth here: instead of "humans," the original reads "moral concerns"!]

[84] See Johann Heinrich Ferdinand v. Autenrieth, "Bemerkungen über die Verschiedenheit beider Geschlechter und ihrer Zeugungsorgane, als Beytrag zu einer Theorie der Anatomie," *Archiv für die Physiologie* 7.1 (1807): 1–139.

otherwise characteristic of Romantic physicians. Autenrieth criticized Brown for knowing only about more or less and nothing about polarity.

Autenrieth articulated his theory of disease in lectures that were later published in two volumes, the first dealing with acute illnesses and the second with chronic ones.[85] In the first volume he dealt with infectious diseases, including nervous fever, which in turn included typhus. Autenrieth distinguished sporadic typhus (today's typhoid fever) from contagious epidemic typhus, which arose only *en masse* as a result of some catastrophe. Although recognizing both forms, including the intestinal ulcers of typhoid fever, he was not at all inclined to investigate locally in either the intestines (typhoid fever) or the brain (epidemic typhus), for the localization of morbid processes was not a primary diagnostic criterion. This is understandable given his theory of metastasis. Furthermore, sharply distinguishing between illnesses was not a matter of concern to him. A clear illustration of this was illnesses involving skin rashes, all of which Autenrieth considered to be linked in a single chain. As far as he was concerned, the altered "typhoid" consciousness was the key nosologic principle. He maintained that any fever could become typhoid, and even sporadic typhus could initially beset the patient's head. It afflicted mainly businessmen, who would spend their evenings gambling and, to be able to work nights, would drink wine and coffee. The result presented as typhus encephalicus. Autenrieth was certainly not the first to bring order to this then still obscure field. But his views help us understand those of Carl August Wunderlich, his student, godchild, later head of the medical clinics in Tübingen and Leipzig, and friend to Wilhelm Griesinger. In his dissertation on *The Nosology of Typhus* in 1839,[86] Wunderlich concluded that there was only one kind of typhus and that every attempt to delineate different kinds was misguided and purely speculative. For our purposes, Wunderlich's study is especially important given that Autenrieth's students bequeathed to us both unitary typhus and unitary psychosis.

In the second volume, Autenrieth argues that most chronic illnesses are nervous illnesses. As to their cause, he writes:

> The nervous system affects nourishment through the vascular system. Without the influence of the nerves, passive congestion results. If the humors thus thicken in one region, they can give rise to acrimony, a direct result of a nervous ailment. Over the further course of the illness, nourishment is disrupted and disorganization occurs. Even hypochondria is initially a nervous ailment. Over time arthritic discharges or arthritic disorganization, or malconfigurations in the body arise. Prosopalgia therefore often results in a herpetic rash or cancer. Simple adynamia in women who, although otherwise not sick, have lain in bed for years, evolves into haemorrhoids or chronic rashes [*Frieseln*].[87]

[85] Johann Heinrich Ferdinand v. Autenrieth, *Specielle Nosologie und Therapie. Nach dem Systeme eines berühmten deutschen Arztes und Professors*, edited by Carl Ludwig Reinhard, 2 vols. (Würzburg: Etlinger, 1834–1835). The volumes were based on Reinhard's notes of Autenrieth's lectures.

[86] Carl August Wunderlich, *Die Nosologie des Typhus: Eine Beleuchtung der wichtigsten Ansichten über dieselbe* (Stuttgart: Rieger, 1839).

[87] Autenrieth, *Specielle Nosologie und Therapie*, vol. 2, 2.

This simple example illustrates how Autenrieth understood the shifting nature of illnesses. No one trained in this environment could possibly place much value in sharply delineating disease entities.

As for Autenrieth's views about actual mental illnesses, or as he saw it, illnesses of the *sensorium commune*, he has been accused of having had very little personal experience. Autenrieth himself claims that in the 10 years up to 1807, he treated only 28 mentally ill patients.[88] And yet he had a keen diagnostic and therapeutic interest in the insane and experience with asylums. He was well aware of the conditions in the Zwiefalten asylum, at the time home to some 160 patients, and had observed patients in Bad Teinach in the Black Forest. He wrote about asylums:

> Asylum statistics always overestimate the number of patients cured because one interprets extended lucid intervals as cures. In newer asylums, the ratios are better, but in older ones cures sink to zero. Although at times only custodial, conditions in new asylums are better because, of all nervous illnesses, lunacy [*Narrheit*] is the most intractable because it becomes habitual [....] Most nervous illnesses become more intractable the more often a person is afflicted [....] Add to this woe the two factors tormenting lunatics, one afflicting the soul, the other the body, then interrupting the habit from the soul's perspective is only possible if one redirects its attention to other objects. This is the first step in freeing the soul. But it can be achieved only by working constantly with the lunatics. And of course, one person can treat only as many lunatics as he can keep occupied throughout the day. But this is impossible in any large asylum, especially for lunatics, since for them the mental factor [*psychische Faktor*] predominates. Now in every new asylum, each new physician does his best, but no one can sustain their élan for years on end. Sooner or later everyone grows weary and falls into a rut, and as Goethe says of doctors: *Durchstudiert die groß und kleine Welt und gehen lassen am Ende, wie es Gott gefällt.* If one wishes to heal the lunatics, it is therefore necessary to treat each one individually. In every asylum, alongside the senior physician, one should introduce a young one to succeed him in ten years, because no alienist can last longer without flagging. Hence, I have recommended to the [Württemberg] Estates that this be implemented in the future asylum in Winnenthal. If this is not done, then it will soon become nothing more than a detention center like [the asylum in] Zwiefalten.[89]

Autenrieth was therefore responsible for having a junior physician added to the staff in Winnenthal, and this physician was none other than Wilhelm Griesinger.

Autenrieth's classification lacked consistency. Catalepsy and ecstasy are ranked as convulsive disorders. Among the diseases of the *sensorium commune*, he counts (1) hypochondria; (2) mental illness or lunacy, which he tries to classify by cause, attributing it to intemperance, recurrent scabies, or constricted secretions of the veins; (3) the manias, including nostalgia, melancholia, and religious delusions; and (4) dementia and cretinism.

It is all rather confused and confusing, and Autenrieth himself had little interest in classification:

> The differences between lunacy, epilepsy, catalepsy, and other nervous illnesses are very small, although in the case of lunacy the causes appear to reside more often in the brain itself. But if lunacy has its seat in other parts of the nervous system, then it will doubtless

[88] Gaupp, "Ferdinand Autenrieth," 57; Stübler, 99. Among these patients was Hölderlin, although Autenrieth never wrote anything about his illness.

[89] Autenrieth, *Specielle Nosologie und Therapie*, vol. 2, 124–126.

ultimately be idiopathic brain-lunacy [*Hirnnarrheit*], and this is especially the case for dementia.[90]

Autenrieth emphasizes that true mental illness begins with physical illness:

It is noteworthy where lunacy's boundary between mental and physical cause lies. A passionate lunatic is not yet a true lunatic until the brain is physically affected. Ambition and arrogance are the easiest roads to lunacy among men. People only become truly crazy when actual signs of cerebral distress appear, such as headaches and cerebral blood congestion [....] Likewise for religious delusions, the body begins to suffer when the patient dulls his brain, resulting in melancholia. Then the brain turns itself around, the patient sees the Third Heaven and angels, or hell and the devil, and then all reasoning is fruitless. In women, lovesick lunacy is similar. If a man is turned down, there are still always enough women in the world. Yet girls are in the majority and some fraction of them can easily wind up without a husband. Women's heightened sensitivity and fragile vanity are also important, because every woman believes that men consider her to be an angel. But true lunacy begins when the body suffers. The illness first manifests as melancholia, but one-sided morbid activity can also arise, i.e. lunacy.[91]

Consider now what the student Albert Zeller could have learned about mental illness and the mentally ill from his teacher Autenrieth:

(a) The forms in which mental illness manifests itself are manifold and often behave like links in a chain.
(b) Suffering often begins with hypochondria or melancholy and later evolves into lunacy and dementia. Most cases of delusion end in dementia once the brain is entirely blunted.
(c) This course corresponds anatomically to the disease process's transition from the elastic nervous system, the ganglion system, to the brain.
(d) Mental and physical causes must come together to create mental illness. Reactively disturbed people [*reaktiv Verstimmte*] become mentally ill only when a physical illness arises.
(e) Physical and mental therapies must therefore be joined together.
(f) Curative and custodial asylums must be separated.
(g) The physical suffering that leads to mental illness evolves according to the laws governing metastasis, the metaschematism of sickness, i.e., in accordance with general pathology.

Knowledgeable readers will already recognize great similarities to Zeller's later systematically articulated concepts, but another connection also comes to mind, namely, that between Autenrieth and Reil.

[90] [Ibid., 117.]

[91] [Ibid., 116.]

Personality and Teachings of J. C. F. Reil

Johann Christian Friedrich Reil (1759–1813) was born the son of preacher in East Frisia and died of Typhus while inspecting military hospitals during the Battle of Leipzig.[92] Full of fire and ingenuity, Reil remained devoted to the *Sturm und Drang* spirit of his youth. But he was also a man of moderation and cultivation who claims always to have renounced public quarrels, and that in a blossoming era of pamphlets, when scholars indulged in ugly and vicious feuds like that between F. W. J. Schelling and H. E. G. Paulus.[93] In 1782 Reil received his doctorate in medicine in Halle, where he became professor of internal medicine in 1787 and municipal physician in 1789, before becoming professor of internal medicine in Berlin in 1810. Although active in nearly all areas of medicine, our focus must remain on his psychiatric influence.[94] Reil was essentially a follower of the analytic method of Condillac (1714–1780) and Pinel (1745–1826): "I have examined all the teaching of physicians young and old and am at times a disciple of one system, at times of another. But I can honestly say that none of them provided me with the reassurance I sought."[95] Reil therefore recommended shunning all hypotheses and relying instead on empirical observation. But as Kierkegaard said, the era of differentiation was gone, overcome by the system, and Reil could not escape the influence of this Zeitgeist and, hence, in many respects, became a speculative systematizer.

All of Reil's thought revolved around the concept of metabolism, specifically intermediate metabolism. Writing the inaugural article of his new *Archive for Physiology*, Reil distinguishes physical force, a general material phenomenon in both organic and inorganic nature, from vital force.[96] The vital force was found only in the living plant and animal world and suggested a relationship between more specific phenomena and a particular kind of matter. The most general attribute of this matter was a kind of crystallization, i.e., a chemical process in both plants and animals. Reil was no adherent of Stahl's animism but rather a metabolism researcher who lacked the ability to conduct research in pathophysiology:

> Illness always has its immediate cause in a change of internal bodily forces, and the body's relationship to external things can never directly and immediately result in illness. Chance illnesses are animal effects that can only ever actually result from animal forces, animal organs. Regular phenomena are the effects of regular forces, anomalous ones the effects of morbid forces [….] The immediate cause of all maladies of the animal body is therefore either an unnatural organization or mixture of animal matter.[97]

---

[92] [On Reil, see also Gerhart Zeller, ed., *Albert Zellers medizinisches Tagebuch*, vol. 2, 11–13.]

[93] [The reference here is to the rationalist theologian H.E.G. Paulus (1761–1851). See Gerhart Zeller, ed., *Albert Zellers medizinisches Tagebuch*, vol. 2, 19–21, 26–28.]

[94] Adalbert Gregor, "Johann Christian Reil (1759–1813)," in *Deutsche Irrenärzte: Einzelbilder ihres Lebens und Wirkens*, edited by Theodor Kirchhoff (Berlin: J. Springer, 1921), 28–42.

[95] Johann Christian Reil, *Über die Erkenntnis und Kur der Fieber*, vol. 4, 2nd ed. (Halle: Curtschen Buchhandlung, 1805), iii.

[96] Johann Christian Reil, *Von der Lebenskraft* (Leipzig: Johann Ambrosius Barth, 1910 [1795]).

[97] Ibid., 91.

Because humoral pathologists also believed that illness was caused by an unnatural mixture (dyscrasia), there was no principle disagreement between Reil and Autenrieth; the two were friends and later coeditors of the *Archive for Physiology.*

Reil's hypotheses were more influential than his analyses. It was Reil who provided Romantic anthropologists their blueprint for the nervous system:

> We can think of our bodies as hollow spheres with a sensitive internal and external surface. The internal surface is like the workshop of the soul, where voluntary movements develop and imaginations play their lawful games. The external surface is exposed to the world, which at the same time is reflected in it. Between both surfaces is a network of nerves and strands, equipped with two sensitive extremities: the one peripheral ending responds to the stimuli of the world and our body; the other core ending [*Centralendigung*] responds to the operations of the soul.[98]

According to Reil, the ganglion system's plexus-like formation, without a center, lacked direction; it was like republican government, in which no single member was allowed to assume the throne. By contrast, the cerebral system was comparable to the monarchy, its throne indestructible thanks to its inner sovereignty. The ganglion system was the seat of the somatic pole of the self and the main source of the passions. The brain was the seat of the pneumatic pole; without it, sensations would remain unconscious. Not until they reached the brain were the organs' diverse sensations united in a harmonious feeling [*Einheit des Gefühls*]: "The sense in us that perceives the body, I have called *sensorium commune* [*Gemeingefühl*]."[99] Elsewhere, in what has been called the first textbook of psychotherapy, Reil had already defined this concept:

> We look with our outer sense upon the things outside of us, upon the world and our bodies; and we look with our *sensorium commune* upon things as our own, in space and in our bodies. The *sensorium commune* is an intermediate thing [*Mittelding*] between inner and outer sense. Although it sees the body as something external, it also sees it as our body and its condition as our condition.[100]

Reil need not have been a true child of his era to be satisfied with dualism as polarity and sought unity as an escalation or compensation. He writes that "the real or ideal sides of man are expressions of an essence in the organism, an essence that develops in two directions, thereby constituting the profound dependency of one side on the other. In this case there would be a higher natural science [*Naturlehre*], subsuming

[98] Reil, *Über die Erkenntnis*, §18, 41. In a later article he described this polarity in greater detail. See Johann Christian Reil, "Über die Eigenschaften des Ganglien-Systems und sein Verhältniss zum Cerebral-System," *Archiv für die Physiologie* 7.2 (1807): 189–254.

[99] Ibid., 240.

[100] Johann Christian Reil, *Rhapsodieen über die Anwendung der psychischen Curmethode auf Geisteszerrüttungen* (Halle: Curt, 1803; reprint, Amsterdam, Bonset, 1968), 162–163. See also the review by Arthur Kronfeld, "Einige Bemerkungen über die ersten psychotherapeutischen Veröffentlichungen insbesondere J. C. Reil," *Allgemeine Zeitschrift für Psychotherapie* 1 (1928): 46–51.

physiology and psychology, insofar as physiology develops the objective side, and psychology the subjective side [of the One fundamental cause of nature]."[101]

It would be strange if this basic understanding of polarity and unity was not found in his concept of mental illness, and yet it is difficult to come to a consensus about his views. Kahlbaum counted Reil among the researchers who had created a simplex system [*wenigerstelliges System*], like Esquirol and Pinel, as opposed to the multiplex systems [*mehrstellige Systeme*], with large numbers of individual forms, of Plater, Guislain, and Flemming and the "non-systems" of Heinrich Neumann, J. B. Friedreich, and Maximilian Jacobi.[102] Kahlbaum discerned four components to Reil's system: (1) fixed delusions, (2) fury, (3) lunacy, and (4) dementia. However, this is not quite correct, and to explain why, we must further examine Reil's views in relation to one of his contemporaries, Johann Christian Hoffbauer.

Hoffbauer was a professor of philosophy and Reil's close associate and friend in Halle.[103] Reil argued that Hoffbauer sought to classify mental illnesses "according to the specific faculties of the soul that have suffered injury, to the abnormal relationship of those faculties with one another, and to the soul's disturbed fellowship with the body. Consequently, he distinguishes three genera of mental illness: mental breakdown [*Geisteszerrüttung*], derangements [*Verrückungen*], and mental illnesses [*Seelenkrankheiten*] in a narrow sense."[104] But Reil disagreed: "Can this classification grasp the entire system of illnesses? Is it not based on symptoms, in so far as the injuries to the faculties are not illnesses, but the product of illnesses? And are the faculties, as far as their necessary conditions are concerned, as heterogeneous as they appear to be based on their manifestations?"[105] Reil then wants to allow Hoffbauer's views to be merely an introduction to the study of different kinds. Based on everything Reil writes here, it is clear that he is searching for a natural system of illnesses corresponding to Linné's system. Yet Reil is too astute to restrict himself to such a model:

> Which differences are essential and which arbitrary? How do kinds differ from varieties? Kinds relate to injured qualities unique to an animal species, varieties are modifications of those qualities in individuals of the given species. Kinds of mental breakdown [*Geisteszerruttungen*] are specific and unique injuries to the brain's dynamic as it relates to its function as an organ of the soul. As such they must manifest essential and enduring symptoms [*Inbegriff steter Symptome*]. The symptoms of these illnesses must present as the disrupted work of the soul [*gestörtes Geschäft der Seele*] in so far as the brain, according to its differ-

---

[101] Reil, *Über die Erkenntnis*, viii–ix.

[102] K[arl] Kahlbaum, *Die Gruppierung der psychischen Krankheiten und die Einteilung der Seelenstorungen* (Danzig: A. W. Kafemann, 1863).

[103] Johann Christian Hoffbauer (1766–1827) was a professor of philosophy in Halle. Together with Reil he published *Beyträge zur Beförderung einer Kurmethode auf psychischem Wege*, 2 vols. (Halle: Curt, 1808–1812). Hoffbauer's major publications include Johann Christoph Hoffbauer, *Untersuchungen über die Krankheiten der Seele und die verwandten Zustände* (Halle: Hahn, 1802); idem, *Psychologische Untersuchungen über den Wahnsinn, die übrigen Arten der Verrückung und die Behandlung derselben* (Halle: Hahn, 1807).

[104] Reil, *Rhapsodieen*, 300–301.

[105] Ibid., 301.

> ent states, participates in bringing forth this work. Varieties arise from the derangement's relationship to its many remote causes, from its different intensity and duration, from its combination with other mental or physical illnesses, and finally from modifications that the abstractly conceived illness incurs when it actually takes hold in an individual.[106]

From these passages we see how strongly Reil leaned toward the assumption of there being just one mental illness.[107] And we see that Kahlbaum was wrong to describe Reil as the founder of a simplex system. Reil clearly articulated his general view on taxonomy [*Systematik*]:

> Given the very real deficits in our knowledge, I am for now content to posit only a few certainties about the chaos of mental breakdown for use by practicing physicians. I wish to choose only specific and unique conditions—ones with enough inherent qualities that they must fit, as kinds, in every system. They must have characteristics allowing them to be recognized everywhere by everyone [….] As kinds of derangement I posit, for the time being, fixed delusions, fury, lunacy, and dementia.[108]

Elsewhere in his work on nervous illnesses,[109] Reil provides similar categories, albeit more detached from systemic strictures. He distinguishes illnesses afflicting (1) the *sensorium commune* (pain, rheumatism, prosopalgia, gout, numbness in the limbs), (2) external sense (photophobia, nervous double vision, amaurosis, deafness), (3) internal sense (maladies of imagination, memory, attention, consciousness), and finally (4) deranged states affecting multiple faculties of the soul simultaneously.

This syndromal classification and its implicit and abstract notion of one disorder, namely, derangement [*Verrücktheit*], were important for the development of Zeller's unitary psychosis. But still more important was the mechanism that Reil conceived to explain the emergence of derangement. That mechanism drew on the polarity of the ganglion and cerebral systems in claiming that the ganglia were afflicted primarily and the brain secondarily.[110] Reil is certainly not dogmatic about this, but he often cites examples of it: "In all cases of mental breakdown related to a false idea about the body's condition, the *sensorium commue* appears to play a major role, acting as an irritant that makes the brain sick. Almost all derangements arising in this way are accompanied by a kind of melancholia."[111] Additionally, "Craziness [*Tollheit*] has its fuse in the solar plexus, where it excites burning, pounding, and fear, until the accumulated irritation crosses over to the brain in the form of an aura, robbing patients of all their senses and driving them to violent actions."[112]

---

[106] Ibid., 299.

[107] See Gregor.

[108] Reil, *Rhapsodieen*, 302, 305.

[109] Reil, *Über die Erkenntnis*, xiii–xiv.

[110] Reil's views on the secondary affliction of the brain are most clearly articulated in Reil, "Über die Eigenschaften."

[111] Reil, *Über die Erkenntnis*, 302.

[112] Reil, "Über die Eigenschaften," 248.

Reil also uses the polar model of cerebral and ganglion systems to explain animal magnetism. In magnetic sleep, Reil argued, all of the brain's vital force is redirected to the ganglion system, which assumes control and functions with cognitive abilities.

Before concluding this section on Reil's significance for the history of unitary psychosis, we should note again that Reil was the actual founder of mental therapy [*psychische Kurmethode*]. He was a robust advocate for the separation of curative and penal institutions. And he also wrote about the organization of asylums for curable patients and custodial institutions for incurable ones.[113] Here we find a clear historical trajectory, beginning with Reil and proceeding through Autenrieth to Zeller, that aimed to create separate curative and custodial institutions. Unfortunately, this trend was disrupted by Heinrich Damerow's highly influential book on the "Relative Connection of Curative and Custodial Institutions for the Insane," which ended up serving as a model for the construction of all new asylums.[114]

To briefly summarize the ideas of Reil that influenced Albert Zeller and hence the development of the concept of unitary psychosis:

(1) There is only one kind of mental illness.
(2) The nervous system has two poles: the cerebral and the ganglion system. In mental illness, the cerebral pole is often afflicted secondarily.
(3) In magnetic sleep, the ganglion system assumes control, in place of the cerebral system, which dominates when awake.
(4) Mental therapy is necessary in spite of the mostly somatic cause of mental illness.
(5) Curative and custodial institutions must be established separately.

After this retrospective on Reil, we now return to Albert Zeller's intellectual evolution. We left him as a student in Tübingen in the summer of 1824 working on his manuscript about the "Consensus of Internal Organs and Systems." Based on his lost correspondence with Jacobi, we know that in 1825 he visited the asylum Sonnenstein in the kingdom of Saxony and thought highly of its director Dr. Pienitz and his wife, its overseer, the Saxon minister Nostitz und Jänkendorf, as well as the head of the nearby custodial asylum in Colditz, the excellent Dr. Hayner.[115]

But did Zeller's visit to Saxony influence the development of his views? Pienitz (1772–1853) and Hayner (1775–1837) had both trained under Esquirol and Pinel.[116] Yet as we shall see later, the ideas of neither Esquirol nor Pinel had any pronounced impact on Zeller. However, the spirit and treatment methods in Sonnenstein and

[113] Johann Christian Reil, "Anhang über die Organisation der Versorgungsanstalten für unheilbare Irrende," in *Joseph Mason Cox: Praktische Bemerkungen über Geisteszerrüttungen* (Halle: Renger, 1811).

[114] Heinrich Damerow, *Über die relative Verbindung der Irren-Heil- und Pflege-Anstalten in historisch-kritischer, so wie in moralischer, wissenschaftlicher und administrativer Beziehung. Eine staatsarzneiwissenschaftliche Abhandlung* (Leipzig: Otto Wigand, 1840).

[115] A[lbert] Zeller, "Irrenanstalten, Irrenhäuser," in *Allgemeine Encyclopädie der Wissenschaften und Künste*, edited by J. S. Ersch and J. G. Gruber (Leipzig: Brockhaus, 1845), 138.

[116] [On Hayner, see Gerhart Zeller, ed., *Albert Zellers medizinisches Tagebuch*, vol. 2, 17–18.]

Colditz certainly resonated with him.[117] In 1817 Hayner had published a catechism on the humane treatment of the insane in which he, as Zeller too later would, abandoned all mechanical restraints except the straight jacket. Although Reil had still believed in the therapeutic benefits of timely corporal punishment, Hayner condemned "every blow administered to this lamentable class of sufferers."[118]

In 1826, Albert Zeller wrote his doctoral thesis in Tübingen under the botanist G. Schübler entitled "Studies on the Effects of Different Organic and Inorganic Matter on the Life of Plants."[119] If any further proof were needed of the enormous influence that Autenrieth had on Albert Zeller, this thesis provides it. Zeller studies the growth of different plants after administering toxic and nontoxic substances. He found one result of his experiments to be especially significant, namely, that poisonous plants are harmed by their own toxins. Fontana's law, according to which poisonous animals were supposedly immune to their own toxins, was thus disproved, at least for plants. Zeller compared plant toxins with animal discharges that were harmful if prevented from exiting animals' bodies. As we know, this was a central theme of Autenrieth's pathology.

Georg Andreas Reimer and His Circle

After completing his studies in Tübingen, Zeller embarked on a second scientific trip, this time to Berlin. On the trip he met by chance the wife of the Berlin publisher Georg Andreas Reimer, whose home and publishing house were focal points of late Romantic literary and artistic life in Berlin. Reimer published works by Fichte, Steffens, Tieck, Novalis, Kleist, Arndt, Fouquè, Jean Paul, the brothers Grimm, Humboldt, and Ritter. Reimer's palatial residence in Berlin became Zeller's new home, where the renowned Protestant theologian Friedrich Schleiermacher also resided. Even before arriving in Berlin, Zeller had read Schleiermacher's writings, and it was Schleiermacher who married Zeller to Reimer's daughter in Berlin's Trinity Church.[120]

Zeller was profoundly influenced by the stimulating intellectual exchanges he experienced in Reimer's circle. In a diary begun in 1827, he describes his readings

[117] [On Sonnenstein and Colditz, see Gerhart Zeller, ed., *Albert Zellers medizinisches Tagebuch*, vol. 1, 195–205, 209 and vol. 2, 170 f. Underscoring the influence of Sonnenstein and its director Pienitz, Gerhart Zeller describes the Winnenthal asylum as a "subsidiary of Sonnenstein." Ibid., vol. 2, 171.]

[118] Christian August Fürchtegott Hayner, *Aufforderung an Regierungen, Obrigkeiten und Vorsteher der Irrenhäuser zur Abstellung einiger schweren Gebrechen in der Behandlung der Irren* (Leipzig: Göschen, 1817), 35. [Abridgement (ca. 60 words): Bernhard v. Gudden's views on Hayner.]

[119] A[lbert] Zeller, "Untersuchungen über die Einwirkung verschiedener Stoffe des organischen und unorganischen Reichs auf das Leben der Pflanzen" (Medical Dissertation, University of Tübingen, 1826).

[120] [Abridgement (ca. 220 words): Biographic details on Reimer.]

and research in Berlin.[121] He mentions Bichat's work on death and life, Schleiermacher's Dogmas, and Friedrich Heinrich Jacobi's writings. Zeller was enrolled as a student at the university and conducted galvanic experiments on animals and plants using methods developed by [Johann Wilhelm] Ritter (1776–1810). Ritter had been one of the more eccentric Romantic natural scientists who, even more so than Autenrieth, promoted the theory that the processes of animal life involved galvanic forces and that the *vis vitalis* itself was likely galvanic.

Albert Zeller and the Seeress of Prevorst

After his wedding, the 25-year-old doctor of medicine set up practice in Stuttgart and soon published anonymously his most famous work, an impassioned critique of animal magnetism and of a book published by Justinus Kerner about the Seeress of Prevorst.[122] The book reveals how much Zeller's experiences in Berlin, and especially Friedrich Schleiermacher's philosophy of religion, had changed him and set up a confrontation with Swabian theosophists and spiritualists. Understanding Schleiermacher's influence helps explain Zeller's dismay in the face of the naively serious and uncritical description of the apparitions purportedly witnessed by the Seeress of Prevorst, Frau Hauffe.[123]

Like Zeller, Schleiermacher too had been raised as a Pietist, albeit under the Moravian Brethren in Barby. He was a pronounced anti-rationalist who advocated the complete autonomy of religion from moral and philological theology. At once both pietistic and mystical, Schleiermacher placed the importance of religious experience at the center of his thought. His philosophy of religion has nothing to do with divine doctrine but rather with religious feeling. Religion is an affair of the heart; a "pious feeling" brings about a direct awareness of the absolute. The relationship between finite nature and the infinite is that of dependency—a dependency that is synonymous with being embraced, protected, and absorbed in the absolute. This is what Schleiermacher calls the feeling of absolute dependence [*Gefühl schlechthinniger Abhängigkeit*], the seat of all religious feeling and the essence of religion itself. [The twentieth-century German philosopher] Nicolai Hartmann rightly suggested that, within this feeling, there still existed a certain knowledge about the essence of God. And so both Spinoza's *amor dei intellectualis* and German

---

[121] Albert Zeller, Studientagebücher.

[122] [Albert Zeller], *Das verschleierte Bild zu Sais oder die Wunder des Magnetismus von einem Freunde der Wahrheit* (Leipzig: Weidmann, 1830). [The book was a critique of the account given by Justinus Kerner. See more extensively, Gerhart Zeller, ed., *Albert Zellers medizinisches Tagebuch*, vol. 2, 24–57, where the seeress is described as a "genius of empathy." Ibid., 25. Furthermore, G. Zeller suspects that while writing his treatise, A. Zeller may have "consulted" with the theologian H. E. G. Paulus. Ibid., 28, 31.]

[123] [On Zeller's close relationship with Schleiermacher, see also Gerhart Zeller, ed., *Albert Zellers medizinisches Tagebuch*, vol. 2, 56–62.]

mysticism's universal feeling [*Allgefühl*] echo in Schleiermacher's work when he characterizes God as the infinite, which permeates all things and is identical with their totality. Schleiermacher's philosophy of religion thus crosses over into the pantheistic metaphysics that dominated nearly all philosophical systems at the time. For Schleiermacher, Romanticism's unified life feeling [*Einheit des Lebensgefühls*] converges with religion.[124]

We can assume that the strong impulse toward unity in Zeller's thought was rooted in an understanding of religion as developed by Schleiermacher. We emphasize this because it underscores the point that Zeller's and Griesinger's unitary psychosis was an outgrowth of the unitive aspirations of Romanticism.

But Schleiermacher impacted Zeller's worldview and anthropology in other ways as well, because he dared to reintroduce the traditional concept of divine causality. We sense our dependency on God by feeling him to be the foundation of our world, i.e., the ultimate cause of all things outside of us and all actions within us. While religious feeling binds a person to the universe, this partaking of the universe does not obliterate the person but instead entails an escalation, as the fully developed individual grows into the absolute. Schleiermacher's individualism pushes him away from pantheism, which as such holds no place for individuals. Nicolai Hartmann rightly argues that Schleiermacher's individualism is rooted not in Leibniz's monads but rather in early Christian ideas about the absolute value of the individual soul, the target of redemptive works. This growth of the finite into the absolute echoes throughout Zeller's poetic writings. It can be experienced in life, in a sense of oneness with God, and be accomplished in death. It strips individual immortality of all naivete and pettiness.

To anyone as immersed as Zeller was in Schleiermacher's theology, especially his understanding of immortality, the spiritualist world of Frau Hauffe was an affront. It prompted from Zeller a response that drew heavily on Novalis and the Romantic ideas circulating in Berlin at the time.[125]

Zeller began his rebuttal with a sketch of normal psychology: "Only someone who knows the *straight* line can determine the deviation of the *crooked* one. Only someone familiar with *health* can judge the *sick*. Only someone who discerns the causality of *sickness* can recognize where *sickness* departs from its *characteristic*, lawful *particularity*."[126]

Of course Zeller grounds this psychology on the idea of God as the cause of all being. He expands on Stahl's idea of the soul as an invigorating principle in true Romantic fashion. For Albert Zeller, God is the invigorating principle and the ultimate cause of unity [*Urgrund der Einheit*]: "The power of the mind and of life are one, the soul builds its body."[127] Drawing on Schleiermacher, Zeller writes that "a

[124] [Abridgement (ca. 130 words): Quote from Paul Kluckhohn, *Das Ideengut der deutschen Romantik* (Tübingen: Niemeyer, 1953), 142 illustrating Schleiermacher's affinity with Novalis and Romanticism.]

[125] Albert Zeller, *Das verschleierte Bild zu Sais*.

[126] Ibid., 1.

[127] Ibid., 20.

being of infinite power, wisdom, and love, in its omnipotence, created everything that exists; we and all around us live, move, and exist always and only in him."[128] Just as God is omnipresent in creation and everywhere whole, so too is the creative power in us everywhere whole and undissipated, although this power operates in each part of us in a specific way. This implies that Zeller has no need for an intermediary between body and mind, no intermediate force, no nervous ether—no intermediary like the one that dominated the Seeress's thought and that gladly served as an explanation for all manner of absurdities. Zeller probes rhetorically:

> Do we need such intermediaries to explain the actual essence of life, does life itself need them to build, preserve, and govern the body? Are mind and matter so foreign to one another, or are not both destined and created for one another by one almighty will. Do we solve riddles with new riddles? Is the neural spirit [*Nervengeist*][129] father, son, or brother of the nerves? Isn't the mind present before the nerves? Electrical and magnetic forces serve life, who will or can deny this? But neither the strongest electricity, nor the most intimately powerful magnetism produce life, not even in its simplest form. They explain just as little as the air we need to breath explains life. However many forces may be at work in a human life, together they do not comprise that life. They are guests of that life and serve it amicably; let us not dismiss them from their service.[130]

Zeller also unites faculty psychology's distinctions of emotion, cognition, and volition [*Begehren*], recognizing no separate faculties but instead only basic actions of the unified mind [*Grundtätigkeiten des einen Geistes*]. He follows Reil in apportioning these actions to certain parts of the body such that "what appears to be the mental fragmentation of the *one* spiritual force [*Seelenkraft*], in fact corresponds to a division and limitation of the flesh. The mind does not therefore come to exist in space, adjacent to other things. For this can never be the case because the mind would then cease to be what it is."[131] Likewise, the five senses are merely expressions of a perceiving power, the sensory power of the mind. Again we find Zeller drawing on Reil's cerebral system: "we feel that the sun of our free-thinking life shines in the brain."[132] The faculty of emotion corresponds to the nervous system, i.e., the ganglion or plexus system and, at its core, the sympathetic nervous system. The emotional faculty itself is divided into faculties for one's own entire body and mind. Here again we encounter Reil's *sensorium commune*. The faculty of desire is associated with the chest and abdomen. In magnetic sleep, the life force appears to have left the entire brain and shifted to the pit of the stomach. Zeller coins the term "somnambulant insanity" to describe the affliction of Frau Hauffe, the Seeress of Prevorst. His description of the condition, which reminds one of later accounts of Charcot's hysterical hypnotees, is worth citing at length:

---

[128] Ibid., 3.

[129] [Schiller uses the term *Nervengeist* in his dissertation. See Schiller, "Philosophie der Physiologie".]

[130] Ibid., 24–25.

[131] Ibid., 26.

[132] Ibid., 32

> The entire aim of the healing force [*Heilkraft*] is to lead *magnetic* life back to a *customary* waking condition. But just like other illnesses can be halted or interrupted in their development, the same can happen here. However it is rare for the magnetic condition, contrary to the law governing its own development, to extend itself or to lose its periodicity, such that individual episodes can hardly be distinguished and instead flow together and intermingle with sleep and wakefulness.[133]

Zeller goes on to explain that the mental image of such a patient becomes more or less a farce. Confused by magnetic sleeping and waking, the somnambule must ultimately go insane:

> Such an unfortunate soul no longer knows whether she is awake, asleep, or dreaming. There then easily ensues a purposeful voluntary extension of the condition, although the somnambule is not at all somnambulant. This explains why, all told, at the end of such a life, we find so much derangement, both self-inflicted and otherwise, even though initially the magnetic life remains true to its original character. If a magnetic illness thus afflicts a person's entire life, ordinary and somnambulant wakefulness will time and again be mixed up. Body and soul together must then succumb, deviating to complete ruin rather than leading to salvation. We are witness to such a totally discordant life in the history of the unfortunate Frau Hauffe, the inevitable victim of so much cruel treatment and all the misery of magnetism.[134]

Zeller concludes his book hoping that it has dug a deep grave for superstition: "The veil of Isis has not been lifted, the gates to the spirit-world have not been breached [....] What paralyzes us from spreading joy in the world is sin [....] Let us work as long as it is day, for the night is coming, when no one can work."[135]

Upon publication, Zeller's book quickly circulated and met with the immediate rebuttal of C. A. Eschenmayer,[136] who had observed Frau Hauffe for 3 years until her death in the summer of 1829.[137] Eschenmayer was a professor of medicine and philosophy in Tübingen and Zeller almost certainly heard him lecture there. And yet his work, especially his spiritualistic interest in magnetism, does not seem to have influenced Zeller. Indeed, Zeller's very public attacks on the doctors treating Frau Hauffe undoubtedly contributed to him being appointed to head the new asylum in Winnenthal castle in 1832 at the age of 26.[138] Before he assumed his position, as was common for prospective superintendents at the time, he embarked on a year-long trip throughout Europe to visit the most prominent mental asylums and their directors. During his trip, Zeller kept a diary that contains important clues about the development of the concept of unitary psychosis.

---

[133] Ibid., 82.

[134] Ibid., 82 f.

[135] Ibid., 168 f.

[136] Carl A. Eschenmayer, *Mysterien des innern Lebens: erläutert aus der Geschichte der Seherin von Prevorst* (Tübingen: Zu-Guttenberg, 1830).

[137] [Abridgement (ca. 860 words): Eschenmayer's rebuttal and a short biographic sketch about him.]

[138] [See Gerhart Zeller, ed., *Albert Zellers medizinisches Tagebuch*, vol. 1, 23 f. Kreuser draws the same conclusion. See [Heinrich] Kreuser, "Zu Albert Zellers Gedächtnis," *MCBlWÄV* 74.45 (1904): 936.]

Psychiatric Journey 1832–1833[139]

Doubtless the most lasting impact of Zeller's journey was his visit to the Siegburg asylum and the intimate friendship which he enjoyed over the next 25 years with that asylum's director, Maximilian Jacobi. Although that friendship grew from a common admiration for Schleiermacher, from the outset they held different views on several scientific questions. It is generally known that Jacobi was a convinced somaticist. For him, there was no mental illness but merely symptoms—like frenzy, depression, delusions, dementia, and lunacy—that accompanied physical illnesses. The manifestations of mental illness were just symptoms. He recognized only what we today call symptomatic mental illnesses. It has long been suspected that this strict one-sidedness was a result of his religious views. Evidence for this can be found in the introduction to his most famous book *The Main Forms of Mental Disturbances as they Relate to Medicine* (1844).[140]

There we encounter Jacobi, a decided advocate of body-soul dualism, insisting on a substantive concept of the soul. But that substance is simply independent, indestructible, and therefore cannot fall ill. For precisely this reason, Maximilian Jacobi had to become a somaticist. In his critique of Jacobi's monograph,[141] Wilhelm Griesinger astutely and coolly exposed all the shortcomings of this conception. Jacobi necessarily fell victim to somatic speculation and reification, especially since his general pathology—an eclectic mix of Brunonian and traditional humoral medicine that struggled to account for pathological anatomy—was in no position to explain all of the questions thrown up by physical illness. Jacobi was also at risk of overlooking psychological effects and had to draw a sharp distinction between mental health and illness. Griesinger assumes that he would have to abandon his principles in order to treat his patients effectively. Echoing Albert Zeller's views, Griesinger rightly noted that most of the difficulties in Jacobi's system would disappear if one took seriously the principle of the unity of body and soul. For example, it would then be self-evident that whenever insanity arises, i.e., abnormal mental phenomena occur, an illness is certainly present. Ever perceptive, Griesinger had identified the key difference. Jacobi was a dualist and Zeller an idealistic pantheistic monist.[142]

---

[139] [Abridgement (ca. 1900 words): Descriptive passages about Zeller's trip and the alienists he met along the way, including Friedrich Groos, C. F. W. Roller, Friedrich Nasse, Maximilian Jacobi. For details about the trip, see Gerhart Zeller, ed., *Albert Zellers medizinisches Tagebuch*.]

[140] Maximilian Jacobi, *Die Hauptformen der Seelenstörungen in ihren Beziehungen zur Heilkunde* (Leipzig: Weidmann, 1844). Jacobi dedicated the book to his friends Albert Zeller and C. F. W. Roller. [Abridgement (ca. 330 words): Several quotes from the introduction to ibid., xxvi–xxviii.]

[141] [Wilhelm] Griesinger, "[Rezension von] M. Jacobi: *Die Hauptformen der Seelenstörungen, in ihren Beziehungen zur Heilkunde nach der Beobachtung geschildert*. Erster Band: Die Tobsucht," *Archiv für physiologische Heilkunde* 3 (1844): 278–296.

[142] [Abridgement (ca. 2820 words): Zeller's encounters with Karl Wilhelm Ideler, J. G. Langermann, and Ernst Horn, as well as his visits to the Quaker "Friends Retreat" in York and to the Parisian

Albert Zeller and Jean-Étienne Dominique Esquirol

During his stay in Paris, Zeller had numerous conversations with the most prominent figure of the day in French psychiatry, Dr. J. E. Dom. Esquirol (1772–1840).[143] Esquirol was a student of Pinel and had become his successor at the Salpêtrière in 1822.[144] In his conversations with Esquirol, Zeller could not escape his influence, and yet the differences between them could not be papered over. Unlike Pinel, Esquirol was not a serious analytical thinker but an eclectic one. He grasped what was important without relying on conceptual principles. Like all prominent French psychiatrists of his day, he shared Gall's phrenologic views. For Esquirol, mental illnesses were brain diseases. He was a phenomenologist, concerned first and foremost about clarify existing clinical evidence. He published no system of mental diseases. Although he distinguished monomanias, mania, dementia, and imbecility, he viewed these conditions as nothing other than combinations of symptoms. Kahlbaum rightly noted that Esquirol never managed to publish a mature account of his views. His monograph *Des Maladies Mentales* was simply a loose summary of his earlier monographs.[145] In his own study, Kahlbaum attempted to sort through and organize Esquirol's categories.[146] According to Kahlbaum's account, Esquirol distinguished mental illnesses with *partial delusions* (*Folie avec délire partiell*), including lypemania, i.e., melancholia, demonomania, and true monomania, from those manifesting *universal delusions* (*Folie avec délire universelle*), such as mania, dementia, and idiocy. The fact that such a passionate systematizer like Kahlbaum was needed to order Esquirol's system demonstrates, we believe, how indifferent Esquirol himself seems to have viewed any such efforts. It appears as though in his conversations with Zeller, the question of classification never arose.

[Among the most significant clues about the development of Zeller's concept of unitary psychosis revealed in his travel diaries involved his encounter with the work of François Joseph Victor Broussais (1772–1838).] At the time of Zeller's visit to France, shortly after the July Revolution of 1830, Broussais had only recently assumed an academic chair in Paris, where his influence among students and practitioners was strong.[147] Broussais's ideas and polemical attacks against specific kinds of disease, which he mocked as "ontologies," undoubtedly found favor with Zeller.

All of Autenrieth's students at some point sympathized with Broussais. Karl August Wunderlich's dissertation on the *Nosology of Typhus* was a polemic against

hospitals Salpêtrière and Bicêtre.]

143 [On Esquirol see Gerhart Zeller, ed., *Albert Zellers medizinisches Tagebuch*, vol. 1, 151–154 and vol. 2, 127–129, 131.]

144 [Abridgement (ca. 140 words): Esquirol's career and private asylum in Ivry-sur-Seine.]

145 Jean Étienne Dominique Esquirol, *Des maladies mentales: considérées sous les rapports médical, hygiénique et médico-légal* (Paris: Baillière, 1838).

146 [See Kahlbaum, *Die Gruppierung*.]

147 [On Broussais, see Gerhart Zeller, ed., *Albert Zellers medizinisches Tagebuch*, vol. 2, 132 f.]

ontologies in the spirit of Broussais. What they all shared was the idea of a new physiological medicine, about which both of Autenrieth's students Wunderlich and Griesinger were so passionate that they together founded the *Archive for Physiological Medicine* in 1842. In the journal, they promoted an understanding of pathology based neither on a natural system of disease along the lines of Linné nor solely on postmortem evidence but rather on deeper knowledge of vital processes in the illness. Considering that the special methods of modern natural science have only recently begun to reveal some of the secrets of pathological physiology, it is clear that Broussais's heuristic approach was correct, although at the time it could not yet be evaluated. Since actual pathophysiological results were still unattainable, speculation had to fill the void. One prospective candidate was the theory of the Scottish physician John Brown (1735–1788) who sought to reduce all of pathology to the relationship between stimulation and excitation. Based on the reaction to stimulation, Brown classified illnesses as either sthenic or asthenic. Brown's powerful influence on Romantic natural philosophy in Germany, especially on Schelling and the Bamberg school of Adalbert Markus (1753–1816) and Andreas Röschlaub (1768–1835), is well known.[148] However, Autenrieth was no friend of Brown's theories, even after meeting one of Brown's most ardent advocates, Benjamin Rush (1745–1813), on a trip to the United States. Broussais argued that the difference between individual illnesses was determined by the degree of stimulus. For him, pathoanatomic changes were secondary—consequences of the infection that the stimulus had elicited. The stimulation then sympathetically takes hold of other organ systems, which can be distant from the site of the primary stimulation. An infection of the digestive system, gastroenteritis, is usually the first consequence of the primary stimulation, i.e., the underlying pathology. Given such a reductive theory of pathology, the therapy was necessarily also simple and hence very ineffective, involving only diets and bleedings.[149] And as Wunderlich surmised, Broussais ultimately simply replaced the old ontologies with a new one: irritation and gastroenteritis.[150]

In his diary, Zeller recorded an excerpt from Broussais's study *De l'irritation et de la folie*[151] that illustrates just how similar Broussais's views were with those of Reil and Autenrieth, albeit based on different assumptions:

> Because of an overly stimulating dietary regime (*régime irritant*), many people suffer from chronic stomach ailments—ailments that, after burdening the patients with hypochondria and nervousness for years, finally lead to mental illness. And others lose their sanity for the

[148] [See Werner Leibbrand, *Romantische Medizin* (Hamburg: H. Goverts, 1937), 50–60.]

[149] Henry Sigerist found that in France in [1827] some 33 million leaches were applied. See Henry E. Sigerist, *Grosse Ärzte: Eine Geschichte der Heilkunde in Lebensbilder* (Munich: Lehmann, 1932), 214.

[150] [See Wunderlich, *Geschichte der Medizin*, 304.]

[151] François Joseph Victor Broussais, *De l'irritation et de la folie: ouvrages dans lequel les rapports du physique et du moral sont établis sur les bases de la médicine physiologique* (Brussels: Melle Delaunay, 1828). [On Broussais, see Gerhart Zeller, ed., *Albert Zellers medizinisches Tagebuch*, vol. 1, 156 f.]

> same reason, but much more quickly. If the affliction is especially brief and the gastric symptoms especially severe, then the delirium is no longer called mental illness [*Geisteskrankheit*] and belongs in the realm of frenzy (*phrénesie*) and febral deliria (*délir fébriles*). Especially remarkable is the fact that it is often the moral causes—i.e. those which affect the brain most directly—that first give rise to the mental illness, after they have led to gastric infections. It is as though certain patients need a visceral reaction in order to reach a high degree of excitation. One should not be surprised by this because many moral convulsions, although they affect the brain, have less subconscious effect on its organization than on the organization of the heart, lung, or stomach. The brain never suffers alone.[152]

One might surmise based on this quote that Broussais was familiar with the idea of unitary psychosis. But this would be incorrect because he rejects more generally the concept of specific diseases. For him, there is no essential difference to be found in illness. In any case, Zeller's engagement with Broussais likely reinforced his acceptance of Autenrieth's conviction that it took an illness to turn a passionate lunatic [*Leidenschaftsnarr*] into a mentally ill one. Zeller also found his rejection of brain-based concepts confirmed by Broussais. For Albert Zeller, mental illness was never only brain illness. He viewed the essence of mental illness as lying in an individual convergence [*Zusammengreifen*] of physical and mental conditions, and throughout his life Zeller remained committed to Reil's schema of cerebral and abdominal systems. As a consequence, he could have no deeper appreciation of pathological anatomy, which at the time was rapidly developing in France. He tried to assess this work, but for him the contradictions and inconsistencies of the young science were more important than its actual results. And so he rightly complained about the autopsies he witnessed at the Salpétrière, which could produce only artifacts, not facts.[153]

As with Broussais, Zeller's encounter with the work of Étienne Jean Georget (1795–1828) likewise helped him clarify his own views.[154] He criticizes Georget for recognizing only a brain—which thinks, feels, is full of wishes, and suffers—but not a soul. Georget believed that thoughts were products of the brain just as urine was of the kidneys, thus vastly overestimating the importance of the brain for organic and intellectual life. Zeller adds that Esquirol had told him in person that in his final years Georget had fundamentally changed his views. Zeller agreed when Georget rejected the independence of mental life, but Georget had forgotten that life and the soul drew on the same source for their existence and that they were not simply a dual manifestation of one common human nature. "In general, in our observations and conclusions, we far too often divide what nature has combined and

152 [Gerhart Zeller, ed., *Albert Zellers medizinisches Tagebuch*, vol. 1, 156.]

153 [Abridgement (ca. 60 words): Contradictory interpretations of postmortem evidence.]

154 Étienne Jean Georget, *De la physiologie du système nerveux et spécialement du cerveau: Recherches sur les maladies nerveuses en général et en particulier sur le siège, la nature et le traitement de l'hystérie, de l'hypochondrie, de l'épilepsie et de l'asthme convulsif* (Paris: Baillière, 1821). [On Georget, see Gerhart Zeller, ed., *Albert Zellers medizinisches Tagebuch*, vol. 1, 158–160 and vol. 2, 134–135. In Albert Zeller's engagement with Georget, Gerhart Zeller sees something "intensely confessional, but unresolved. It drives him toward a Christian interpretation of Spinozism ..." Ibid., vol. 2, 135.]

united, or even made identical. Above all, our research on mental illnesses is lost if we forget that humans are not just comprised of body and soul, but instead are together (*ensemble*) both body and soul."[155]

[¶] In these his reflections on Georget, Zeller for the very first time clearly articulates his own opinion about the origins of mental illness:

> If, prior to falling mentally ill, a person doesn't pay careful attention to their senses and powers of imagination, then their body's derangement can often seize the opportunity to take up bad habits. These habits, together with the body's agitation, can culminate in mental illness (*aliénation mentales*). And very often it becomes extremely difficult to make a full recovery, either by suspending those bad habits or eliminating them to resolve the body's illness.[156]

[The final weeks of Zeller's trip took him to Leipzig and were dominated by a vehement and passionate exchange of views with J. C. A. Heinroth about morality, freedom, and sin.][157] Reading Zeller's account of their intense confrontation begs the question of what the true basis and driving impetus of their scientific disagreement could have been.[158] Ackerknecht interprets the dispute between Somatiker and Psychiker as an expression of the era's speculative bent.[159] Wolfgang de Boor interprets the dispute as a revival of the hotly disputed scholastic problem of universal concepts and their validity.[160] However, both of these interpretations are incorrect, and for the first time in Zeller's diary, we find a key to understanding the dispute. Albert Zeller writes:

> For some people, enormous somatic transformations produce no emotional change whatsoever, even though their general sensibility is highly developed. For other people, a slight fever elicits delirium, a bit of wine intoxication.[161]

And to this he then adds that among others Jacobi and Roller had

> personally experienced things differently than Mr. Heinroth. When I told Mr. Heinroth about such powerful moods, he seemed not to understand me because he himself enjoys such good health, with his body and soul in harmony, the feelings in one eliciting no response in the other. This kind of person knows nothing of the internal struggles we must overcome.[162]

---

155 [Ibid., vol. 1, 158.]

156 [Ibid., 162.]

157 [Abridgement (ca. 150 words): Quote from Zeller's travel diary about the meeting. On Heinroth, see ibid., vol. 1, 183–188 and vol. 2, 149–155. G. Zeller describes the exchange with Heinroth as the "intellectual pinnacle" of Albert Zeller's trip. Ibid., vol. 2, 150.]

158 For all of their differences, Zeller concluded his remarks on Heinroth with the words: "I will always remain thankful to this man who adopted viewpoints that were crucial for all of psychiatry." Ibid., vol. 1, 211.

159 [See Ackerknecht, 58.]

160 [See de Boor, 3–4.]

161 [Gerhart Zeller, ed., *Albert Zellers medizinisches Tagebuch*, vol. 1, 187.]

162 [Ibid.]

Here Zeller leads us toward the ultimate origin of such contradictory beliefs. That origin lies not in the realm of rationality but in personal experience.[163] Whoever, upon introspection, experiences themselves as free will always argue for freedom, but whoever experiences themselves as unfree will argue for bondage [*Unfreiheit*]. One is reminded of Zeller's contemporary, Arthur Schopenhauer (1788–1860), who argued vehemently against free will.[164] For such a passionate, angry, and ambitious person like Schopenhauer, must not self-reflection have exposed feelings of being unfree? And must not this direct personal experience have been stronger than every logical argument? Let us recall that Albert Zeller was an analyst of the subjective and that from early on, in observations of his own mental condition, he encountered inexplicable mood swings. Zeller must have deemed these moods to be a consequence of somatic processes. As a result of personal experience, Zeller became convinced that one's mood depended on one's overall bodily constitution [*körperliche Gesammtverfassung*]. Zeller's vigorous disagreement with Heinroth was a product of his own personal experience. And thus did Albert Zeller arrive at the modern-sounding concept of a constitution:

> The most enlightened view of mental illnesses is likely to be achieved through a comprehensive assessment of all known phenomena within the soul, of how those phenomena emerge from the organism, of how the psyche is modified by nationality, by the transmission of inner and external familial resemblances, by temperament and constitution (two terms that correlate like body and soul, or vice versa, like soul and body, force and organ), of how the prognosis of an illness can be derived from an individual's character, of how the development of body and soul run parallel to each other, and of how emotions can be influenced by eat, drink, rest, activity, and sleep [....] One will have thus examined the natural life of the soul, which in an awakened state is constantly producing and which alone comprises the life of most people. Only then might one descend into the night of dreams and wishes, into the night of madness, to see how even there a higher power is at work and how our miserable anthropologies glide along the surface depths, where magical forces play and reign supreme.[165]

We must now leave the travel diary and its rich content, concluding with a short quote encapsulating Zeller's core anthropological conviction: "We humans always divide what God has united; and what God has united, no one should separate."[166]

---

[163] [See ibid., 185–187.]

[164] See Arthur Schopenhauer, "Über die Freiheit des menschlichen Willens," in *Die beiden Grundprobleme der Ethik, behandelt in zwei akademischen Preisschriften* (Leipzig: Brockhaus, 1860 [1840]), 3–106. [On Schopenhauer's influence, see Gerlof Verwey, *Psychiatry in an Anthropological and Biomedical Context: Philosophical Presuppositions and Implications of German Psychiatry, 1820–1870* (Dordrecht: Reidel, 1985), 76–85, 156–175.]

[165] [Gerhart Zeller, ed., *Albert Zellers medizinisches Tagebuch*, vol. 1, 184 f.]

[166] [Ibid., 184.]

The Birth of the Unitary Psychosis Doctrine: Albert Zeller and Joseph Guislain

[Upon returning from his journey across Europe, Zeller took up his position as director of the Royal asylum Winnenthal in March of 1834 and published his first description of the institution].[167] He emphasized how the asylum was fundamentally a therapeutic institution governed by somatic principles. Only bodily disorders could so bind the psyche that error and delusion became insanity, sadness and fear depression, sin and passion craziness, and foolishness dementia. Mental treatment was necessary, and it needed to be based on quiet, determined, and uninterrupted psychological control [*geistiger Einfluß*], as well as a wise and moral daily regime. The aim was essentially to reeducate [*Rückerziehung*] the patient in a way suited to their specific condition.

But it was not until 1837, in his first full report as asylum director, that Zeller addressed topics relating to unitary psychosis. In this report, Zeller for the first time stated that the major forms of insanity were in fact main stages that the illness tended to pass through, even though nature could never be reduced to static forms. [It is worth citing the report's key passage in full:]

> In general, it is moral and intellectual weaknesses and mistakes that first enable physical illnesses to usurp the mind [*Überwältigung des Geistes*]. In many cases, these weaknesses may well be the result of corresponding congenital and acquired weaknesses and imbalances of the organism. In the vast majority of case histories of mental illness we recognize anguish [*Schmerz*] to be the mother of all morbid phenomena. This anguish is deep-seated, it permeates the entire person, and it arrives either suddenly and violently, or it slowly and relentlessly gnaws away at all of one's powers. It has its origins in the loss of some actual or perceived good at the center of the person's world. The loss can be of material property, or of honor, love, friendship, innocence, peace, or of one's good conscience. The anguish can also be caused by the fear of losing that good, by the despair of never being able to acquire it, or by an absence of support in the face of misfortune. This anguished mood is the fundamental tone of most mental disturbances. Its unpleasant, tormenting bodily sensations lead to a general sadness of the soul and thus a dimming of mental lucidity. In most cases, this mood also reverberates in all of the blissful intoxication [*selige Trunkenheit*] of delusional patients. Indeed, the delusion of never ending happiness is often simply this mood's inversion, adopted by the soul in its inherent urge to be happy. If a full cure is to ensue, usually more than just the physical disturbance accompanying or causing the mental disturbance must be removed; the distressing inner conflict must also be resolved. The lost world must be replaced with something good that cannot be taken away.[168]

In this 1837 report, Zeller articulates for the first time two essential components of the unitary psychosis doctrine. First, that primary manifestations are only stages that the illness tends to traverse without sharp transitions; and second, that mental

---

[167] [Albert Zeller, "Mitteilungen über die neu errichtete Irrenheilanstalt Winnenthal," *MCblWÄV* 3.5/14 (1834): 34–36, 108.]

[168] Albert Zeller, "[Erster] Bericht," 327. [Zeller's next sentence is worth noting: "One must come to the aid of the unfortunate and nothing can demonstrate and provide more assistance than religion."]

anguish is the mother of all morbid phenomena. Although we find the idea of a single mental illness that manifests itself differently at different stages already preconceived in the work of Reil and Autenrieth, in this report we encounter the first instance of Zeller recognizing anguish as a fundamental mental disturbance. Of course, Zeller's recognition was not out of the blue. Both Reil and Autenrieth repeatedly claimed that mental illness begins with melancholia, i.e., with an irritation of the abdominal ganglion system, and later proceeds to insanity by way of an irritation of the cerebral system. Nevertheless, Zeller's concise expression of the view that anguish over the loss of an important subjective good comprised the fundamental disturbance of mental illness is entirely new.

To help clarify how Zeller arrived at this view, it is useful to review the work of Joseph Guislain (1797–1860), especially his book *Traité sur les phrénopathies*,[169] which we know Zeller read and critiqued after it was published in 1833.[170] Typical of Guislain's psychopathologic thought was his search for an *altération fondamentale*. He found it in mental anguish [*Seelenschmerz*], i.e., in the morbid stimulation of sensibility. In the first chapter of his study of phrenopathic disorders, Guislain articulates his position:

> All tissue, once its sensibility has been stimulated, expresses its sensation through an inherent vital process [*Lebensverrichtung*]. The sensation elicited by an overly strong stimulus manifests itself as pain; and this pain has more or less the same character across the different organs experiencing the stimulation. The soul has its own stimulants, and also its own pain. But this pain manifests itself differently than physical pain. It involves worry, frustration, fright, in a word, an affliction of the soul [*Seelenleiden*] [….] If one insults an individual, or allows them to endure some affliction, a series of phenomena will ensue: tears of frustration or rage will flow; threats will be met with defiance, insults rebutted; disquiet will spread. The person will muster all of their resources to kill, remove, or destroy the agent that is imposing the burden. This is the psychological reaction that follows from a physical reaction.[171]

Consequently, for Guislain all manifestations of mental disturbance are reactions to the *altération fondamentale*, and these reactions are governed by laws. The reactions lead to (1) increased organic activity, (2) the participation of the nervous system in the expression of symptoms,[172] (3) a decline in mental powers, and (4) their destruction. Guislain calls the first two reactions primary and the second and third

---

[169] Joseph Guislain, *Traité sur les phrénopathies, ou doctrine nouvelle des maladies mentales, basée sur des observations pratiques et statistiques, et l'étude des causes, de la nature, des symptomes, du pronostic, du diagnostic et du traitement de ces affections* (Brussels: Établissment Encyclographique, 1833).

[170] Zeller deemed the book so important that he had it translated into German. Cf. Joseph Guislain, *Abhandlung ueber die Phrenopathien*. [Abridgement (ca. 730 words): Deliberation on who translated Guislain's monograph and that it could not have been Carl August Wunderlich (1815–1872). Also a brief synopsis of Guislain's career.]

[171] [Joseph Guislain, *Abhandlung ueber die Phrenopathien*, 37 f.]

[172] Here Guislain confesses his allegiance to Gall's phrenology and argues that the brain is the seat of mental disorder.

ones secondary. These reactions result in four constitutive elements of mental disorders:

(1) Excitement (exaltation of brain activity)
(2) Aberrations (aberration of cerebral processes)
(3) Suppression (suppression of cerebral processes)
(4) Destruction (exhaustion of mental powers)

From these mental elements, or due to the participation of certain somatic circumstances, emerge the following basic forms of mental illness:

A. Manifestations of stimulation (mental anguish, phrenalgia)

  (1) *Lyperophrenia* (melancholia, simple affliction of sensibility)

B. Manifestations of reaction

  (2) *Hyperphrenia* (mania, heightened mental activity)
  (3) *Paraphrenia* (insanity, delusion, aberration of mental activity)
  (4) *Hyperplexia* (stupidity, melancholia stupida)
  (5) *Hyperspasmia* (epilepsy, Huntington's chorea)
  (6) *Ideosynchysia* (delirium, illusions, hallucinations, delusion [*Wahnwitz*], aberrations of thought)
  (7) *Anacoluthia* (confusion, incoherent thought)

C. *Noasthenia* (dementia, incomprehension)

Guislain would later eliminate hyperspasmia and anacoluthia from this classification, leaving six basic forms. Each of the forms can remain simple and become what Esquirol called monomania and Guislain called monopathy. However, several basic forms can also combine into one illness, arising either simultaneously or in sequence. Combined forms are more frequent, and it is they, in their myriad variations, that comprise the actual kinds of mental disorder. Guislain thought he could identify over 100 specific forms.

To judge by his 1837 report, Zeller was an enthusiastic reader of Guislain's book, which appears to have helped him clarify his own like ideas. But Zeller was also a critical reader, and he formulated his reservations in an introduction and commentary to the German translation of Guislain's *Phrénopathies*.[173] Zeller's critique took aim at two central claims: Guislain's advocacy of the psychogenesis of mental illness, as well as his acceptance of Gall's hypothesis that mental illness was a brain malady. In elaborating his objections to these two ideas, Zeller for the first time clearly formulates his own psychopathological views.

Zeller proceeds from the assumption that mental disturbances must be studied anthropologically. Research should adopt an approach that is neither one-sidedly cognitive or psychological nor one-sidedly somatic but that instead takes into account human nature as a whole, overlooking neither the inner, dynamic structure,

[173] Joseph Guislain, *Abhandlung ueber die Phrenopathien*, 1–28, 440–518.

nor the outer bodily one. But the thread of life is sewn by the nervous system. It can be defined by physical conditions, by all the body's solid and fluid structures. Furthermore, the entire nervous system can, from any given point in the system, be drawn into the most profound conflict. But within the entire nervous system, it is the ganglion system that directly stimulates our bodily and mental personality and our inner awareness of these stimulations and conditions (Guislain's *sens affectif*). It is thanks to Reil's inner sense that the human personality becomes truly subjective, it acquires a heart, and a kind of thought entity [*Gedankending*][174] is transformed into an actual individual. But the nature of this sensibility, the character of feeling, predominated as it is by the involuntary, means that humans stand much closer to the unfree, to the bondage imposed by suffering and passion, than to the more objective sensations of the rest of the nervous system. The human personality and all of its actions come about only within the healthy entanglement of the free and unfree, of mind [*Geist*] and nature. And because this is so, the ultimate cause of a mental disturbance must usually lie in a displacement and destruction of this relationship between the brain and ganglion system. Just as one observes constitutionally disposed individuals in whom body and soul clearly interact, in whom a certain organ or group of organs is regularly affected following strong and unpleasant feelings [*psychische Eindrücke*], so too does one conversely observe in these same individuals that, upon the functional disruptions of these organs, psychological affects ensue. However, the development of the organ's malady is governed by the laws of metastasis, corresponding to the consensus of the organs.

This is what Jacobi first recognized and what we have ever since called an organically elicited feeling [*organische Gestimmtheit*].[175] On the basis of his own experience, Albert Zeller describes this as "bitter, painful, gloomy feelings that we are unable to explain to ourselves or to others, conditions in which every loving glance, every joyous tone, the most peaceful and harmless words injure, sadden, and upset us, provoke fits of anger and malicious ridicule; every consolation can frighten us, we mistrust everything, and everything that we otherwise love and cherish disgusts us, everything we once easily mastered now weighs on us like a ton of bricks."[176] On the other hand, Zeller underscores the fact that the deepest mental anguish still belongs to a healthy and reasonable human life, so long as there are sufficiently reasonable grounds for the suffering. Zeller shares Guislain's view that the somatic path to mental disturbances is much rarer than the psychological path. But he repeatedly insists on the limitations of this claim. For only under certain somatic

[174] [Immanuel Kant, *Kritik der reinen Vernunft* (Hamburg: Meiner, 1956), A489/B517, 22–29: "Possible experience is that which can alone give reality to our concepts; in its absence a concept is a mere idea, without truth, that is, without relation to any object. The possible empirical concept is therefore the standard by which we must judge whether the idea is a mere idea and thought-entity [*Gedankending*], or whether it finds its object in the world."]

[175] Maximilian Jacobi, ed., *Sammlungen für die Heilkunde der Gemütskrankheiten*, vol. 2 (Elberfeld: Schönian, 1825). [Jacobi interpreted mental phenomena *naturhistorisch*: for him, they were "entirely the result of specific conditions of the animal organism." Ibid., 343.]

[176] [Joseph Guislain, *Abhandlung ueber die Phrenopathien*, 16–17.]

conditions can a painful emotional episode [*schmerzhafte Gemütsbewegung*] produce mental disturbances. Hence, it often comes to pass that a psychological moment, which absent any somatic moment would quickly lapse, can over time recede into the background. Indeed, it can recede so much that once the somatic malady—which has evolved independently, even if elicited by the psychological moment—is resolved, the psychological cause will be all but forgotten by the convalescing patient.[177]

Zeller was far less critical of Guislain's classification. He chided only the inclusion of convulsive ailments as mental disorders, and in 1854 Guislain removed them from his system. Zeller also pointed out that course was not at all schematic and that individual deviations regularly occur. He agrees with Guislain that melancholia and mania are closely related conditions. He objects to overly detailed subcategories, identifying transitions everywhere and fixed boundaries nowhere.

Albert Zeller's Asylum Reports and Encyclopedia Articles

We turn now to Zeller's second report on the Winnenthal asylum, published in 1840.[178] The report covers the period just prior to Wilhelm Griesinger's arrival as assistant physician.[179] Much of the report is given over to a discussion of whether curative and custodial institutions should be geographically separated from one another, a hotly debated question at the time and one that to this day has lost none of its relevance. Zeller was a decided advocate of separate institutions.[180] More importantly for our purposes, however, the report also includes Zeller's first classification of mental illnesses and citing his views verbatim is revealing:

> Because we consider the general form of insanity to be more important than its duration, some remarks about the classification of mental disorders that we have used now seem to

[177] [On this, see essentially verbatim Joseph Guislain, *Abhandlung ueber die Phrenopathien*, 18–19.]

[178] [Albert Zeller, "Zweiter Bericht".]

[179] [Abridgement (ca. 50 words): Citing Carl August Wunderlich, "Wilhelm Griesinger: Nekrolog," *Archiv für Heilkunde* 10 (1869): 148, Zeller reflects briefly on the reports and Griesinger's possible influence on them. In fact, however, that influence is revealed not in deviations in the reports published in the *Medicinisches Correspondenz-Blatt des Würtembergischen Ärztlichen Vereins* but rather in the heavily revised and substantially expanded version of the third report published in the *Allgemeine Zeitschrift für Psychiatrie* (*AZP*). Cf. Albert Zeller, "[Dritter] Dreijähriger Bericht" and [Albert v.] Zeller, "[Dritter] Bericht über die Wirksamkeit der Heilanstalt Winnenthal vom 1. März 1840 bis 28. Februar 1843," *AZP* 1.1 (1844): 1–79.]

[180] [See Albert Zeller, "Irrenanstalten, Irrenhäuser," 139–140. Gerhart Zeller would later publish two papers on this theme: Gerhart Zeller, "Von der Heilanstalt zur Heil- und Pflegeanstalt: Ein Beitrag zur Geschichte des psychiatrischen Krankenhauswesens," *Fortschritte der Neurologie und Psychiatrie* 49 (1981): 121–127; idem, "Hat das psychiatrische Reformprogramm Wilhelm Griesingers aus dem Jahr 1868 heute noch eine Bedeutung?," in *Rehabilitationspsychiatrie*, edited by Jürgen-H[elmut] Mauthe (Stuttgart: Enke, 1998), 1–14. Abridgement (ca. 140 words): Zeller expands briefly on the interrupted tradition of separate therapeutic and custodial institutions.]

> be necessary. This necessity is all the greater given the truly Babylonian hubbub and confusion among scholars and laymen alike. Although we are certainly not in a position to claim that our efforts have produced the best true and accurate result, at least our terminology is clear and understandable. For the most part, we have retained the classification used in the first report, simplifying it only slightly. We believe that our classification is a natural one and draws on the wisdom of scholars through the ages. However we don't wish to deny that, in One [sic!] individual patient, we can find the most extraordinary diversity in the basic forms. Nor do we wish to pass judgment over whether one expression or another is the sole best alternative. Instead, we will be satisfied if we have succeeded in establishing and characterizing essential differences in nature. The point of classification is not to discover every last subgroup; instead, at issue are the basic conditions of all mental life, and especially the stages as forms of insanity. Specific groups and changes in individual cases are very easily accounted for in our classification. Accordingly, we have strayed little from the old classification, except for one essential difference: we have divided the traditional description of melancholia into two basic forms that heretofore were thrown together, namely depression [*Schwermut*] and derangement [*Verrücktheit*]. We are convinced that delirium must not be excluded from our assessment of insanity. Instead, it forms a direct bridge between common illnesses and mental disturbances. Very often, true mental disturbances evolve solely out of febrile delirium. And studying delirium can often reveal the physical causes of insanity most clearly. And yet, the many other pathological symptoms that characterize delirium are too predominant for it to be placed alongside the other, clearer forms of mental disturbances, at least for now. We therefore believe that the best choice of a straightforward classification includes four basic forms or stages of insanity: 1) depression [*Schwermut*], melancholia, 2) craziness [*Tollheit*], mania, 3) derangement [*Verrücktheit*], partial insanity, *Wahnwitz*, paranoia, 4) imbecility, amentia, dementia with its gradual transitions from mere silliness to the demise of all conscious sensibility.[181]

Albert Zeller then provides very detailed descriptions of these conditions. He again explicitly mentions that, for him, depression [*Schwermut*] is the true basic form and first stage of all mental disturbances that, even partially, appear to evolve over time. It can, but need not evolve into other forms of illness, and it is governed by its own laws of development. Zeller then details how mania and melancholia behave like positive and negative poles, like chills and fever. He draws a distinction between cerebral mania and ganglionic mania. He describes how craziness [*Tollheit*] becomes ever more muddled, dreamlike, incoherent, persistent, and raging the more it involves the brain or mind, as opposed to the ganglion system or emotions [*Gemüt*]. The third main form of insanity, i.e., derangement, partial insanity, *Wahnwitz*, and paranoia, almost never manifests as a primary form, *at least as far as he had seen*, unless by way of jealousy, querulousness, and hallucinations.

And so Zeller's nosology was carefully devised, as it had to be given his vast experience. The fact that he recognized the two classic forms of paranoia, or "primary derangement," namely, jealousy mania and querulousness, is testament to that broad experience. Any course of illness that does not improve, ends in dementia. The intensity and causes of dementia vary widely, although the better the patient's general condition, the worse the prognosis.[182]

---

[181] Albert Zeller, "Zweiter Bericht", 132.

[182] [Abridgement (ca. 100 words): Quote on Zeller's therapeutic approach reflecting the influence of Autenrieth's metastatic views about pathology.]

[The basic structure of this nosology remained unchanged in subsequent asylum reports. However, in those reports he occasionally revisited the topic of psychiatric classification.]

His third report[183] appeared as the lead article in the inaugural, 1844 issue of what soon became Germany's flagship professional journal, the *Allgemeine Zeitschrift für Psychiatrie*. Effectively acting as the mouthpiece of emergent alienism in Germany, Zeller expressly retained his categories, again emphasizing that the main forms were different stages, and that depression was the primary disturbance.[184]

And in the fourth report he remarked as follows:

> Concerning the main forms of mental disturbance and their classification, we saw no reason to adopt different categories and terms. Although like every classification it too has its shortcomings, as far as diagnosis and prognosis are concerned, it seems to remain the clearest and most practical alternative. Certainly, in some cases we encounter craziness as a primary form, for example in a mental disturbance arising from gastro-nervous fevers, arthritis, intemperance, sunstroke, fright, and especially apoplexy. But again, the evidence, as compiled in tables, confirms that depression [*Schwermut*] is the primary form of mental anguish. Other observers may well have reached different conclusions, so that while among women we found depression to be the primary form, others instead found frenzy [*Tobsucht*].[185]

[In the fifth and final report, he again concluded, in his last remarks on classification, that his approach seemed to be the most practical and broadly applicable. But he also added the following remarks on melancholia and mania:]

> Regarding the melancholic form, in recent years we have learned to recognize the duality of passive and active forms. We have increasingly been forced to assign many cases of mania to the latter, just as earlier we divided craziness (mania) into subgroups of frenzy [*Raserei*] and lunacy [*Narrheit*]. Most recently and increasingly, we have been led to treat mania, when it originates in derangement [*Verrücktheit*] and delusions (paranoia), as being unique in all its relationships and manifestations, and distinct from primary craziness [*Tollheit* ...].[186]

Interestingly, it is precisely mania—the touchstone of psychiatric diagnosis—that continues to disturb Zeller's classification, although not inducing him to abandon his concept of unitary psychosis.

---

183 See Albert Zeller, "[Dritter] Dreijähriger Bericht" and idem, "[Dritter] Bericht." The version published in the *AZP* was heavily redacted and expanded, likely by Griesinger.

184 [Abridgement (ca. 1120 words): Evaluation of the third (focusing mostly on therapeutics) and fourth reports, especially Griesinger's influence on them. Zeller's 1844 encyclopedia articles and C. F. W. Roller's review of them.]

185 Albert Zeller, "[Vierter] Dreijähriger Bericht", 11. [This quote deviates from the version published in the *AZP*. Cf. [Albert v.] Zeller, "[Vierter] Bericht über die Wirksamkeit der Heilanstalt Winnenthal, vom 1. März 1843 bis 28. Februar 1846," *AZP* 5 (1848): 177–178. Abridgement (ca. 700 words): Evaluation of the fifth report.]

186 Albert Zeller, "[Fünfter] Bericht" (1854), 304.

Section 2.3

Albert Zeller and Wilhelm Griesinger

We can now summarize the intellectual development of the father of unitary psychosis. We have seen the young man, influenced by the "sensitivity" of his mother and the spirituality of Swabian Pietism, grow up to be an acute observer of himself and an analyst of the subjective. Trained in medicine under Autenrieth, Zeller adopted his theory of metastasis and became convinced that there often existed an inner affinity of very different morbid conditions, which were thus interpreted as developmental stages of one disease process. Autenrieth also introduced him to Reil's concept of an inner sense and his theory of ganglion and cerebral systems. In 1824 he became involved with late-Romantic circles affiliated with Georg Andreas Reimer in Berlin and was strongly influenced by the writings of Schleiermacher. In Berlin he was exposed to the unitarian aspirations [*Einheitsstreben*] of his age, which throughout his life infused his anthropology. Body and soul are one; they are expressions of one divine power. He never tired of teaching this doctrine. Whether mental illness had physical or psychological origins was therefore of secondary concern. For the most part, however, Zeller sided with the somatic school of thought because, based on observations of his own mental states, he repeatedly encountered psychologically unmotivated changes in mood. Visits to eminent psychiatric institutions and scholars in Europe solidified his rejection of Gall's theories about the brain and informed his views about the treatment of mental illnesses.[187] Henceforth, his therapeutic goal was to combine individual somatic treatment with individual psychological treatment and to couple this with effective group therapy, all of which he did as the director of the Winnenthal asylum from 1833 until his death in 1877. He treated 3600 patients and was able to discharge two-thirds of them as cured or improved. Profiting from his engagement with Joseph Guislain's *Traité sur les phrénopathies*, by 1840 Zeller had consolidated his theory of unitary psychosis. In light of Zeller's development, his unitary psychosis can plausibly be termed Romantic unitary psychosis. Zeller's unitary psychosis is a legitimate child of Romanticism's unitarian aspirations and obsessions.

Zeller's direct scientific impact was not large. However, through Wilhelm Griesinger and his textbook, Zeller's indirect influence was broad. It is therefore to Griesinger that this study now turns, asking first whether he too can be counted among the Romantics.

Wilhelm Griesinger (1817–1868) was born and raised in Stuttgart and studied medicine under Autenrieth in Tübingen.[188] He was very open to modern ideas,

[187] [See Gerhart Zeller, ed., *Albert Zellers medizinisches Tagebuch*, vol. 2, 64 f.]

[188] Theodor Kirchhoff, "Wilhelm Griesinger," in *Deutsche Irrenärzte*, edited by Theodor Kirchhoff (Berlin: J. Springer, 1921), 1–14; Wunderlich, "Wilhelm Griesinger"; Carl Westphal, "Nekrolog. Nach einer Rede gehalten zur Gedenkfeier für Griesinger," *Archiv für Psychiatrie und Nervenkrankheiten* 1 (1868): 760–774; Georg Stickler, "Wunderlich, Roser, Griesinger: 'Die drei

especially those coming out of France. Together with Carl August Wunderlich and Wilhelm Roser, he established the *Archive for Physiological Medicine* in 1842. No doubt this undertaking was inspired by Broussais, but it would soon outgrow his influence.

We do not know what motivated Griesinger to become assistant physician to Zeller at the Winnenthal asylum in 1840. We know only that Autenrieth had provided that the asylum employ a second physician after 10 years and that it was Griesinger who assumed this new post. We have already cited Griesinger's views about Zeller and his time in Winnenthal.[189] Another account of their relationship has been given by Carl Westphal:

> Winnenthal opened up a new world for Griesinger and he immersed himself in it. He enjoyed a life-long friendship with the asylum's director and privy councilor, Dr. Zeller, and often remembered his days in Winnenthal as the happiest of his life [….] The friendship is all the more extraordinary given their very different beliefs, especially when it came to religious matters.[190]

As tragic fate would have it, Griesinger soon departed Winnenthal at the end of 1841. To understand Griesinger's psychiatric work, it is necessary to emphasize how influential Zeller and his asylum were. In fact, up until the publication of the first edition of his *Pathology and Therapy of Mental Illnesses* in 1845, all of his psychiatric publications were nothing but a discourse on the ideas of his teacher Albert Zeller.

Griesinger's critique focused on two issues that linked Zeller most closely to his times. The first was Reil's model of a cerebral and ganglion system, a model that comprised the foundation of Zeller's unitary psychosis. The primarily afflicted ganglion system produced morbid feelings and moods. And if the illness, governed by the laws of metastasis, crossed over into the brain, then secondary morbid ideas would result. Griesinger could no longer accept this key assumption of Romantic anthropology. He had to create a new conceptual model of mental illness, albeit without abandoning the traditional doctrine of primary depression and secondary disturbances of thought and cognition. Just as Zeller was impressed by the physiological views of his time, Griesinger too needed to draw on the modern results of physiological research and did so in two key articles. In the first article published in 1843,[191] he argued that in the spinal cord, at the very aphelion of consciousness, a response was generated to the centripetal signals of sensory nerves. This response corresponded to the equilibrium—or more precisely the intermediate activity—of the sensory and motor system, specifically the tension or tonus of muscles, of cellular tissue, as well as of the blood and lymph vessels. Similarly, the brain generated

Schwäbischen Reformatoren der Medizin'," *Sudhoffs Archiv* 32/33 (1939/40): 32: 217–274 and 33: 1–54. [Gerhart Zeller, "Welcher psychiatrischen Schule hat Wilhelm Griesinger angehört?," *Deutsches Medizinisches Journal* 19 (1968): 328–334.]

[189] [Cf. Griesinger, *Die Pathologie und Therapie*, vi.]

[190] [Westphal, 761.]

[191] Wilhelm Griesinger, "Ueber psychische Reflexactionen. Mit einem Blick auf das Wesen der psychischen Krankheiten," *Archiv für physiologische Heilkunde* 2 (1843): 76–113.

a response to the massive flow of diffuse impressions from the organs, namely, a state of apparent equanimity that regulated the force and direction of mental movement or impulses [*psychische Bestrebungen*]. This relationship of the aggregate sum of all impressions to the force, fluency, and direction of potential mental impulses Griesinger called mental tonus [*psychischer Tonus*], a term that, for the most part, corresponded with terms like character and emotional disposition [*Gemüt*]. But just as centripetal stimuli in the spinal cord were not just dispersed throughout the entire organ but also put into centrifugal action, so too did impressions arriving in the brain—some directly from sensory organs, others indirectly from the spinal cord—result not only in subconscious impulses in the mental tonus but also crossed over into conscious impressions and then impulses. Impressions evoke and become impulses, and in turn, impulses evoke and become movements, i.e., muscular action. Just as spinal reflex can be inhibited by the brain, so to, within the brain, can the transition from impressions to impulses be inhibited. That inhibition is due to the common effect of all other impressions on the currently active impression. This forms the basis of what Griesinger calls sanity [*Besonnenheit*]. Insanity results from anomalies in the dispersal of impressions and their transition into impulses. Inhibitions in the free flow of impressions both throughout the organ and in the transition into impulses produce mental displeasure [*Unlust*], sadness, and even despair or, in other words, depression and melancholia. It became an inviolable principle for Griesinger that, in the vast majority of cases, mental depression was the point of departure for numerous other changes that constituted insanity. And Griesinger claims to have himself witnessed several hundred such cases in Winnenthal in which depression was the primary affliction.

This state of inhibition could arise under the influence of various external experiences. But it could also result primarily from the brain, as an organ of impressions and impulses [*Vorstellungs- und Strebungsorgan*], or secondarily via sympathetic stimulation from other organs (often the genitalia). Due to the reduced or inhibited flow of impressions and especially impulses, an affliction of the brain would result.

Griesinger expanded his efforts to construct a new conceptual model that could support unitary psychosis in a second article published a year later in 1844. In the article's revealing introduction, Griesinger wrote that he was continuing[192] his "comparison of the physiological sensory and motor phenomena in the spinal cord with the mental phenomena in the brain, under morbid and healthy conditions. Just as Goethe's hypothesis and Oken's proof that common laws governed the development of the bones of both the vertebrae and the scull were extremely fruitful in understanding cranial structure, so too we may hope that a comparison of the vital activities of the spinal cord and the brain will provide important clues to help understand mental phenomena."[193]

---

[192] [See ibid.]

[193] Wilhelm Griesinger, "Neue Beiträge zur Physiologie und Pathologie des Gehirns," *Archiv für physiologische Heilkunde* 3 (1844): 69.

This passage reveals Griesinger as the transitional figure he was. Otherwise reticent about all things ideological, interested only in positive knowledge, here he waves the magic Romantic wand of analogy, expressly citing Oken! We can be certain that many of the difficulties he faced can be attributed to his internal balancing act on the threshold between natural philosophy and positivism.

The second article begins with an avowal of the pathophysiological interpretation of mental illness and a lament about the unsatisfactory results of pathoanatomy. Zeller too had written about the entirely negative results of pathoanatomic research on insanity.[194] Griesinger introduces the term spinal irritation and defines it as a malady with no visible lesion. From it, he then constructs by analogy the term cerebral irritation. Depressive conditions are defined as cerebral irritation with the pronounced symptom of anguish, which is seen as being analogous to neuralgic pain. Just as neuralgia is characterized by subjective pain, objective contraction, tremors, and paralysis, so too was cerebral irritation characterized subjectively by anguish, objectively by inhibition and excitation. Griesinger understands mania as a psychoconvulsive condition. Secondary forms (delusion, partial derangement, lunacy) are juxtaposed with chronic spinal irritation. As with spinal illnesses, here too debility—a mental debility [*psychische Schwächezustand*]—is the most prominent characteristic. Finally, dementia is mental paralysis and corresponds to the residual palsy of spinal irritation.

Using the analogy of spinal irritation and neuralgia, Griesinger had found his conceptual model—a model that was able to explain the course of mental illness from the anguish of depression to complete paralysis in dementia and that correlated with Zeller's classification based on stages.

[¶] However, this model also contradicted the views of Griesinger's mentor. For Zeller had waged a lifelong campaign against Gall's cerebral doctrines and was convinced that mental illness was never only a matter of the brain, since the entire body was the soul's organ [*Seelenorgan*]. Zeller had criticized Guislain for overemphasizing the role of the brain in causing insanity. Now Zeller was confronted with the fact that his own student, Griesinger, had promptly defined mental illness as cerebral irritation. Indeed, at the beginning of his *Pathology and Therapy of Mental Illnesses* in 1845, Griesinger posed the rhetorical question: "Which organ must everywhere and always be afflicted in cases of insanity?" Answering it thus: "Since physiological and pathological facts demonstrate that this organ can only be the brain, we must recognize that mental illnesses are always *brain maladies*."[195] The two men would certainly have departed ways had not Griesinger otherwise, at least at the time, remained a loyal student of his mentor.

We catch a glimpse of this loyal disciple, indeed this spokesman of Zeller's, in a review that Griesinger wrote about Jacobi's monograph *The Main Forms of Mental Disturbances*. In the review, Griesinger commits above all to Zeller's anthropology and his belief in the unity of body and soul. Griesinger writes:

---

[194] See Albert Zeller, "[Vierter] Dreijähriger Bericht", 14.

[195] [Griesinger, *Die Pathologie und Therapie*, 1]

> The dualistic hypothesis contradicts the empirically supported and much more likely hypothesis of a direct unity of somatic and psychic phenomena. Until now, this view has been far less examined and developed compared to the dualistic one, not least because of timidity in the face of the term 'materialism'.[196]

Furthermore, Zeller had always argued that the mind [*Geist*] had its body [*Physis*] and its physics and that its most advanced and freest actions were bound to this organic and dynamic causality. Adopting this position as his own, Griesinger wrote:

> In our view, psychology must relate to psychiatry just as physiology relates to pathology and medicine. Both must demand of each other the most profound insight. However we needn't belabor the point that psychology is nothing other than an empirical, an observational, a natural science. But for such a science, the mechanics of brain activity are axiomatic, which even the most abstract spiritualism must recognize. In this field, one can finally take seriously the proposition—so often proclaimed, but so rarely adhered to in psychiatry—that body and soul are one.[197]

Wilhelm Griesinger and Johann Friedrich Herbart

We must assume that Griesinger engaged, indeed had to engage, psychology as the foundation of psychopathology. But Zeller had not engaged it and did not need it. The psychological insights that Zeller had acquired through empathy and subjectivist analysis were no longer available to the younger natural scientist Griesinger. Zeller's method must have seemed prescientific to him. Yet if Griesinger wished to remain true to the physiological medicine that he, Roser, and Wunderlich passionately believed in, he had to construct his textbook *Pathology and Therapy of Mental Illnesses*, which he had begun writing after leaving Winnenthal, on a psychological foundation. In the introduction to that textbook, Griesinger wrote:

> In many regards, I found myself in disagreement with the traditional psychological analysis of insanity. This demanded that I develop my own interpretation and preface my study with some remarks about the healthy life of the mind [*Seelenleben*]. It was not my intention to write a textbook on psychology, but simply to underscore several key points relevant to mental illness. At times I found myself having to suppress my own views about psychological phenomena because they couldn't be addressed with the brevity required in this book. I have therefore needed to rely on the terminology of the well-respected psychologist Herbart. At a later date I will expand on my own views.[198]

Because the first edition of Griesinger's *Pathology and Therapy of Mental Illnesses* is so rare, some readers have overlooked the fact that his use of Herbartian psychology was expressly provisional. Attempts to derive all of Griesinger's psychiatry from Herbartian psychology are therefore unproductive or at least less productive than tracking Griesinger's evolution out of the teachings of his mentor Albert Zeller.

---

[196] Griesinger, "[Rezension von] M. Jacobi," 296.

[197] [Ibid.]

[198] [Griesinger, *Die Pathologie und Therapie*, iv–v.]

That said, and as we shall see, Herbart's psychology had much to offer, and Griesinger found in it results that corresponded to conclusions he had reached along other paths.

Two works published by Herbart in 1816 and 1825 count among the first textbooks on psychology as a science in its own right.[199] The subtitle of Herbart's second work must have attracted Griesinger's attention, promising as it did a "scientific psychology, newly founded on experience, metaphysics, and mathematics." Herbart was actually still an adherent of associationism; his mental units were impressions [*Vorstellungen*], not faculties [*Vermögen*]. Griesinger too in his work on mental reflex had emphasized impressions. However, Herbart was little concerned with physiology; his work contains no explanations that rely on neurological concepts. The idea of supplementing Herbart's work neurologically must have appealed to Griesinger. However, Herbart's "impressions" were fundamentally different from Griesinger's. They were dynamic units that battled one another for a place in consciousness and that interacted with one another according to certain quantitative laws. According to Herbart, impressions could either merge into a harmonious whole or displace one another. Were the impressions of equal strength, complete stalemate resulted. If two or more competing impressions of equal strength inhibit one another, they transmit their results to consciousness, where their content finds expression in the play of competing impressions. Famously, Herbart attempted to quantify this relationship. If consciousness could thus be explained in terms of impressions that were not, or not fully, present in consciousness, then the unconscious would necessarily be especially significant. Herbart distinguishes three levels of consciousness: first, the conspicuous impressions that can be clearly discerned and understood; second, peripheral impressions that are blurred and not clearly present; and third, impressions that have been entirely displaced out of consciousness. An impression that has been displaced does not cease to exist; it simply joins the large number of other displaced impressions and can resurface, either when the countervailing impression weakens or when the impression combines with a similar one, since combined forces can overcome the resistances they face. We leave it to readers to connect Griesinger's concept of mental tonus with Herbart's interpretation of consciousness. However, we are thoroughly convinced that Herbart was not the inspiration for Griesinger's work. Instead, in search of a conceptual model for mental illness and a psychology that could support his psychopathology, i.e., in an attempt to free himself from Zeller's influence, Griesinger necessarily, for lack of alternatives, had to return to Herbart.

Now that we have illustrated the basic principles informing Griesinger's *Pathology and Therapy of Mental Illnesses*, we need not delve into his other publications, for it is not our task to fully describe Griesinger's importance for

[199] Johann Friedrich Herbart, *Lehrbuch der Psychologie* (Königsberg: 1816); idem, *Psychologie als Wissenschaft* (Königsberg: 1824/25). Our treatment of Herbart's psychology relies on the German translation of John Carl Fluegel, *Probleme und Ergebnisse der Psychologie: Hundert Jahre psychologischer Forschung* (Stuttgart: Klett, 1947).

psychiatry. Although we have already dealt with Griesinger's nosology, we can add here that it remained unchanged through its fourth edition published in 1876.

It appears that Griesinger's description of unitary psychosis differs from Zeller's only in the apodictic manner in which he stated it. Writing about the third main form of insanity, i.e., derangement [*Verrücktheit*], Zeller had maintained that it "almost never manifested as a primary form, a least as far as he had seen, unless by way of jealousy, querulousness, and hallucinations."[200] These caveats have disappeared in Griesinger. Griesinger's subgroups are more differentiated. He distinguishes depression and exaltation as two primary mental conditions. Among the depressive conditions he counts hypochondria, melancholia, melancholia with dullness, melancholia with violence, and melancholia with continuous excitation of the will. Among the exaltation conditions he counts frenzy [*Tobsucht*] and delusion [*Wahnsinn*]. Secondary conditions are defined, analogous to neuralgia and spinal irritation, as mental debilities [*psychische Schwächezustände*] and include partial derangement, confusion, and apathetic dementia. In later editions of the textbook, Griesinger adds idiocy and cretinism.

Wilhelm Griesinger and Ludwig Snell

In spite of its broad and mostly favorable reception, Griesinger's textbook did not escape criticism. Indeed, that criticism echoed some of the reservations and concerns that Zeller himself had expressed.

Certainly the most consequential critique was delivered by Ludwig Snell (1817–1892), head of the asylum in Hildesheim, in an address to the annual meeting of German natural scientists in 1865 entitled "On Monomania as a Primary Form of Mental Disturbance."[201] In his lecture, Snell presented eight cases that, today, we would easily diagnose as paranoid-hallucinatory schizophrenia. On the basis of his observations, Snell drew five conclusions: (1) monomania (delusion) develops in pure form as a primary mental disturbance; (2) the morbid conditions evolving out of mania and melancholia differ from pure monomania in that they afflict the entirety of mental life; (3) monomania evolves in two ways, most often gradually, but rarely also accompanied by the turbulent phenomena of acute suffering; (4) delusions of persecution with self-aggrandizement comprise the fundamental characteristics of this psychiatric form; and (5) overconfidence is usually secondary, but it can also precede paranoid ideas or arise simultaneously with them.

Snell's critique represented the first serious threat to the broad consensus about Griesinger's and Zeller's concept of unitary psychosis, and Griesinger's response to it is instructive. It came not in a new edition of his textbook, which he should have

[200] [Albert Zeller, "Zweiter Bericht," 135.]

[201] Ludwig [Daniel Christian] Snell, "Über Monomanie als primäre Form der Seelenstörung," *AZP* 22 (1865): 368–381.

revised to account for Snell's findings. For Griesinger had interpreted the so-called secondary conditions as debilitated conditions and embedded them as such into his system. In addition, the notion of a primary debility was incompatible with the conceptual model of neuralgia and spinal irritation. Snell's critique was a heavy blow to Griesinger, who saw himself forced to reevaluate the foundations of his psychiatric ideas.

Griesinger first went public with his still inchoate and evolving views at the beginning of his clinical lectures in Berlin in 1867. In the first lecture, he clearly sets out his overarching priority: "Let us steer clear of the so-called 'forms' of psychiatry; let us return to the elements we observe, to our 'primordial deliria'."[202] Primordial deliria, which Griesinger also called typical or fundamental deliria, were recurrent false associations [*Gedankenverbindungen*] afflicting seven in ten patients. And in approximately five of ten patients they represented the predominant and persistent delirious form throughout their illnesses.

Griesinger believed he could distinguish several main groups of primordial deliria. For one group, the delirious content involved suffering, impairment, and suppression. A second group manifested active, expansive, and amplified qualities. Among the primordial deliria, Griesinger also counted bodily delusional ideas [*körperliche Wahnvorstellungen*], sexual deliria, as well as the peculiar emotional and cognitive awareness of overall otherness. The first and second groups were the main ones and could combine with others. Hence, a mixture of delusions of grandeur and paranoia would produce the clinical pictures that Snell had described and to which Griesinger assigned the new term "primary derangement" [*primäre Verrücktheit*]. Still embedded in that term was the temporal dimension of the old unitary psychosis, whereby affective conditions preceded deeper cognitive and volitional ones. However in 1867 Griesinger effectively broke up that system. In his first clinical lecture of the semester he announced: "Now I too doubt whether primordial deliria *evolve* out of pathological affect [*pathologische Gemütsbewegungen*]. [...] Recent observations have convinced me that, at the very least, this is not as generally true as I once believed."[203]

We have used the term "tragic" to describe Griesinger's career, and we now see how appropriate that description was. One year prior to his death he published the third, unrevised edition of his textbook in which he reproduced his long-standing system of mental illnesses, and yet simultaneously in his lecture, he destroyed that very system.

We can only speculate how Griesinger imagined his research proceeding. Apparently he hoped to use statistics to isolate a series of initial syndromes and then study them over the course of the illness. No doubt this would have been a methodologically sound way to proceed and would have produced results similar to those of Kraepelin. Griesinger's unexpected death from appendicitis cut off further

---

[202] W[ilhelm] Griesinger, "Vortrag zur Eröffnung der psychiatrischen Klinik zu Berlin am 2. Mai 1867," *Archiv für Psychiatrie und Nervenkrankheiten* 1 (1867): 148.

[203] [Ibid., 150.]

development. But because Griesinger's reputation rests mainly on his textbook, he lives on as an advocate of unitary psychosis, even though he destroyed it at the end of his life. If only for this reason, in the future it would be better to speak not of a Zeller-Griesinger unitary psychosis but rather of the Romantic doctrine of unitary psychosis. This development was not entirely unanticipated in Griesinger's thought: in the first edition of his textbook he was already attempting to isolate elementary disturbances by analyzing clinical symptoms. In this he was doubtless inspired by Joseph Guislain, who in essence sought exactly such elementary disturbances, as typical reaction forms that could arbitrarily interact with each other. In this sense, Guislain was not searching for any unity of the psychoses; instead, his work is better understood as a precursor to a psychiatric syndrome theory. As such, Guislain stands at the beginning of a development that led to Erich A. Hoche's [critique of Kraepelinian psychiatry][204] and that continues to this day.

Systematically pursuing this quest for the ultimate elementary particles of mental illness would have required a cooler, analytic mind. Griesinger, however, was a transitional figure and hence destined to fail in this endeavor. He remained devoted to his mentor, Albert Zeller; he viewed his 2 years working in the Winnenthal asylum as the highlight of his life; he waved the magic wand of analogy just as Oken and Gall had; and he strove passionately to advance science. Griesinger's significance in the history of psychiatry has to do with his advocacy of a truly anthropological psychiatry, i.e., a psychiatry that pays as much attention to the mental and spiritual aspects of mental illness as it does to its somatic ones.[205]

Section 2.4

Heinrich Neumann and Positivism

[If after decades of promoting the concept of unitary psychosis in his textbook Griesinger had finally all but abandoned it in 1867, another of his contemporaries, Heinrich Neumann, reenvisioned the concept in a positivist key, publishing a rival textbook to Griesinger's *Pathology and Therapy of Mental Illnesses* in 1859.][206]

To read Neumann's analytical, skeptical, and positivistic textbook alongside Griesinger's is to be struck by just how far psychiatry was moving away from Zeller's Romantic, pantheistic, and synthetic worldview. Neumann's rendering was cold and clear, scientistic, nonreligious, and everywhere confined to the positively knowable. Neumann's language is precise, and he decisively stakes his claim on the

---

204 Alfred Erich Hoche, "Die Bedeutung der Symptomenkomplexe in der Psychiatrie," *Zeitschrift für die gesamte Neurologie und Psychiatrie* 12 (1912): 540–551.

205 [Abridgement (ca. 220 words): Remarks about Friedrich Wilhelm Hagen (1814–1888).]

206 Heinrich Neumann, *Lehrbuch der Psychiatrie* (Erlangen: Enke, 1859). [Abridgement (ca. 390 words): Biographic sketch of Heinrich Neumann (1814–1884).]

very first pages of the textbook: "The science of human existence in space we call anatomy, that of human existence in time we call physiology. A third kind of knowledge about humans doesn't exist, at least as a natural science."[207] The term soul [*Seele*] is absent from Neumann's text: "A living whole that becomes fully or partially conscious of its own inner workings is called an animated entity [*beseeltes Wesen*]. One should no longer say that humans have a soul, but rather that humans are animate beings."[208] "The trajectory of science leads neither to nor from God; it crosses the path of religion at no junction whatsoever."[209]

Considering that these lines were written just 5 years after Zeller's last asylum report, one becomes acutely aware of the enormous intellectual change that transpired in the first half of the nineteenth century, and one understands why Albert Zeller ceased publishing the results of his scientific research in 1854.[210]

Neumann described the positivist method he used to explain psychological phenomena as "analytical," and at the very beginning of his textbook he drew on an example from analytic chemistry to elaborate this point. However, he deduces logically that analysis always presumes a whole, a totality that can be dissected. The psychiatric unit to be dissected was the human being, specifically its functions.

One of the basic functions that justified the term "animated entity" was metamorphosis, i.e., the activity whereby humans transformed their sensory impressions into conscious states.[211] Neumann spoke of hypermetamorphosis to describe a condition when metamorphosis was so active, constantly commanding all resources of attention, that it displaced other mental activity.[212] This condition is synonymous with erethism and excessive wakefulness (pervigilium). The excitation leads to irritation, so that all sensations become unpleasant and painful. Hypermetamorphosis progresses to frenzy [*Tobsucht*], although Neumann did not consider this a specific disease but rather "only an invitation to diagnosis, i.e. to an investigation of the causal elements and necessary consequences of the frenzy."[213] Hypermetamorphosis is nevertheless also the breeding ground for illusions.

Hypermetamorphosis's complementary condition is ametamorphosis.[214] Whereas in hypermetamorphosis consciousness is dominated by sensory perception and hence by the outer world, ametamorphosis shuts patients off from the outer world; they turn inward, and their mental powers decline. Patients sense nothing, want nothing, and neglect themselves, and hallucinations and delusional ideas arise. Ametamorphosis incorporates both melancholia and ecstasy or, in today's terminology, retarded depression and stupor.

---

[207] [Ibid., §3, 4.]

[208] [Ibid., §20, 9.]

[209] [Ibid., §6, 5.]

[210] [Abridgement (ca. 170 words): Short quote about Auguste Comte's Positivism.]

[211] [Neumann, *Lehrbuch*, §91, 40.]

[212] [Ibid., §159, 71.]

[213] [Ibid., §162, 75.]

[214] [Ibid., §176, 91.]

And so we see how Neumann derives, from the two basic conditions of hypermetamorphosis and ametamorphosis, all so-called elements, which themselves are by no means evidence of a disease. A disease arises only when, out of one element, others progressively evolve, i.e., when a disease process occurs.[215]

Wherever such a process occurs, we have a mental disturbance. Neumann emphasizes: "There is only one kind of mental disturbance [*Seelenstörung*] and we call it *insanity* [*Irresein*]."[216] In other words, insanity has different stages rather than different forms. And those stages are called delusion [*Wahnsinn*], confusion, and dementia. It follows from this that a patient who suffers from delusions and remains uncured will descend into confusion and dementia.

For anyone delving into Neumann's system, it seems strange how he deals with affective psychoses. Whereas Griesinger and Zeller had clearly distinguished between affective and non-affective conditions, Neumann makes no such clear distinction. Certainly, Neumann concedes that, in many cases, delusional states are *in fact* often preceded by a *stadium melancholicum.*[217]And yet Neumann also insists that melancholia, as a type of illness, is useless.[218] Despondent mood could accompany every form and every stage of insanity.

We conclude with an account of what Neumann himself believed to be his specific contribution. In his textbook, Neumann emphasizes two points: First, he had sought to parse concrete morbid mental states to the point where no further subdivision seemed possible. What he found he called elements. Hypermetamorphosis was an element, as were frenzy and hallucinations. Yet elements alone can yield no classification. Second, a real classification of mental illnesses had to involve cognitive processes [*geistige Verrichtungen*]. But in fact these processes could not be as easily subdivided as those in psychological systems. For Neumann, it is simply a matter of having the courage to admit that no classification is better than a false classification: "One needs to accept that *human illnesses* are the category under which *mental illnesses* appear as a *genus*. But the individual cases represent the *species* [....] Common to all species, however, is that they begin with delusions [*Wahnsinn*], evolve into confusion [*Verwirrtheit*], and end in dementia [*Blödsinn*]."[219] Neumann excludes from this course only congenital dementia (idiocy, cretinism).

---

[215] [Ibid., §155, 69.]

[216] [Ibid., §247, 167.]

[217] Ibid., §255, 170–171.

[218] Ibid., §267, 182–184.

[219] Ibid., §266, 182.

The Romantic and Positivistic Unitary Psychosis

If we have described Zeller and Griesinger as representing a Romantic understanding of unitary psychosis, then Neumann represents a positivist and skeptical one. Certainly, both share some basic ideas, for example, Neumann's concept of metamorphosis and the idea of mental reflex that Griesinger posited in 1843. Nevertheless, we must clearly distinguish Romantic and positivistic unitary psychosis, above all due to the different assessments of affective states. Whereas Zeller places those states at the center of his analysis, for Neumann they are insignificant baggage. Neumann is able to achieve his unity only by daring to eliminate Zeller's primary forms.

This unusual move, which distorted factual evidence, was certainly a result of personal factors. Zeller's temperament swung harmoniously between happy and sad, while Neumann's temperament appears to have been built to psychaesthetic proportions.[220]

Section 2.5

From Unitary Psychosis to Karl Ludwig Kahlbaum's Vesania Typica

No one recognized just how lopsided Neumann's system was better than Karl Ludwig Kahlbaum (1828–1899).[221] And yet Neumann's work was a key point of reference in Kahlbaum's own important and influential 1863 study on *Groups of Mental Illness*.[222] Throughout that book, Kahlbaum praises Neumann's work and never doubts that his theory of stages is correct, even subscribing to the view that the course of mental illness as depicted by Neumann was typical. Citing Zeller, Griesinger, and Guislain, Kahlbaum proceeds to construct a class of mental illnesses that he defines using the old-fashioned term *vesania*. He defines it as an idiopathic mental disturbance that afflicts more or less the entirety of mental life.

Kahlbaum then distinguishes three types of *vesania*

(1) *Vesania acuta*, i.e., febrile insanity without etiological involvement of extracerebral diseases.

---

[220] [G. Zeller is drawing here on Ernst Kretschmer's theory of temperaments, retrospectively diagnosing Neumann as "schizothymic," which involves sensitive and cold poles in "psychaesthetic proportion" to each other, and Zeller as "cyclothymic." See Ernst Kretschmer, *Körperbau und Charakter: Untersuchungen zum Konstitutions-Problem und zur Lehre von den Temperamenten*, 11th and 12th edition (Berlin: Springer, 1936), 136–140.]

[221] [Abridgement (ca. 630 words): Biographic sketch of Karl Ludwig Kahlbaum (1828–1899) and Hermann Reimer (1825–1906).]

[222] Kahlbaum, *Die Gruppierung*.

(2) *Vesania typica*, i.e., idiopathic mental disturbances with certain and regular stages of development. These stages are:

I. *Stadium melancholicum (incrementi)*
II. *Stadium maniae (acmes)*
III. *Stadium perturbationis (decrementi)*
IV. *Stadium dementiae (defectus)*

Here we again have the old unitary psychosis as Zeller described it, except that it is now only one—albeit the most common—course, among others. Alongside *vesania typica* Kahlbaum then also places [(3)] *vesania progressiva*, i.e., progressive paralysis. Later he also added *vesania catatonica*. Of all human mental illnesses, Neumann had allowed only insanity [*Irresein*] and had completely ignored the affective psychoses, theoretically and descriptively. But Kahlbaum's rigorous and unbiased empiricism kept him from following Neumann.

[¶] Alongside the category *vesania*, Kahlbaum placed the category *vecordia*, defining it as an idiopathic mental disturbance with well-defined symptoms that usually emerge after puberty. Within the *vecordia* group, Kahlbaum distinguishes *vecordia dysthymia*, which manifests mainly emotional disturbances at onset. Kahlbaum subdivides this group into *dysthymia meläna* and *dysthymia elata* manifesting sad and happy affect, respectively. In addition to *vecordia dysthymia*, Kahlbaum adds *vecordia paranoia* and *vecordia diastrephia* manifesting cognitive and volitional disturbances, respectively. A final member of the *vecordia* category is *vecordia insania*, a partial disruption with no specific direction, but one manifesting other symptoms—a rather opaque category.

The entire *vesania* group is characterized by a certain continuity of symptoms throughout the illness as well as by a favorable prognosis.

In addition to *vesania* and *vecordia*, Kahlbaum also introduces the category *dysphrenia*, a sympathetic and symptomatic disturbance that follows a specific physiological or pathological somatic condition and that afflicts the entirety of mental life. This category includes *neophrenia* (a mental defect acquired at birth or in the first year of life) and *paraphrenia* (a defect associated with biological transitions such as puberty (*hebetica*), old age (*senilis*), and sleep (*hypnetica*, including somnambulism).

While it is tempting to further explore Kahlbaum's nosology, we must be content simply to recognize that he has taken unitary psychosis and made it one of five different categories. In other words, it is Kahlbaum who finally overcame the doctrine of unitary psychosis. He blazed a trail to the ever-clearer delineation of disease entities. This achievement was not limited to psychiatry: it was happening elsewhere in medicine as well, especially once in bacteriology Robert Koch (1843—1910) began demonstrating the specificity of certain illnesses.

With that, one might conclude that unitary psychosis had died a natural death in the face of expanding clinical evidence. But this judgment would be premature. For Rudolf Gottfried Arndt, a professor of psychiatry in Greifswald, resuscitated unitary psychosis in a textbook he published in 1883,[223] the same year in which the first edition of Emil Kraepelin's *Compendium of Psychiatry* appeared in print.[224]

Section 2.6

Rudolf Arndt and the Fundamental Law of Biology

Rudolf Arndt[225] was a modern natural scientist yet with a strong inclination to generalize the causal relationships he observed. To this day, Arndt is known for his discovery and formalization of the so-called Arndt-Schulz rule which states: "Weak stimuli arouse vital activity, stronger and moderate stimuli accelerate and promote it, strong stimuli inhibit it, and the strongest stimuli end it." Arndt's colleague in Greifswald, the pharmacologist Hugo Schulz, believed this rule was the fundamental principle of pharmacology. And to prove it, he conducted experiments with so-called yeast toxins, which in small doses sped up yeast growth. For Arndt, the rule was a fundamental law of biology that could be applied universally to explain the most heterogeneous phenomena, from flat-footedness and clubfoot, to giants and dwarfs, to black and white pigmentation in animals and humans, to body temperature and fever. Of course, such broad application of a general rule was bound to return some hits. Arndt's attempt to explain Pflüger's law of twitching was just such a hit and has since garnered him a place in the annals of neurophysiology.[226]

Given Arndt's luck in applying his fundamental law of biology to fatigued and dying nerve cells, it must have seemed obvious to apply the same law to mental illness, especially seeing that Griesinger had drawn an analogy between mental illness and neuralgia. In his textbook, Arndt writes:

> It seems that every psychosis is nothing other than the expression, i.e. the reaction of the undernourished and therefore compromised nervous system, especially the brain. Accordingly, the undernourished nervous system is nothing other than the expression of the twitching law that governs undernourished and damaged nerves. Hence, the course of every psychosis follows the twitching law of fatigued or dying nerves. And so it is in fact! One must recognize, however, that nerve-cell death can take a long time, years and decades, as is the case for what we call involution. Involution is simply a death march [....] *Early*

---

[223] Rudolf Arndt, *Lehrbuch der Psychiatrie für Aerzte und Studirende* (Vienna and Leipzig: Urban und Schwarzenberg, 1883).

[224] Emil Kraepelin, *Compendium der Psychiatrie: Zum Gebrauche für Studirende und Aerzte* (Leipzig: Abel, 1883).

[225] On the life and work of Arndt, see W[illy] Vorkastner and Pophal, "Rudolf Gottfried Arndt 1835–1900," in *Deutsche Irrenärzte*, edited by Theodor Kirchhoff, vol. 2 (Berlin: J. Springer, 1924), 138–142. [Abridgement (ca. 100 words): Biographic sketch of Rudolf Arndt.]

[226] [In 1859 Eduard Pflüger (1829–1910) described muscular twitching when Galvanic current was used to stimulate motor neurons. Abridgement (ca. 170 words): Quote illustrating the neurophysiological relevance of the law drawn from Johann Gottschick, *Die Leistungen des Nervensystems* (Jena: Fischer, 1955), 32.]

> *melancholia* corresponds to the reaction of the simple, tired nerve, the reaction of the tiring mental organs. *Mania* corresponds with the initial stage of the dying or slightly tired mental organ, and *secondary melancholia* to the somewhat tired and hence somewhat paralyzed mental organ. [….] Just as the twitching law can manifest itself in numerous ways in the undernourished and damaged nerve, so too the psychoses. This explains the variety and case-specific presentation of the psychoses. Certainly, if the individual stages of a psychosis are fairly regular in terms of their duration and strength, such that mania presents itself just like initial and secondary melancholia did, and a distinct course becomes visible, then we follow Kahlbaum in calling the psychosis *vesania typica*. Otherwise we call the psychosis by a different name: *dysthymia* or also *melancholia*, *mania*, *lypemania*, *chaeromania*, *frenzy*, etc. But if a given stage of the psychosis lasts for a long time, seems to become habitual, and in any way involves paresthesia, parabulia, paralogia, or parergasia, then it becomes a psychosis quasi sui generis and we call it derangement [*Verrücktheit*] or lunacy [*Narrheit*], *paranoia*, *idiocy*, *dementia*.[227]

And so in every full-blown psychosis one can discern three stages: an initial or primary melancholic stage, a manic stage, and a secondary melancholic stage. Every mental illness begins and ends with melancholia.

And so we see Arndt continuing along the path that Griesinger had embarked upon in the early 1840s.[228] Furthermore, he is in agreement with Griesinger that mental illnesses are functional illnesses, i.e., disturbances of brain function. Yet at the same time, he agrees with Zeller that the entire body is the soul's organ [*Seelenorgan*]: "Every bodily process is a source of mental life. The question is only whether these processes are conveyed, in one form or another, to the cerebral cortex and there become elements of thought, of consciousness."[229]

Arndt is therefore in fact the last representative of unitary psychosis as conceived by Zeller and Griesinger. The individual clinical presentations of mental illness are simply phases in the course of a comprehensive process. The course of all mental illnesses proceeds according to the same schema, even progressive paralysis. The variations in clinical presentation are the result of the varied intensity of the different phases and the peculiar qualities of the patient's personality. The clinical symptoms of paranoia appear when *vesania typica* develops in a patient with a paranoid predisposition. These kinds of patients can also suffer primary paranoia.

After characterizing Zeller's unitary psychosis as Romantic unitary psychosis, can we also count Arndt among the Romantics? Certainly not. There exists a fundamental difference in Arndt's thought and that of Romantic physicians. In Romantic thought, everything interrelates, connections are seen everywhere, and everything is part of a living, evolving whole. By contrast, Arndt's totality is achieved by way of a generalization and universalization of an otherwise correct fundamental rule. These are antithetical paths. Of Romantics one could say that the particular is interesting only as part of a whole. But for Arndt, even the most general case is just an example of a particular rule. Were it not so disrespectful, one could say that Arndt had a monomanic conception of unitary psychosis.

---

227 Arndt, *Lehrbuch*, 253 f.

228 Griesinger, "Ueber psychische Reflexactionen"; idem, Griesinger, "Neue Beiträge".

229 [Arndt, *Lehrbuch*, 4.]

Section 2.7

Concluding Summary

We have now carefully examined the broad spectrum of pre-Kraepelinian phenomena related to the idea of unitary psychosis, which progressively evolves through typical stages from melancholia, to mania, to deranged thought, and finally to dementia. We have clearly distinguished three different conceptions of unitary psychosis:

A Romantic one (Albert Zeller)
A skeptical, positivistic one (Heinrich Neumann)
A monomanic one (Rudolf Arndt)

The doctrine of unitary psychosis ends with Karl Ludwig Kahlbaum, who reduced it to just one (albeit typical) course among many courses of psychosis. He called it "*vesania typica completa*."

Let us briefly summarize the development of unitary psychosis. We found that Sydenham, Reil, and Autenrieth had already described mental illnesses that manifested a course corresponding to what later came to be known as unitary psychosis. Autenrieth's student, Albert Zeller, became the first to clearly articulate this doctrine in 1840. We explored in detail some of its personal and intellectual roots. We found that the unitarian aspirations of the Romantic era were key to Zeller's unitary psychosis. Zeller's upbringing, his personality, and his ties to a circle of intellectuals in Berlin associated with the publisher Georg Andreas Reimer, especially Friedrich Schleiermacher, all contributed to his deeply Romantic sensibilities. These sensibilities, combined with the results of his own self-observations, led him to posit the problem of mood [*Gestimmtsein*] as the starting point for his psychopathological investigations. Joseph Guislain's concept of mental anguish [*Seelenschmerz*] as a fundamental disturbance of mental illness helped to focus Zeller's own similar ideas. One can therefore say that *the concept of unitary psychosis was born when Zeller engaged with Guislain's ideas*. Neither is the precursor of the other; their mutual encounter enriched both.

Zeller's student, Wilhelm Griesinger, then further advanced the concept of unitary psychosis, to the point that it was accepted by most alienists. Griesinger formulated it more forthrightly than Zeller had; he allowed for no exceptions and sharply separated primary, affective conditions from secondary, non-affective ones, which were characterized by mental debility.

But in Griesinger's apodictic rendering, the doctrine of unitary psychosis became extremely vulnerable to attack. That attack ensued in September of 1865 at the annual meeting of German natural scientists in Hannover, where Ludwig Snell described eight cases that we would today diagnose as paranoid, hallucinatory schizophrenia. Snell explained that the cases were primary, with no prior melancholic stage. Snell's evidence was so convincing that in 1867, in his first clinical lecture of the semester, Griesinger completely abandoned unitary psychosis and proposed a research program to investigate mainly the initial stages of what he called primordial deliria. That Griesinger failed to revise the 1867 third edition of his *Pathology and Therapy of Mental Illnesses* represents one of the truly tragic moments of his life. Griesinger's early death in 1869 left the contradictions in his own work unresolved.

We have described Griesinger as a transitional figure, lodged on the threshold of enormous changes between the first and second halves of the nineteenth century. He was still half a Romantic natural scientist and already half a positivist one as well. And in the history of unitary psychosis itself, Griesinger is also a transitional figure: he ensured the concept's broadest recognition but was also the first to abandon it.

We encountered the skeptical, positivistic form of unitary psychosis in the work of Heinrich Neumann. Neumann's thought built on Griesinger's research, but he rejected any attempt at systematization. For him, no system at all was better than a false one. Neumann was thus, as Kahlbaum rightly saw, the founder not of a unified system but of a non-system. If he was nevertheless able to arrive at a unified understanding of mental illness, then he did so in a rather contrived manner: he equated mental disease [*Geisteskrankheit*] with insanity [*Irresein*], discounting all of Zeller's and Griesinger's primary affective conditions. For Neumann, melancholia was only an accompanying symptom that could arise at any stage of insanity and had no autonomous nosological standing. And so this study has clarified, for the first time, that Zeller's and Neumann's unitary psychosis was essentially different and they should not be associated with one another.

The third form of unitary psychosis that we encountered prior to Kraepelin was that described in Rudolf Arndt's textbook of 1883. Together with the pharmacologist Schulz, Arndt had discovered the so-called Arndt-Schulz rule and provided experimental evidence of its validity. Arndt reinterpreted this important rule as a universal biological law, using it to explain a panoply of phenomena. Mental illness represented just one more example of the validity of the law. Arndt basically retained the structure of disease course described by Zeller and Griesinger, drawing an analogy between the different stages and the behavior of fatigued and dying nerves, thus rendering them subject to Pflüger's twitching law. Arndt followed the path Griesinger had embarked upon to its conclusion. In essence, he understood mental illness as simply a special, extenuated case of his basic rule—or as we have called it, a monomanic form of unitary psychosis.

Kahlbaum then harmoniously incorporated unitary psychosis into emerging research on disease entities. For him, unitary psychosis became one typical course, among others, and it became "*vesania typica*."

In this study, our aim has been primarily to elucidate the intellectual and biographic context from which the different forms and versions of the doctrine of unitary psychosis evolved prior to Kraepelin. In doing so, it was certainly not our intent to dispute all the empirical evidence supporting this doctrine. However, today, cases manifesting these courses are quite rare. And so at the conclusion of our study, we wish to raise the question of whether they could have been more frequent in Albert Zeller's day. Albert Zeller repeatedly stated that in his experience, things were as he had described them. He even wondered why elsewhere different forms were more frequent. In his first asylum report he wrote: "But it remains curious that lunacy [*Narrheit*], which in France is more prevalent than all the other forms, is so rarely seen here, and that depression [*Schwermut*] in women, and partial derangement are so predominant."[230]

To this day, as every experienced observer knows, the character of the Swabian people is marked by a subdepressive mood. And we may associate this with the high percentage of pyknic constitutional types in the Swabian population. Prior to the migration unleashed by the industrial revolution, which increasingly blurred the different tribal characteristics, the percentage of pyknic types in Swabia was likely higher. As a result, in the Swabian patient population they saw, Zeller and Griesinger must have seen mainly cases of depression or substantially retarded schizophrenia [*stark gebremste Schizophrenien*]. This likely was not the case for Ludwig Snell, whose population in Hildesheim contained more cases of full-blown schizophrenia. Snell's objection might thus have been based on empirical observation just like the doctrine of unitary psychosis had been in Swabia.[231]

This historical study has reexamined the full range of issues surrounding unitary psychosis. Given the intensive interest of past physicians in a single psychosis with a uniform course, one hopes the problem will again be revisited on a new and broader foundation with the aid of modern psychiatric methods, especially those related to constitutional theories of personality, gestalt psychology, and research on somatic psychosis.

[230] [Albert Zeller, "[Erster] Bericht," 334.]

[231] [In his later publications, Zeller modified this epidemiological interpretation of the evolution of unitary psychosis, placing greater emphasis on conceptual differences. See G[erhart] Zeller, "Die Tübinger Psychiater-Schule," in *Wahn*, edited by Walter Schulte and Rainer Tölle (Stuttgart: Georg Thieme, 1972), 102 f.]

Kapitel 3
Die Geschichte der Einheitspsychose vor Kraepelin

Gerhart Zeller and Eric J. Engstrom

TEIL 3.1

Einleitung

„Alle Betrachtung der Vergangenheit empfängt ihr Licht und ihre Farbe von der Gegenwart.“[1] Dieser unmittelbar einleuchtende Satz des bedeutenden Tübinger Historikers Johannes Haller gibt uns das Recht, unsere medizinhistorische Studie mit der Frage zu beginnen, woher es wohl kommen mag, daß seit wenigen Jahren plötzlich ein starkes Licht des Interesses auf einen Abschnitt der Geschichte unserer Wissenschaft fällt, welcher bis dahin als hoffnungslos überholt und damit als uninteressant galt, nämlich auf die Lehre von der „Einheitspsychose“.

Es gehört nicht zu der uns gestellten Aufgabe, zu untersuchen, in welcherlei wissenschaftlichem Gewand diese Wendung zum Vorvorgestrigen gegenwärtig auftritt. Lediglich um zu illustrieren, mit welchem Ernst und mit welcher Intensität diese Rückwendung erfolgt und in die aktuelle Diskussion um Deutung und Ordnung der Psychosen eingreift, sei hier die Arbeit des Madrider Klinikers Bartolomé Llopis „Das allen Psychosen gemeinsame Achsensyndrom“[2] angeführt. Ganz bewußt wird dort auf den alten Begriff der Einheitspsychose zurückgegriffen, und zwar in der Form, welche von Wilhelm Griesinger in der ersten Auflage seiner *Pathologie und Therapie der psychischen Krankheiten* im Jahre 1845 geprägt wurde.

An Stelle einer nur schwer zu erreichenden Definition, welche zudem als abstrakt die konkrete Untersuchung der sich wandelnden historischen Gestalt wenig fördern

---

Zum Zeitpunkt der Veröffentlichung war der Autor “Gerhart Zeller” verstorben.

---

[1] Johannes Haller, *Die Epochen der deutschen Geschichte* (Stuttgart: Port Verlag, 1950), 15. [Hallers ursprünglich 1923 erschienenes Buch wurde zum großen Publikumserfolg].

[2] Bartolomé Llopis, „Das allen Psychosen gemeinsame Achsensyndrom,“ *Fortschritte der Neurologie und Psychiatrie* 28.2 (1960): 106–129.

G. Zeller et al., *A History of Unitary Psychosis*, Theory and History in the Human and Social Sciences, https://doi.org/10.1007/978-3-031-90182-9_3

würde, möge Griesinger selbst zitiert sein: „Zwei große Gruppen psychisch anormaler Grundzustände ergeben sich aus der Analyse der Beobachtungen als die beiden wesentlichsten Verschiedenheiten des Irreseins. Einmal nämlich beruht dasselbe auf dem krankhaften Entstehen, Herrschen, Fixiertbleiben von Affekten und affektartigen Zuständen, unter deren Einflüsse nun das ganze psychische Leben die der Art und Weise des Affekts adäquaten Modifikationen erleidet. Das anderemal besteht das Irresein in Störungen des Vorstellens und Wollen, die nicht (nicht mehr) von dem Herrschen eines affektartigen Zustandes herrühren, sondern ein, ohne tiefere Gemütserregtheit selbstständiges, beruhigtes falsches Denken und Wollen (meist mit dem herrschenden Charakter psychischer Schwäche) darstellen. Die Beobachtung ergibt nun weiter, daß die Zustände, die in der ersten Hauptgruppe enthalten sind, in der außerordentlichen Mehrzahl der Fälle den Zuständen zweiter Reihe vorangehen, daß die letzteren gewöhnlich nur als Folgen und Ausgänge der ersteren, bei nicht geheilter Gehirnkrankheit auftreten. Es zeigt sich ferner innerhalb der ersten Gruppe, bei einer größeren Durchschnittsbetrachtung, wieder eine gewisse bestimmte Aufeinanderfolge der einzelnen Arten affektartiger Zustände, und so ergibt sich eine Betrachtungsweise des Irreseins, welche in dessen verschiedenen Formen verschiedene Stadien eines Krankheitsprozesses erkennt, welcher zwar durch die mannigfachsten intercurrierenden pathologischen Ereignisse modifiziert, unterbrochen, umgeändert werden kann, im Ganzen aber einen stetig successiven Verlauf einhält, der bis zum gänzlichen Zerfall des psychischen Lebens gehen kann.“[3]

Die Frage, in welcher medizinischen Disziplin oder in welchem Zweig der Naturwissenschaft eine solche Renaissance einer über hundertjährigen, seit zwei Generationen als überholt geltenden Theorie, möglich wäre, führt mit Notwendigkeit zur Untersuchung der Ursache einer solchen Entwicklung.

Das Wort „Einheitspsychose“, übrigens recht jungen Datums, das sich bei keinem der später genau zu untersuchenden Begründer dieser Lehre findet, hat für uns einen besonderen Bedeutungsinhalt, der dazu beiträgt, unser historisches Interesse auf diesem Gebiet zu beleben. Aber warum spricht es uns an? Nun, weil viele der heutigen Psychiater der Symptomatik mit ihrer scharfen Abgrenzung einzelner Krankheiten überdrüssig geworden sind. Ernst Kretschmer hat schon 1919 in seiner grundlegenden Arbeit über psychogene Wahnbildung bei traumatischer Hirnschwäche diesen Überdruß in die Worte gefaßt: „Was wir an Systematik gewinnen, das verlieren wir an Verständnis.“[4] Überdrüssig sind wir aber auch einer ins Uferlose fortgeführten Individualisierung, die mancherorts unter dem Titel „no diagnosis at all“ zu einer Auflösung der Wissenschaft geführt hat, welche doch stets System und Ordnung ist.

Die Sehnsucht nach der allseitig befriedigenden einheitlichen Betrachtungsweise der Geisteskrankheiten, welche einem angestrebten einheitlichen Seelenbegriff

---

[3] Wilhelm Griesinger, *Die Pathologie und Therapie der psychischen Krankheiten* (Stuttgart: A. Krabbe, 1845), 151.

[4] Ernst Kretschmer, „Über psychogene Wahnbildungen bei traumatischer Hirnschwäche,“ *Zeitschrift für die gesamte Neurologie und Psychiatrie – Originalien* 45.3/4 (1919): 298.

entsprechen könnte, ist es wohl, welche Licht und Farbe auf unsere psychiatrische Vergangenheit wirft. Einheit als Gegensatz zu Vielheit, wie sie uns wissenschaftlich geordnet im Lebenswerk Emil Kraepelins entgegentritt, ebenso wie in einer Betrachtungsweise, welche nur individuelle Lebensgeschichten sieht und alle systematische Ordnung auflöst.

Deutsche Literatur zum Thema ‚Einheitspsychose'

Ist somit das Interesse an der Lehre von der „Einheitspsychose" weitgehend aus der momentanen Situation der Psychiatrie geboren, so dürfen wir allerdings kaum hoffen, den älteren medizin-historischen Arbeiten allzuviel an konkreten Forschungsergebnissen entnehmen zu können. Der folgende Überblick über das bisher Bekannte oder Vermutete wird sich daher auf knappe Angaben beschränken können.

Sigmund Kornfelds *Geschichte der Psychiatrie* ist mit seinen 127 Seiten bis heute die umfang- und inhaltsreichste Bearbeitung des Themas, und wir finden hier auch wichtige Hinweise, deren Kernstück folgender Passus ist: „Albert Zeller (1804–1877) (Berichte über die Irrenanstalt Winnenthal, insbesondere 2. Bericht 1840) unterscheidet zwei große Gruppen von psychische anormalen Grundzuständen. Die eine Gruppe beruht auf dem krankhaften Entstehen, Herrschen und Fixiertbleiben von Affekten und affektartigen Zuständen …"[5] Es handelt sich hier um den bereits wörtlich zitierten Abschnitt aus Griesingers *Pathologie und Therapie psychischer Krankheiten*, also nicht um ein Zitat oder ein Excerpt aus den fünf Berichten über die Wirksamkeit der Heilanstalt Winnenthal. Diese hatte Zeller über den Zeitabschnitt vom 1. März 1834, dem Eröffnungsdatum der Anstalt, bis zum 28. Februar 1854 im *Medizinischen Correspondenz-Blatt des württembergischen Ärztlichen Vereins* veröffentlicht.[6] Ihr Inhalt ist weiter unten eingehend zu untersuchen, vor allem im Hinblick auf die Ausgestaltung und Abänderung, die Zellers Ansichten bei seinem Schüler Griesinger erfahren haben. Diese Abweichungen sind keineswegs so geringfügig, daß man Griesingers Formulierungen einfach als von Zeller übernommen annehmen könnte, wie das Kornfeld tut, aus dessen Darstellung man schließen muß, daß er die „Berichte" wohl kaum in Händen gehabt haben dürfte.

[5] S[igmund] Kornfeld, „Geschichte der Psychiatrie," in *Handbuch der Geschichte der Medizin*, hg. von Max Neuburger und Julius Pagel (Jena: Fischer, 1905), 688.

[6] [[Albert v.] Zeller, „[Erster] Bericht über die Wirksamkeit der Heilanstalt Winnenthal von ihrer Eröffnung den 1. März 1834 bis zum 28. Februar 1837," *Medicinisches Correspondenz-Blatt des Würtembergischen Ärztlichen Vereins* (*MCblWÄV*) 7.30 (Beilage #11) (1837): 321–335; ders., „Zweiter Bericht über die Wirksamkeit der Heilanstalt Winnenthal vom 1. März 1837 bis zum 29. Februar 1840," *MCblWÄV* 10.17–19 (1840): 129–147; ders., „[Dritter] Dreijähriger Bericht über die Wirksamkeit der Heilanstalt Winnenthal vom 1. März 1840 bis zum 28. Februar 1843," *MCblWÄV* 13.38–39 (1843): 297–310; ders., „[Vierter] Dreijähriger Bericht über die Wirksamkeit der Heilanstalt Winnenthal vom 1. März 1843 bis 28. Februar 1846," *MCblWÄV* 18.2–3 (1848): 9–20; ders., „[Fünfter] Bericht über die Wirksamkeit der Heilanstalt Winnenthal vom 1. März 1846 bis 28. Februar 1854," *MCblWÄV* 24.38 (1854): 297–318].

Nicht viel besser werden wir von Emil Kraepelin in seiner Studie *Hundert Jahre Psychiatrie*[7] belehrt, obgleich er wohl als erster eine, wenn auch nur skizzenhafte, dem Umfang des Gesamtwerkes entsprechende Geschichte der Einheitspsychose gibt. Kraepelin geht dabei von Guislain aus, dessen Lehre er prägnant charakterisiert. Guislain habe die Auffassung vertreten, das die mannigfaltigen klinischen Krankheitsbilder Ausdrucksformen der allmählich immer weitere Gebiete in Mitleidenschaft ziehenden Ausgleichsbestrebungen gegenüber einer eingreifenden seelischen Schädigung seien. So komme es, daß sich zunächst unter der unmittelbaren Einwirkung des Reizes das Gefühl der Betrübnis, der Schwermut einstelle, der dann als Reaktion des „Erhaltungsinstinktes" Anfälle von Jähzorn und Wut, die „Tollheit" folgen. Weitere Entlastungsbestrebungen seien dann „sonderbare Abweichungen in den Entschlüssen", Grillen als Erscheinungen der „Narrheit", „Nervenspannung" in Form der „Ekstase", Konvulsionen und endlich die falschen Vorstellungen, wie sie uns in der „Verrücktheit" entweder als „betrübende" oder als „tröstende" Einbildungen, als Verfolgungs- oder Größenwahn entgegentreten. Die Verschiedenheit der tatsächlichen Krankheitsbilder sei auf die Verschiedenheit der persönlichen Veranlagung zurückzuführen. Kraepelin führt dann wörtlich weiter fort: „Wie es scheint, hat sich an diese Gedankengänge Guislains die später von Zeller aufgestellte, von Hagen übernommene und von Griesinger seiner Darstellung der Seelenheilkunde zugrunde gelegte Anschauung angelehnt, daß die klinischen Formen des Irreseins in der Hauptsache Verlaufsabschnitte darstellen, von denen die mit lebhafter Gemütserregung einhergehenden Bilder, die Schwermut, die Tobsucht und der Wahnsinn, als die ersten, heilbaren Stufen des Leidens betrachtet wurden, während die mehr selbstständig hervortretenden Störungen des Denkens und Wollens, wie sie als Verrücktheit und Blödsinn bezeichnet werden, den Übergang in unheilbare Schwächezustände bedeuten."[8] Diese Zeller-Griesingersche Lehre habe sich, so meint Kraepelin, jedoch als unhaltbar erwiesen, als von Snell und Westphal festgestellt wurde, daß die Verrücktheit durchaus nicht immer den Ausgang einer mit Gemütserregung einhergehenden Geistesstörung darstelle, sondern auch „primär" selbstständig entstehen könne.

Seit diesen Ausführungen Kraepelins gilt Guislain als direkter Vorläufer von Zeller und Griesinger. Es darf indes nicht unbeachtet bleiben, daß diese Verbindung bisher viel zu eng gesehen wurde. Kraepelin hat übersehen, daß Zeller bereits 1838 Guislain eine geprägte eigene Ansicht kritisch entgegenstellte,[9] sodaß man schon hieraus den Schluß ziehen kann, daß es sich bei Guislain und Zeller nicht einfach um das Verhältnis von Vorläufer und Nachfolger handelt. Man darf allerdings vermuten, das Kraepelin Zellers Vorwort und Zusätze zu der Übersetzung von Guislains

[7] Emil Kraepelin, „Hundert Jahre Psychiatrie: Ein Beitrag zur Geschichte menschlicher Gesittung," *Zeitschrift für die gesamte Neurologie und Psychiatrie* 38 (1918): 161–275.

[8] Ebenda, 240.

[9] Joseph Guislain, *Abhandlung ueber die Phrenopathien oder neues System der Seelenstörungen, gegründet auf praktische und statistische Beobachtungen und Untersuchung der Ursachen, der Natur, der Symptome, der Prognose, der Diagnose und der Behandlung dieser Krankheiten. Mit einem Vorwort und Zusätzen von Dr. Zeller* (Stuttgart: Rieger, 1838), 1–28, 440–518.

Abhandlung über die Phrenopathien nicht gekannt hat, sonst hätte er wohl nicht von Zeller als dem Übersetzer Guislains gesprochen.[10]

Auch der durch seine 1921 erschienene verdienstvolle Biographiensammlung Deutsche Irrenärzte[11] bekanntgewordene Theodor Kirchhoff hat sich eigene Gedanken über die historische Entwicklung der Einheitspsychose gemacht. Er schreibt über Griesinger: „Epochemachend war sein Lehrbuch der Geisteskrankheiten, welches, auf Reils Lehre von den Störungen des Gemeingefühls (Zellers Einheitspsychose) fußend, die Herbart'sche Psychologie mit den eigenen klinischen und anatomischen Erfahrungen verband. Hervorgehoben zu werden verdient die auch von Griesinger vertretene einheitliche genetische Auffassung der psychischen Störungen, welche in einer bestimmten gewissen Aufeinanderfolge der verschiedenen Formen nur verschiedene Stadien *eines* Krankheitsprozesses zu erkennen sucht. Diese schon im Altertum wiederholt auftretende Ansicht ist nicht streng durchführbar gewesen, aber sie ist auf die Richtung der Entwicklung psychiatrischer Einteilungen von großem Einfluß geblieben."[12]

Auffallend ist, daß Heinrich Haeser dem Gedanken der Einheitspsychose keine Beachtung schenkt.[13] Man möchte meinen, daß er der Psychiatrie doch wohl etwas zu ferne gestanden hat, um Interesse an der historischen Entwicklung ihrer Probleme im Detail nehmen zu können. Er begnügt sich mit einem eleganten Überblick, der später immer wieder zitiert wurde: „Die Psychiatrie hat seit ihrer Neubegründung im 18. Jahrhundert dieselben Phasen der Entwicklung durchlaufen, wie die Pathologie überhaupt: die rein theoretische, vertreten durch den Animismus von Stahl, die beschreibende, begründet durch Pinel und Esquirol, die pathologisch-anatomische unter der Führung von Spurzheim, und die physiologische, repräsentiert durch Griesinger."[14]

Hatten wir wenig Hoffnung auf die ältere Literatur gesetzt, so vermissen wir auch in der neueren eine eingehende, auf Studium der Quellen fußende Bearbeitung des Themas. Diepgens *Geschichte der Medizin*[15] kennt das Stichwort „Einheitspsychose" nicht. Von Griesinger sagt Diepgen: „Er kam von der inneren Medizin und Neurologie her und war der physiologischen Heilkunde durch und durch ergeben, die man mit naturwissenschaftlichen Denken identifizierte. In jüngeren Jahren war er eine Zeitlang Assistent bei dem bedeutenden Psychiater Albert Zeller (1804–1877) an der Irrenanstalt Winnenthal gewesen. Er hat selbst niemals eine

---

[10] [Vgl. Kraepelin, „Hundert Jahre Psychiatrie," 197].

[11] Theodor Kirchhoff, *Deutsche Irrenärzte: Einzelbilder ihres Lebens und Wirkens*, 2 Bde. (Berlin: J. Springer, 1921/24).

[12] Ders., *Geschichte der Psychiatrie*, in *Handbuch der Psychiatrie*, hg. von Gustav Aschaffenburg (Leipzig und Vienna: Deuticke, 1912), 46.

[13] Vgl. Heinrich Haeser, *Geschichte der Medicin in der neueren Zeit*, 3. Aufl., Bd. 2 (Jena: Fischer, 1881). [Heinrich Haeser war ein Medizinhistoriker, der 1881 ein Lehrbuch veröffentlichte].

[14] Ebenda, 1028.

[15] Paul Diepgen, *Geschichte der Medizin: die historische Entwicklung der Heilkunde und des ärztlichen Lebens*, 2. Aufl., Bd. 2/1: Von der Medizin der Aufklärung bis zur Begründung der Zellularpathologie (etwa 1740 – etwa 1858) (Berlin: Walter de Gruyter, 1959).

psychiatrische Klinik geleitet, auch nicht später in Berlin. Aber die Eindrücke aus seiner Winnenthaler Zeit verbanden sich bei ihm mit seiner internistischen und neurologischen Erfahrung."[16]

In der kurzen *Geschichte der Psychiatrie* von E. H. Ackerknecht, der umfangreichsten Psychiatrie-Geschichte seit Kraepelin und Kornfeld wird auf das Lehrer- und Schülerverhältnis zwischen A. Zeller und W. Griesinger hingewiesen: „Obwohl Griesinger hier seinem Lehrer Zeller in der Annahme einer einzigen Psychose, die in zwei Stadien verläuft, folgt, gibt er doch eingehende Beschreibungen der Hypochondrie, Melancholie, Manie, Monomanie und Geistesschwäche."[17] Ackerknecht verzichtet jedoch darauf, in die Zusammenhänge tiefer einzudringen. Er berührt das Problem nur einmal mit dem Satz: „Als Reaktion auf die Zeller-Griesingersche Einheitspsychose erfolgte eine große Reihe sehr weitschweifiger Klassifikation[en] (Schüle, v. Krafft-Ebing, Meynert, Skae, Maudsley, Tuke, Blandford)."[18]

Wolfgang de Boor streift in seiner Arbeit „Psychiatrische Systematik, ihre Entwicklung in Deutschland seit Kahlbaum"[19] das vorliegende Problem nur; dabei springt die bisher ungeklärt gelassene Frage nach der Beziehung zwischen Heinrich Neumann und Zeller-Griesinger erstmals deutlich ins Auge.

Roland Kuhn faßt dann in seinem Vortrag über Griesingers Auffassung der psychiatrischen Krankheiten und seine Bedeutung für die weitere Entwicklung der Psychiatrie das bisher über Griesinger Bekannte noch einmal zusammen: „Bekanntlich hat Griesinger die vor allem von Guislain und Zeller vertretene ‚Einheitspsychose' übernommen, das heißt, die Auffassung, es gebe nur eine einzige Geisteskrankheit, und die verschiedenen Zustandsbilder, die der klinischen Beobachtung entgegentreten, seien bloß verschiedene Stadien von einem und demselben Prozeß. Dieser könne jederzeit zum Stillstand kommen, er befalle zuerst die affektiven Seiten und sei solange noch reversibel; später aber führe er über Störungen des Gedankenganges zur Verblödung. Das erste Stadium soll in den meisten Fällen ein melancholisches sein, auf das dann die Manie folgt, die nach Griesinger wieder in zwei verschiedene Formen von ‚Exaltationszuständen' zerfällt, nämlich in die ‚Tobsucht' und den ‚Wahnsinn'. Es schließen sich dann die ‚psychischen Schwächezustände' an mit der ‚partiellen Verrücktheit', der ‚Verwirrtheit oder allgemeinen Verrücktheit', dem ‚apathischen Blödsinn', und von der 2. Auflage an ist noch ein Kapitel über ‚Idiotismus und Cretinismus' hinzugefügt. Als ‚Complicationen des Irreseins' werden dann beschrieben die ‚progressive Paralyse' und die ‚Epilepsie'. Bodamer hat in seiner leider erst im Manuskript zugänglichen Untersuchung über

[16] Ebenda, 180.

[17] Erwin Heinz Ackerknecht, *Kurze Geschichte der Psychiatrie* (Stuttgart: Enke, 1957), 66.

[18] Ebenda, 70.

[19] Wolfgang de Boor, *Psychiatrische Systematik: Ihre Entwicklung in Deutschland seit Kahlbaum* (Berlin: Springer, 1954).

Griesinger gezeigt, wie diese Auffassung der Geisteskrankheit sich notwendig aus der Übernahme von Herbarts Psychologie ergab.“[20]

In diesem gedrängten Überblick über die deutsche medizingeschichtliche Literatur erübrigt es sich, auf Heinrich Damerow[21] und C. A. Wunderlich[22] einzugehen weil beide zu unserem Thema nicht Stellung nehmen. Kurz sei wenigstens der medizinhistorische Abschnitt in Jaspers' *Allgemeiner Psychopathologie*[23] gestreift. Bekanntlich teilt Jaspers die psychiatrischen Schriftsteller des letzten Jahrhunderts in die beiden Gruppen der Analytiker und Schilderer. Unter den Analytikern nennt er nur Neumann, Spielmann und Wernicke. Das Gros wird für ihn von den Schilderern gebildet, zu welchen er auch Griesinger rechnet. Allerdings hat sich diese Unterteilung nicht recht durchführen lassen, wie Bodamer schon früher am Beispiel Griesingers gezeigt hat,[24] der ja Schilderer und Analytiker zugleich war. Auch was Jaspers über den Streit der Somatiker und der Psychiker schreibt, ist nicht ganz glücklich. Er übersah dabei, daß der Standpunkt der Somatiker mindestens ebenso von ihrer weltanschaulichen Grundeinstellung abhing wie der der Psychiker. Besonders deutlich wird dies am Beispiel M. Jacobi, für den es undenkbar war, daß die unsterbliche Seele erkranken könne, und der daher aus christlicher Überzeugung heraus die Ursache des Irreseins im körperlichen Bereich suchen mußte.

Fremdsprachige Literatur zum Thema ‚Einheitspsychose‘

Nachdem sich das deutsche medizinhistorische Schrifttum für das Problem der Geschichte der Einheitspsychose im Ganzen als unergiebig erwiesen hat, ist kaum zu erwarten, daß sich eingehendere Untersuchungen dieses vorwiegend deutschen wissenschaftlichen Problems in der außerdeutschen Literatur finden. G. Zilboorgs *History of Medical Psychology*[25] ist ohne Zweifel ein verdienstvolles und umfangreiches Werk, die einzige Psychiatrie-Geschichte, die in englischer Sprache erschienen ist. Doch hat der Verfasser leider einen zu großen inneren und räumlichen Abstand

[20] Roland Kuhn, „Griesingers Auffassung der psychischen Krankheiten und seine Bedeutung für die weitere Entwicklung der Psychiatrie,“ in *Beiträge zur Geschichte der Psychiatrie und Hirnanatomie*, hg. von Alfred Glaus (Basel: Karger, 1957), 49. [Vgl. Joachim Bodamer, „Wilhelm Griesinger und die Entwicklung der Psychiatrie im 19. Jahrhundert“ (Medizinische Dissertation, Universität Heidelberg, 1944).]

[21] Heinrich Philipp August Damerow, *Die Elemente der nächsten Zukunft der Medizin, entwickelt aus der Vergangenheit und Gegenwart* (Berlin: Reimer, 1829). [Über Damerow vgl. auch Gerhart Zeller (Hg.), *Albert Zellers medizinisches Tagebuch der psychiatrischen Reise durch Deutschland, England, Frankreich und nach Prag von 1832 bis 1833*, Bd. 2 (Zwiefalten: Psychiatrie und Geschichte, 2007), 13–14].

[22] Carl August Wunderlich, *Geschichte der Medizin: Vorlesungen gehalten im Sommersemester 1858* (Stuttgart: Ebner & Seubert, 1859).

[23] Karl Jaspers, *Allgemeine Psychopathologie*, 5. Aufl. (Berlin: Springer, 1948), 703–716.

[24] Vgl. Bodamer, „Wilhelm Griesinger“.

[25] Gregory Zilboorg, *A History of Medical Psychology* (New York: Norton, 1941).

von den Problemen, die Europa im beginnenden 19. Jahrhunderts bewegten, als daß man von ihm gerade über diesen Abschnitt der Geschichte mehr als allgemeine Feststellungen erwarten dürfte, Feststellungen, die zudem oft durch ein zu scharfes Schema verfälscht werden. So sind für ihn die Somatiker Materialisten, und Psychiker Romantiker. Von Griesinger meint er, daß er den Streit zwischen den beiden Parteien geschlichtet habe. Es wird sich im Verlauf der vorliegenden Arbeit zeigen, daß diese Meinungen gänzlich unhaltbar sind.

Aus dem französischen Schrifttum nennen wir nur Laignel-Lavastine M., Vinchon J., *Les Malades de l'Esprit et leurs Médecins du XVIe au XIXe siècle.*[26] Das Werk enthält jedoch nichts, was für unser Thema Bedeutung hätte.

Überblickt man die historischen Einsichten und Hinweise der bisher vorliegenden Literatur, so ergibt sich, daß am häufigsten die Lehre von der Einheitspsychose in Zusammenhang mit dem Winnenthaler Psychiater Albert Zeller, dem Lehrer Griesingers, gebracht wird. Es ist vielfach üblich, von der Zeller-Griesingerschen Einheitspsychose zu sprechen. Griesinger selbst sagt im Anschluß an das oben angeführte Zitat „Mittelst dieser – von Zeller am deutlichsten ausgesprochenen – Erkenntnis ist es uns denn möglich, von dem Wege der Symptomatologie her auch den immer in den Vordergrund zu stellenden, Aufgaben der anatomisch-pathologischen Auffassung und Diagnostik der Geisteskrankheiten näher als bisher zu rücken."[27] Er hat auch in den folgenden Auflagen seines Lehrbuchs diesen Absatz nicht geändert und damit seinem Lehrer ein bleibende Denkmal gesetzt. Die erste Auflage seines Lehrbuchs ist Zeller gewidmet: „Übrigens habe ich in der allmählichen Vollendung dieser Schrift, ungeachtet ich viele Mängel an ihr wohl erkenne, den reichhaltigsten Genuß gefunden; ihre Abfassung hat mir umso mehr Vergnügen gemacht, je mehr sie mich an meine frühere Wirksamkeit als ausübender Irrenarzt in einer der besten deutschen Anstalten erinnerte, wo meine ersten praktischen Studien in der Psychiatrie den Vorteil hatten, von einem hochverehrten Freunde, Herrn Hofrat Dr. Zeller in Winnenthal, geleitet zu werden. Möge auch ihm diese Schrift Anlaß zu freundlicher Erinnerung werden."[28]

Gänzlich unbearbeitet blieb jedoch bis heute die Frage nach den Vorgängern Albert Zellers. Am häufigsten wird [Joseph] Guislain genannt und behauptet, Zeller sei Guislain gefolgt oder gar, er habe seine Theorien übernommen. Kirchhoff stellt dann Beziehungen zu Reil her, Gruhle zu Knight, Kuhn, Bodamer folgend, zu Herbart. Bewiesen und begründet wird keine dieser Vermutungen. Gänzlich unklar blieb auch bisher das Verhältnis der Zeller'schen Einheitspsychose zu der Neumanns und welche von beiden dann auf Arndt und Kahlbaum gewirkt hat.

Die Fülle ungeklärter Fragen verlangt nächst Rechenschaft über die Methoden, die zu ihrer Lösung heranführen. Zwei Wege stehen zur Verfügung: der ideengeschichtliche

[26] M. Laignel und Jean Vinchon, *Les malades de l'esprit et leur médecins du 16e au 19e siècle* (Paris: Maloine, 1930).

[27] Griesinger, *Die Pathologie und Therapie*, 151.

[28] Ebenda, vi.

und der biografische. Der erste müßte dem Problem in all seinen Varianten an Hand der vorliegenden Literatur nachgehen. Die Quellen wären daraufhin zu untersuchen, ob sie eine gemeinsame geistesgeschichtliche Wurzel haben oder ursächlich durch Tradition miteinander verbunden sind. Auf diesem Wege kann jedoch eine klare und beweisbare Beantwortung der schwebenden Fragen nicht gefunden und vor allem die Frage der Beziehung zwischen Guislain und Zeller nicht beantwortet werden. Der andere Weg scheint gangbarer. Dem Bemühen, die wissenschaftliche Biografie der Schlüsselfigur Albert Zeller so detailliert zu erforschen, daß seine Konzeption der Einheitspsychose deutlich wird, stellen sich allerdings fast unüberwindliche Hindernisse entgegen. Die größte Schwierigkeit liegt darin, daß Albert Zeller nur wenig veröffentlicht hat.[29]

Handschriftliche Quellen

Deswegen muß die gegenwärtige Arbeit auch auf den handschriftlichen Nachlaß zurückgreifen, wenn der Versuch einer Analyse der Albert Zellerschen Auffassung Aussicht auf Erfolg haben soll. Nun hat es allerdings mit diesem handschriftlichen Nachlaß eine besondere Bewandnis. Er war bisher so gut wie unleserlich. Alle Versuche, ihn zu entziffern, scheiterten und es konnten bisher immer nur Bruchstücke ausgewertet werden.

An handschriftliche Quellen sind zuerst die Tagebücher zu nennen. Das wichtigste davon ist ein umfangreiches Heft von 344 Seiten, überschrieben „Medizinisches Tagebuch der psychiatrischen Reise durch Deutschland, England, Frankreich vom Februar 1832 bis Mai 1833".[30] Dieses Tagebuch, welches Robert Gaupp wiederholt durch Doktoranden entziffern lassen wollte, trotzte bisher allen derartigen Versuchen, nicht nur der Schrift wegen, sondern auch deshalb, weil es in Frankreich französisch, in England englisch und zwischendurch lateinisch abgefaßt ist. Es ist nun erstmals gelungen, die Manuskripte zu übersetzen und in Maschinenschrift zu übertragen. Ein zweites Tagebuch ist wesentlich geringer an Umfang.[31] Es lag bereits maschinenschriftlich vor und wurde daher auch von R. Gaupp als Unterlage für seine biografischen Arbeiten benutzt.[32] Es ist in der Studienzeit Albert Zellers entstanden. Ein drittes Tagebuch gibt die Eindrücke eines Studienaufenthaltes in Berlin im Jahre 1827 wieder, auch dieses lag bisher nur handschriftlich vor.[33]

---

[29] [Auslassung (ca. 575 Worte): Annotierte Bibliografie von Albert Zellers Veröffentlichungen. Siehe die mit Sternchen (*) gekennzeichneten Titel in der Bibliografie].

[30] [Kurz nach Gerhart Zellers Tod 2006 ist dieses Tagebuch in zwei Bänden mit Kommentar herausgeben worden. Vgl. Gerhart Zeller (Hg.), *Albert Zellers medizinisches Tagebuch*].

[31] Albert Zeller, Studientagebücher, 1824–1827, Albert Zeller Papers, Berlin.

[32] [Robert Gaupp, „Ein zyklothymer Psychiater über seine seelischen Krankheitszeiten," *Zeitschrift für die gesamte Neurologie und Psychiatrie* 166 (1939): 705–710; ders., „Albert Zeller," *Schwäbische Lebensbilder* 1 (1940): 574–582].

[33] Albert Zeller, Studientagebücher.

An Briefen ist leider so gut wie nichts von Wert mehr erhalten. Im letzten Kriege wurde der gesamte Zeller-Jacobi'schen Briefwechsel vernichtet.[34] Er bestand aus 162 Briefen von Jacobi und 151 von Zeller. Er begann mit dem Jahre 1832 und endete mit einem Brief Jacobis, den er am 8. Mai 1858, 10 Tage vor seinem Tode, schrieb. Dieser Briefwechsel wurde leider nie vollständig ausgewertet, obwohl er einmal für längere Zeit der Forschungsanstalt für Psychiatrie in München ausgeliehen war.[35] In seinem Buch über *Carl Wigand Maximilian Jacobi, ein deutscher Arzt* hat Johannes Herting Teile des Briefwechsels benutzt und auch Hermann Zeller zitiert in seiner Biografie wenigstens Bruchstücke daraus.[36] Außerdem ist ein kleiner handschriftlicher Versuch, der unvollendet blieb, aus dem Sommersemester 1824 „Über den Consens der inneren Organe und Systeme" erhalten geblieben.[37]

Wieweit es uns gelingen wird, auf Grund dieses bisher unerschlossenen Quellenmaterials neue Erkenntnisse über die Geschichte der Einheitspsychose zu fördern, werden die folgenden Abschnitte zeigen.

TEIL 3.2

Albert Zellers Abstammung, Familie, Kultur und geistesgeschichtlicher Hintergrund

Will man sich über die geistige Entwicklung eines Menschen Klarheit schaffen, dann wird man gut daran tun, zunächst einmal die Frage „wo kommt er her?" zu stellen, eine Frage, welche zwei bedeutsame Teilaspekte hat, nämlich die Ascendenz und die Kulturlandschaft mit ihren stammesmäßigen Besonderheiten. Danach wird man sorgfältig prüfen: wo und von wem hat er gelernt? und zuletzt: wie hat er sich auf Grund der gegebenen Voraussetzungen selbstständig entwickelt? Gehen wir so an die Persönlichkeit Albert Zellers heran, dann fällt es uns zunächst nicht schwer, eine klare Antwort auf die erste Frage zu bekommen.[38]

Die Familie Zeller läßt sich bis zum Jahre 1521 zurück verfolgen. Der Urgroßvater war Prälat, der Großvater Arzt und Physikus in Laufen am Neckar. Sein Vater (1769–1846) Johann Friedrich heiratete Johanna Regine Andreae, deren Vater Jakob

[34] [Lediglich Abschriften von Jacobis Briefe an Zeller sind erhalten geblieben. Vgl. Archiv des Landschaftsverband Rheinland (Pulheim-Brauweiler), Nr. 31557 und 31656].

[35] [Gemeint ist das heutige Max-Planck-Institute für Psychiatrie].

[36] Johannes Herting, *Carl Wigand Maximilian Jacobi: Ein deutsche Arzt (1775–1858)* (Görlitz: C. A. Starke, 1930); Hermann Zeller, „Ernst Albert Zeller," in *Deutsche Irrenärzte*, hg. von Theodor Kirchhoff (Berlin: J. Springer, 1921), 208–218.

[37] Albert Zeller, „Versuch über den Consens der inneren Organe und Systeme, 1824," Albert Zeller Papers, Berlin.

[38] [Im überarbeiteten Preisschrift hat Gerhart Zeller die Behandlung der Familiengeschichte radikal gekürzt. Zur Geschichte der Familie Zeller, vgl. auch Gerhart Zeller (Hg.), *Albert Zellers medizinisches Tagebuch*, Bd. 1, 10–14].

Eberhard Hofmedikus in Stuttgart war. Dem Vater Albert Zellers, dem späteren Oberjustizrat Johann Friedrich v. Zeller, war eine wichtige Aufgabe im Rahmen der Eingliederung der Neuerwerbungen in dem württembergischen Staatsverband zugefallen, und zwar dadurch, daß er zum ersten württembergischen Oberamtmann der ehemaligen freien Reichsstadt Heilbronn und zum Nekarschiffahrtskommissär ernannt wurde. Er war eine damals bekannte Persönlichkeit, ein weltgewandter, realistischer Politiker von aufrechter und energischer Art. Wir haben sein Bild, gemalt von Johann Baptist Seele (1774–1814), der ab 1789 der Hohen Carlsschule angehörte und dem wir auch sonst charakteristische Porträts und lebendige Genrebilder verdanken.

Von Zellers Mutter, einer tiefempfindenden Frau, ist ein Brief erhalten, in welchem sie dem erwachsenen Sohne Albert auf seine Bitte mitteilt: „Wie ich meine Kinder erzog."[39] Es ist ein wohlbekannter Ton, der uns aus diesem Brief entgegenklingt: das Lebensgefühl der deutschen Empfindsamkeit, die sich aus dem Pietismus heraus und in ständiger Wechselbeziehung mit ihm entwickelte. Hier ist der Grund und Boden der geistigen Persönlichkeit Albert Zeller und vielleicht auch der modernen Psychiatrie und Psychologie.[40] Es sind dies beinahe vergessene historische Zusammenhänge. Haeser wußte noch von diesen und erwähnt sie kurz bei seiner Besprechung von August Hermann Francke (1663–1772), dem Prediger und Professor der Theologie und dem Gründer eines Waisenhauses sowie der damit verbundenen Anstalten in Halle. Auch Max Dessoir – dem wir hier vorwiegend folgen – hat in seiner „Geschichte der neueren deutschen Psychologie"[41] immer wieder auf die Bedeutung des Pietismus hingewiesen. In der neueren Literatur zum Thema erscheint kaum mehr das Stichwort. Dies hat seinen Grund in erster Linie darin, daß der Pietismus, wie er uns heute noch in Württemberg entgegentritt, aus Enge, Ressentiment und moralisierendem Konventiklertum zu bestehen scheint. Man muß den Pietismus aber als Teil jener gewaltigen geistesgeschichtlichen Bewegung sehen, der von der deutschen Mystik des Mittelalters bis zur deutschen Romantik reicht, um seine Bedeutung richtig würdigen zu können. Zunächst noch durch die starke Betonung von Verstand und Wille gegenüber Wahrnehmung, Gefühl und Fantasie unabsichtlich der Aufklärung verbunden – wie man gerade bei Philipp Jakob Spener (1635–1705), dem Vater des Pietismus, sehen kann, der trotz dieses aufklärerischen Wesens selbst noch „Däumeln", das Aufschlagen der Bibel, zum Zwecke persönlicher Belehrung übte – wurde der Pietismus immer mehr Reaktion auf die starre Äußerlichkeit und Engherzigkeit der herrschenden Theologie und

---

[39] [Der Brief ist im 2. Weltkrieg verschollen. Im Originalmanuskript werden daraus länger Zitate aus Abschriften angeführt. Doch bei der Überarbeitung hat Gerhart Zeller diese Zitate gestrichen. Vgl. aber Gerhart Zeller (Hg.), *Albert Zellers medizinisches Tagebuch*, Bd. 1, 14].

[40] [Auch später unterstrich Gerhart Zeller den entscheidenden Einfluß des Pietismus auf die Entwicklung der Psychiatrie in Deutschland. Vgl. Gerhart Zeller, „Bonhoeffers wissenschaftliches Werk. Entwicklung und Bedeutung," in *Karl Bonhoeffer: Zum hundertsten Geburtstag am 31. März 1968*, hg. von Jürg Zutt, Erwin Straus und H. Scheller (Berlin: Springer, 1969), 119–121].

[41] Max Dessoir, *Geschichte der neueren deutschen Psychologie*, Bd. 1, 2. Aufl. (Berlin: Duncker, 1902).

einer Philosophie, welche die Bedeutung der Fantasie und das Geheimnisvolle im Glauben mißachtet hatte. Der hallische Pietismus besann sich wieder auf den sittlichen Gehalt des Christentums, auf die innere Offenbarung im Gewissen. So entstand die Lehre, jeder in Christo Wiedergeborene solle sich unaufhörlich mit Gott und seiner eigenen Unwürdigkeit beschäftigen und alles gegen die innere Selbstversenkung gering achten. Hieraus entwickelte sich schließlich eine Bewegung, welche den Wissenschaften, der Kirche, ja selbst dem Unterschied der Religionen gleichgültig gegenüber stand und nur im Genuß des inneren Lichtes Heilsgewißheit und Befriedigung finden konnte. Dieser Vorgang im religiösen Bewußtsein des Volkes wirkte sich auf das Seelenverständnis in drei Beziehungen aus.[42]

Die erste Folge war die Betonung der inneren Erfahrung und Bevorzugung der subjektivistischen seelischen Tatsachen. Es entwickelte sich ein intimer Sinn für das innere Leben. Tersteegen (1697–1769) schrieb 1748 an eine Freundin: „Alles, was in mir ist, neigt sich zur Abgeschiedenheit, Stille, Bildlosigkeit und Einigkeit zu und mit Gott."[43] „O das heißt Leben, so leben zu können."[44]

Die andere Wirkung bestand in dem wiedergewonnenen Verständnis für das Unwillkürliche im Menschen. So mahnt Bengel: „Der Einfluß der göttlichen Kraft durch die einfachsten Wahrheiten, welche ohne eigenes Bemühen in das Herz eingelassen werden, breitet sich hernach selbst mannigfaltig aus. Dabei suche man nicht diese und jene sinnliche Erfahrung in sich zu erzwingen, sondern halte nur in wahrer Treue aus."[45]

Als dritte Folge ist das Interesse für psychologische Lebensbeschreibungen frommer Menschen, gleichviel welchen Standes, aufzufassen.

Zur selben Zeit, als der hallische Pietismus erstarrte, regte er sich in Württemberg, welches im 18. Jahrhundert eine etwas abseitige Rolle im deutschen Geistesleben innegehabt hatte. Dadurch, daß dem Adel im Lande außerhalb des Hofes keine Bedeutung zukam, blieb im gesellschaftlichen Leben die aus Geistlichkeit und Beamten zusammengesetzte Ehrbarkeit tonangebend. Es entstand der „Pfarrer- und Schreiberstaat", wie ihn Schelling einmal voll Verachtung nennt. Diese Struktur hatte deshalb so große Festigkeit, weil durch ein weitreichendes System der Begabten-Förderung fast die ganze Intelligenz des Landes in den Pfarrerstand hineingeleitet wurde. Herzog Christoph, der Sohn des umstrittenen Reformationsherzogs Ulrich, bereicherte sich nicht so wie andere am Kirchengut, sondern unterstellte es einer eigenen Rentkammer, aus welcher die Pfarrer besoldet und die ehemaligen Klosterschulen sowie das Tübinger Stift unterhalten wurden. Die Ausbildung auf diesen Seminarien war kostenlos für alle begabten Kinder, welche das Landexamen bestanden hatten. Der Ausbildungsgang wurde im Tübinger Stift mit dem Studium der Theologie fortgesetzt.

---

[42] Dessoir.

[43] [Die Originalquelle dieses Zitats ließ sich nicht ermitteln].

[44] [Die Originalquelle dieses Zitats ließ sich nicht ermitteln].

[45] [Die Originalquelle dieses Zitats ließ sich nicht ermitteln].

Die auf diesem Wege sich ständig erneuernden bürgerliche Ehrbarkeit Württembergs war der Aufklärung ebenso abhold wie der höfischen Bildung. Sie öffnete sich dafür breit der Aufnahme des Pietismus. Die Bewegung wurde in Württemberg so mächtig, daß es sogar notwendig wurde, sie durch Gesetz und Verordnung zu regeln. Dies geschah in dem sogenannten Generalreskript vom Jahre 1773. Das Gemeinschaftswesen konnte sich so in Württemberg auf dem Boden und im Schoße der Evangelischen Landeskirche entwickeln.

Durch Christoph Friedrich Ötinger (1702–1782) und Albrecht Bengel (1687–1752) kam neues Leben in die Bewegung. Ötinger knüpfte an Jakob Böhme an, er wirkte hauptsächlich auch auf Schelling. In ihm verband sich die pietistische Seelenauffassung mit schwäbischem Wirklichkeitssinn. Sein Zug zur Natur und zum Leben läßt ihn in eine Linie treten mit dem Künstlergeschlecht des Sturm und Dranges. Die Stimmung des Pietismus wandelte sich zum Originalismus, der Gläubige wurde zum Seher, die Religion zur göttlichen Kunst. Aus der im Gegensatz zur „Politik“ stehenden Abwendung vom Leben wurde ein gleichfalls der „Galanterie“ feindlicher Trieb nach Leben.

Kommen wir auf Zeller zurück, so wissen wir von ihm, daß er vom Vater, mit seinen Brüdern zusammen, zunächst einem Pfarrer in Horkheim bei Heilbronn zur Ausbildung übergeben wurde. Nach der Zurückberufung seines Vaters nach Stuttgart besuchte er dann dort das Gymnasium. Er legte das Abitur ab und ging anschließend an die Landes-Universität Tübingen, um einem schon lange feststehenden Wunsche entsprechend Medizin zu studieren.

Wir haben aus dieser Zeit, vorwiegend aus dem Jahre 1824, von ihm ein in Abschrift 54 Schreibmaschinenseiten umfassendes Tagebuch und den 19 Seiten langen „Versuch über den Consens der verschiedenen Organe und Systeme“ aus dem Sommersemester 1824. Beide Quellen sind von besonderer Wichtigkeit. Das schon seit langem bekannte und häufig zitierte Tagebuch gibt uns Einblick in die innere Entwicklung seines Wesens und seiner Denkart. Der „Versuch über den Consens der Organe“ zeigt, aus welcher wissenschaftlichen Schule Zeller seine Anschauungen bezog. Beginnen wir mit dem Tagebuch:

Steige nur hinab in dich!
Kräfte, welche lange schliefen,
hält dein unergründlich Ich
tief in seinen innren Tiefen.[46]

Diese Verse hat Zeller 1825 in sein Tagebuch eingetragen. Sie könnten als Motto über demselben stehen. Der 20 Jahre alte Student tritt uns in diesen und überhaupt in dem ganzen Tagebuch entgegen als „subjektivistischer Analytiker“,[47] welche eine nach Selbstkenntnis strebende, auf das eigene Ich beschränkte Zergliederung des inneren Befundes erstreben und nicht allgemeingültige wissenschaftliche Erkenntnis. Man wende nicht ein, diese Neigung zur Selbstbeobachtung sei bei ihm noch altersspezifisch und ein Symptom der Reifezeit, denn wir haben genug Zeugnisse

[46] Albert Zeller, Studientagebücher.

[47] Dessoir, 301–302.

dafür, daß er zeitlebens dieser Denkrichtung verbunden blieb. Mit 72 Jahren, 1 Jahr vor seinem Tod, erwarb er noch das Musterstück dieser Art von psychologischer Literatur, das zu diesem Zeitpunkt völlig vergessen und hoffnungslos unpopulär geworden war, nämlich Adam Bernds „eigene Lebensbeschreibung".[48] Mit welchem Eifer Zeller noch in seinem Alter dieses klassische Denkmal seelischer Selbstzergliederung des ersten dekadenten Psychologen, wie Dessoir mit Grund Adam Bernd nennt, las, zeigen die dicken roten Striche, mit welchen er das, was ihm wichtig erschien, bei der Lektüre hervorhob. Den dicksten Strich trägt der Abschnitt: „Diese Bestie, der Jach-Zorn, hat in mir zu wüten auch nicht eher aufgehört, bis Gott endlich einen Affect mit dem andern vertrieben, und durch schreckliche Furcht und Melancholie dem Zorn ein Ende gemacht, oder denselben doch sehr geschwächt; und bis ich die Wurzel der unmäßigen Affecten im Leibe gefunden, und durch Medikamente dem feurigen und hitzigen Geblüte des Leibes widerstanden habe."[49] Wir werden erst später sehen, wie sehr sich Albert Zeller in diesen Worten bestätigt finden mußte.

Der subjektivistisch-analysierende Student teilt über sein eigenes Wesen mit: „Es ist curios, daß ich fast in allem zurück war, im Anfang gegen meine Mitschüler vom ABC an bis zur Logic im Schachspielen, im Rechnen bis zum heutigen Tag, im Zeichnen und Sprachen, in allem, was die reine Verstandestätigkeit erfordert besonders, und doch war ich nicht dumm und übertraf die anderen dann in Kurzem, wenigstens in Manchem. Es geht mir heute noch nach und noch weiß ich nicht, was für ein Fehler in meinem Erkenntnisvermögen liegt. Aber das Schöne und Gute erfaßte ich leichter, nur keine Verstandesformen und -formeln."[50] Wer würde bei diesen Zeilen nicht an Goethes „Trennen und Zählen lag nicht in meiner Natur"[51] erinnern, oder an Bengels Kritik an der Mathematik: „Die Mathematik gibt in gewissen Stücken eine gute Beihilfe, aber in solchen Wahrheiten, die ihrem Forum fremd sind, verliert man durch sie die Auffassungskraft. Indem man lauter bestimmte Vorstellungen haben will, verliert man die lebendigen."[52] Wir sehen, daß die Verstandesart Albert Zellers geeigneter war, ein Ganzes lebendig zu erfassen als Details zu analysieren. Es lag in ihm eine starke Bereitschaft, an dem Ganzheits- und Einheitsstreben seiner Epoche, nämlich der Romantik, teilzunehmen, welche Leibbrand mit viel Berechtigung geradezu „einheitssüchtig" nennt.[53] Er brachte

---

[48] Adam Bernd, *Eigene Lebens-Beschreibung Samt einer aufrichtigen Entdeckung, und deutlichen Beschreibung einer der grösten, obwohl großen Theils noch unbekannten Leibes- und Gemüths-Plagen, Welche Gott zuweilen über die Welt-Kinder, und auch wohl über seine eigene Kinder verhänget: Den Unwissenden zum Unterricht, Den Gelehrten zu weiterem Nachdencken, Den Sündern zum Schrecken, und Den Betrübten, und Angefochtenen zum Troste* (Leipzig: Johann Samuel Heinsius, 1738).

[49] Ebenda, 103.

[50] Albert Zeller, Studientagebücher.

[51] Johann Wolfgang Goethe, „Der Verfasser teilt die Geschichte seiner botanischen Studien mit," in *Sämtliche Werke* (Leipzig: Insel, 1917 [1817]), 259.

[52] [Die Originalquelle dieses Zitats ließ sich nicht ermitteln].

[53] [Die Originalquelle dieses Zitats ließ sich nicht ermitteln].

aber auch viel Talent zur romantischen Vertiefung mit, eine Vertiefung, die bei ihm einer „anima naturaliter christiana“,[54] wie ihn Bodamer nennt, religiöse Bahnen suchen mußte. Im Tagebuch schreibt er: „Wenn ich Gott nicht fände in der Natur, sie läge reizlos für mich.“[55] Zeller erlebte in echt mystischer Weise die Geheimnisse der Seele mit Gott, und es nimmt so nicht wunder, daß seine ganze Liebe dem Evangelisten Johannes gehört. Er sieht aber auch die Entgleisungslinie, welche sich hier für ihn als Arzt auftut, deutlich, und so trägt er als Mahnung in sein Tagebuch ein: „Vor dem Mystizismus habe ich mich sehr zu hüten.“[56] Wie sich bei ihm romantisches Einheitsstreben mit christlicher Denkweise verbindet, zeigt das Tagebuch fast in allen Stücken, zum Beispiel in dem Satz: „Einheit fehlt dem Menschen, solange er kein Christ ist, er mag ringen und streben, solange er will.“[57]

Über welche gefühlsmäßige Feinheit der Einfühlung Zeller verfügte – wohl die stärkste Wurzel seiner seelenärztlichen Wirksamkeit -, zeigt sich in folgender Selbstbetrachtung: „Es ist mir schon oft begegnet, daß ich Gedanken anderer erriet, wenn gar kein Grund da war, daß ich darauf fallen konnte. So fand ich schon die sonderbarsten Wörter, die ein anderer suchte, ohne daß ich nur wußte, welcher Art sie waren, besonders bei Personen, die ich leiden mochte. So geht es mir auch, wenn jemand ein Gedicht verliert, und ich kann oft ganze folgende Sachen sagen, die noch nicht ausgesprochen wurden. Es kommt mir auch natürlich vor. Ich setze mich in das Gefühl und die Stimmung und die ganze Situation des Dichters und dann kann die weitere Entwicklung in mir ebenso vor sich gehen, wie sie im Dichter ihren Verlauf nahm.“[58] Bei diesem ständigen Streben nach Erkenntnis seiner selbst mußte er dann auch auf seine depressive Anlage stoßen, auf welche Robert Gaupp [aufmerksam machte].[59] Albert Zeller schreibt selbst über sich: „In den Augenblicken der höchsten Lust schwebt mir das Bild des Todes vor. Ich verlor als Knabe kurz nacheinander einen Bruder und zwei Gespielen, die ich zärtlich liebte. Der Gedanke an den Tod kam mir daher in meinen Kindheitsspielen schon sehr oft, besonders, weil der eine plötzlich erkrankte mitten unter uns und in drei Tagen schon begraben wurde. Ich sah sie im Sarge, ich kann sie immer noch sehen, die holden bleichen Knaben, und mein eigener früher Tod schien mir ganz gewiß. So wurde der Grund zur Melancholie schon in die erste Zeit meines Lebens gelegt und wuchs mit mir zum Jüngling mit der gesenkten Fackel. Ich muß und will sie frisch abschütteln und die Fackel, ehe die Flamme erlöscht, emporschwingen, damit das Senken nur dazu gedient, sie heller anzufachen.“[60]

---

[54] [Joachim Bodamer, „Zur Entstehung der Psychiatrie als Wissenschaft im 19. Jahrhundert,“ *Fortschritte der Neurologie, Psychiatrie und ihrer Grenzgebiete* 21 (1953): 523].

[55] Albert Zeller, Studientagebücher.

[56] Ebenda.

[57] Ebenda.

[58] Ebenda. [Für Albert Zeller soll die Einfühlung bzw. die Sympathie „das Hauptthema seines Lebens“ gewesen sein. Vgl. Gerhart Zeller (Hg.), *Albert Zellers medizinisches Tagebuch*, Bd. 2, 38].

[59] Gaupp, „Ein Zyklothymer Psychiater“ und ders., „Albert Zeller“.

[60] Albert Zeller, Studientagebücher.

Es will uns scheinen, daß Albert Zellers Temperament zu echten ernsten depressiven Schwankungen neigte, und wir können diese Tatsache für die spätere Entwicklung seiner psychiatrischen Systematik nicht hoch genug anschlagen. Mußte sich ihm nicht die Frage nach der Grenze zwischen krankhafter und noch nicht krankhafter Melancholie schärfer stellen als seinen Zeitgenossen? Auf der anderen Seite mußte er aus der Beobachtung an sich selbst das Gefühl ständiger unverschuldeter psychischer Gefährdung ableiten. Hieraus ergab sich eine scharfe Ablehnung jeder überspitzten moralischen Betrachtung der Geisteskrankheiten. Dadurch wurde der Weg frei zu echter menschlicher Begegnung mit den Kranken. Wir brauchen nur noch auf die zeitliche Nähe zwischen Albert Zeller und Kierkegaard hinzuweisen. Kierkegaard sagt in „Der Begriff der Angst" 1844: „Der Arzt in einer Irrenanstalt, der dumm genug ist zu glauben, er sei für alle Ewigkeit klug und seine Portion von Verstand sei dagegen versichert, je im Leben Schaden zu nehmen, ist in gewissem Sinne wohl klüger als die Wahnsinnigen, ist aber zugleich dümmer als sie und wird auch nicht viele heilen."[61] Vor einer solchen „Dummheit" war Albert Zeller durch seine Selbsterfahrung zeitlebens geschützt.

Vermittelt das Tagebuch einen Einblick in das innere Wesen des jungen Mannes so führt der handschriftliche unvollendete Versuch aus dem Sommersemester 1824 „Über den Consens der verschiedenen Organe und Systeme"[62] mitten hinein in das Studium an der Tübinger Universität und direkt hin zur beherrschenden Figur des damaligen Tübingen, zu Johann Heinrich Ferdinand v. Autenrieth (1772–1835), da dieser Versuch nichts anderes darstellt als ein Excerpt aus Autenrieths *Handbuch der empirischen menschlichen Physiologie*.[63]

[J. H. F. Autenrieth,] die Universität Tübingen und die Hohe Carlsschule

Hier verweilen wir bei einer kurzen Schilderung der Universität Tübingen zu dieser Zeit sowie der Persönlichkeit und der Lehre Autenrieths.[64] Autenrieth war Schüler der Hohen Carlsschule in Stuttgart ebenso wie Schiller. Er hatte dieselben Lehrer wie er. Seine Studienzeit fällt in die Blütezeit der 1770 gegründeten und bereits 1794 aufgehobenen Carlsschule, welcher 1775 eine medizinische Abteilung angegliedert worden war. Autenrieth gehörte der Carlsschule als Oppidaner, das heißt als

[61] Søren Kierkegaard, *Der Begriff Angst* (Leipzig: Fr. Richter, 1844), 50.

[62] Albert Zeller, „Versuch".

[63] Johann Heinrich Ferdinand v. Autenrieth, *Handbuch der empirischen menschlichen Physiologie*, 3 Bde. (Tübingen: Heerbrandt, 1801–02).

[64] Vgl. Gustav Schleich, *Ein Stück aus der Geschichte der medizinischen Fakultät der Universität Tübingen* (Tübingen: Schnürlen, 1910); Eberhard Stübler, *Johann Heinrich Ferdinand v. Autenrieth (1772–1835)* (Stuttgart: Schröder, 1948). [Zu Autenrieth, vgl. auch Gerhart Zeller (Hg.), *Albert Zellers medizinisches Tagebuch*, Bd. 1, 14–18 und Bd. 2, 14–17. Dort wird Autenrieth als „Vitalist und Zeller als Animist" beschrieben. Ebenda, Bd. 1, 15].

Stadtschüler an, er war nie, wie Schiller, im Internat. Am 9. Oktober 1785 trat Autenrieth in die Carlsschule ein, um auf die Dauer von sieben Jahren an deren Unterricht teilzunehmen. Während Schiller dort einem Dichterkreis um sich sammelte, so gehörte Autenrieth einem naturwissenschaftlichen Verein an. Das Haupt bzw. der Gründer dieses naturwissenschaftlichen Vereins war Georges Cuvier (1769–1832), mit welchem Autenrieth auch später noch in Verbindung blieb. Der medizinische Unterricht in Stuttgart unterschied sich von dem damals allgemein üblichen durch die pädagogisch wichtige Eigenart, daß im Unterrichtsbetrieb ausgiebig ältere Schüler als Lehrer verwendet wurden und daß alle Schüler, auch die Mediziner, bis zu ihrem Ausscheiden philosophische Kurse besuchen und Prüfungen in Philosophie ablegen mußten. Noch immer stand trotz des Vorbilds, welches der große Herman Boerhaave (1668–1738) in Leyden durch Begründung eines klinischen Unterrichts gegeben hatte, die Theorie für die Studierenden im Vordergrund, allerdings auch in Stuttgart nicht mehr ausschließlich und vielleicht besser als in Tübingen; geht doch aus dem Vorlesungsverzeichnis hervor, daß Stadtchirurgus Rossnagel in den Stuttgarter Krankenhäusern und Geburtszimmern Entbindungskunst lehrte und daß die Professoren Reuss und Plieninger praktische pathologische Unterweisungen in den öffentlichen Krankenhäusern abhielten.

Christian Klein gab Unterricht in Anatomie. Als Hilfe war ihm Johann Heinrich Morstatt seit 1786 beigegeben. Die Vorlesungen über die Gebiete der inneren Medizin teilten sich Johann Friedrich Consbruch, der Lehrer Schillers und Theodor Plieninger (1756–1840) seit 1785. Die Medizingeschichte kennt kaum mehr die Namen dieser Männer. Nur Christian Friedrich Jäger, der vor seiner 1784 erfolgten Berufung nach Stuttgart Professor der Medizin in Tübingen gewesen war, machte eine gewisse Ausnahme dadurch, daß er für gerichtliche Medizin interessiert und auf diesem Gebiet literarisch tätig war.

Es ist nicht leicht, sich ein Bild davon zu machen, was der Student J. H. F. Autenrieth von seinen Lehrern gelernt hat. Dies ist erst annähernd durch ein Druckschriftenverzeichnis der Carlsschule möglich.[65] Johann Friedrich Consbruch, geboren 1736 in Stuttgart, gestorben 1810 ebenda, war der wirkungsvollste medizinische Lehrer der Akademie. Wenn die von Ernst Müller angekündigte Übersetzung der lateinisch abgefaßten Dissertationen vorliegen wird, läßt sich die Frage leichter klären, welche der später von Autenrieth vorgetragenen medizinischen Theorien schon bei seinen Lehrern vorgebildet sind. Im gegenwärtigen Augenblick muß man sich auf die Titel der Arbeiten und den Inhalt der publizierten medizinischen Schriften Schillers beschränken.[66]

Folgende von der medizinischen Fakultät der Carlsschule verfaßten Arbeiten scheinen wichtig zu sein: Johann Friedrich Consbruch „Tentamen circa doctrinam de crisi et metastasi“ (1781, 28 Seiten) und G. Kerner: „Animadversiones quaedam

---

[65] Vgl. Ernst Müller, „Forschung, Erziehung und Lehre untersucht nach den Druckschriften der Carlsschule,“ in *Die Hohe Carlsschule [Ausstellungskatalog]* (Stuttgart: Turmhaus, 1960), 48–55.

[66] [Gemeint ist Friedrich Schiller, *Medizinische Schriften: eine Buchgabe der Deutschen Hoffmann-LaRoche AG aus Anlaß des 200. Geburtstages des Dichters, 10. November 1959* (Berlin: Fischer, 1959)].

circa metastases“ (1791, 28 Seiten). Beide Arbeiten zeigen, daß die später für Autenrieth so wichtige Metastasenlehre, die auch noch auf Autenrieths Schüler Zeller wirkte, schon von Consbruch erörtert wurde.

Aus Schillers Arbeiten[67] geht deutlich hervor, daß Thomas Sydenham (1624–1689) und Boerhaave die großen Autoritäten der Schule waren. Schiller bezieht sich in seiner Arbeit über die Fieber besonders auf Sydenhams Krisenlehre; im übrigen ist man für Friedrich Hoffmann (1660–1721) und gegen Georg Ernst Stahls (1659–1734) Animismus, den man in den Bereich der Spekulation glaubt verbannen zu können. Hoffmanns Lehre vom Nervenäther wird von Schiller in seiner Arbeit über den Zusammenhang der tierischen Natur des Menschen und seiner geistigen klar und überzeugend formuliert.

Wir legen auf die Feststellung der Bedeutung Sydenhams über den Unterricht auf der Carlsschule großen Wert. Zieht sich doch durch Sydenhams Werk als Grundton der Gedanke einer tiefen inneren Verwandtschaft der Krankheiten. Dies wird auch in seiner Lehre von den Infektionskrankheiten deutlich. Der Genus epidemicus ist wandelbar, nicht alle Erkrankungen in einer Epidemie haben trotz ihrer Zusammengehörigkeit dieselben Symptome. Wenn eine Epidemie herrschte, zum Beispiel die Pocken, so pflegte Sydenham alle gleichzeitig vorkommenden fieberhaften Erkrankungen ebenfalls als Pocken zu diagnostizieren. Bei Sydenham findet sich aber auch schon der Gedanke, daß eine Krankheit, zum Beispiel ein Fieber als Nachkrankheit, Symptome eines ganz anderen Organsystems hervorrufen könne. Heinrich Laehr zitiert in seinen Gedenktagen der Psychiatrie einen Fall, den Sydenham in seinem Werk über Hysterie und Hypochondrie erwähnt: Als Nachkrankheit eines Wechselfiebers sei Manie aufgetreten, welche in Blödsinn ausgegangen sei.[68]

Wir möchten dieses Thema nicht verlassen, ohne noch kurz den philosophischen Geist zu streifen, der auf Carls Hoher Schule herrschte. Ernst Müller nennt die Schule mit Recht: „[… eine schöne Frucht der protestantisch bestimmten Aufklärung und des Absolutismus in seinem Ausklang als Wohlfahrtsstaat.“[69] Diese geistige Grundverfassung der Schule bildet sozusagen den festen Boden, auf welchem sich zwei doch recht verschiedene Geisteshaltungen behaupteten. Auf der einen Seite stand der „Tübingensche Senior der herzoglichen Philosophie“, der hochbedeutende und in der Schulphilosophie des 18. Jahrhunderts als originaler Kopf gewürdigte Gottfried Ploucquet (1716–1790), der, selbstständig den spekulativen Rationalismus weiterbildend, die cartesianischen und leibnizianischen Gottesbeweise kritisierte und an Hand calvinistisch-reformierter und auch schwäbisch-pietistischer Vorstellungen für falsch erklärte. Auf der anderen Seite stand als Denker aus

[67] Vgl. Friedrich Schiller, „De discrimine febrium inflammatoriarum et putridarum,“ in *Medizinische Schriften* (Miesbach: W. F. Mayr, 1959 [1780]), 63–134; ders., „Versuch über den Zusammenhang der thierischen Natur des Menschen mit seiner geistigen,“ in *Medizinische Schriften* (Miesbach: W. F. Mayr, 1959 [1780]), 135–180.

[68] Heinrich Laehr, *Gedenktage der Psychiatrie und ihre Hilfswissenschaften in allen Ländern*, 4. Aufl. (Berlin: G. Reimer, 1893).

[69] Müller, 41.

Erfahrung und Beobachtung, auch wenn er noch starke spekulative Züge aufweist, Jakob Friedrich Abel (1751–1829), dem Schiller Zeit seines Lebens verpflichtet blieb. Ernst Müller, auf welchen wir auch hier verweisen müssen, weist nach, daß Abels erkenntnistheoretischer Ausgangspunkt die Theorie der Erfahrung der Engländer von Locke über Reidt bis Ferguson bildete. Indem er diese Grundanschauung mit nachleibnizianischen Vorstellungen von Seelenkräften verband, kommt Abel fast zu einem System des Mechanismus von wirkenden Kräften (*vires*) des Denkens, Fühlens, Empfindens, der Fantasie, der Reproduktion von Vorstellungen u. ä. diese vires werden auch bemüht, wenn Abel sein Hauptthema abhandelt: den Einfluß der Seele auf den Körper und umgekehrt. E. Müller vermutet, daß dieses Thema zwischen Medizinern und Philosophen an der Carlsschule in gemeinsam abgehaltenen Kolloquien behandelt wurde, da Abels große Abhandlung über Sympathie und den Ursprung des Charakters auf weiten Strecken den Arbeiten Consbruchs gleiche. Müller meint, der eine habe dem anderen das Problem zur Weiterforschung übergeben und beide hätten auf denselben Autoren, zum Beispiel Haller, Boerhaave, Gaubius, Hume, de Wytt gefußt.[70]

Wir sehen hier deutlich die zweite Quelle Autenriethschen Denkens. Bei aller Spekulation, welche ihm anhaftete, bleibt er nüchterner und sachlicher Empiriker; schreibt er doch in den *Tübinger Blättern*, welche er von 1815 bis 1870 mit dem Physiker J. G. Bohnenberger zusammen herausgab, es sollte ein „Geist [herrschen], der die Natur zu erkennen wünscht, wie sie ist, und nicht, wie sie etwa sich träumen ließe, der Untersuchungen des Einzelnen liebt, um von ihnen aus einer sichern Kenntnis des Allgemeinen sich zu nähern, soll in diesen Blättern herrschen."[71] Man spürt aus diesen Zeilen, daß die Kantsche Denkweise des transzendentalen Kritizismus an der Carlsschule nicht mehr oder vielmehr zu spät, erst 1791, mit dem Einzug von G. Bardili (1761–1800) Eingang gefunden hatte. Autenrieths naiver Rationalismus hatte noch nicht an sich selbst zu zweifeln gelernt. Auf der anderen Seite liegt hier auch die Wurzel dafür, das Autenrieth das Interesse an philosophisch-theoretischen Themen nie mehr verlor. Hat er doch Aufsätze über „Die Verbindung der Seele mit den organischen Kräften", „Über den Menschen und seine Hoffnung einer Fortdauer vom Standpunkt des Naturforschers" (Tübingen 1823) und 1823 „Über das Buch Hiob" verfaßt.[72]

Es ist merkwürdig, daß bis heute selbst bei Diepgen Autenrieth als Schüler von Johann Peter Frank (1745–1821) gilt.[73] Autenrieth war gerade ein halbes Jahr, von 1792 bis 1793, in Pavia. Er wurde dort nicht warm. In einem ausführlichen Brief vom 27.2.1793 an seinen ehemaligen Lehrer an der Hohen Carlsschule, den Chirurgen Christian Klein, übt er scharfe Kritik an Frank. Stübler hat in seiner verdienstvollen

---

[70] Ebenda, 45.

[71] [J. H. F. Autenrieth and J. G. v. Bohnenberger, „Vorrede," *Tübinger Blätter für Naturwissenschaften und Arzneykunde* 1.1 (1815), 1].

[72] Johann Heinrich Ferdinand v. Autenrieth, *Ansichten über Natur- und Seelenleben* (Stuttgart: Cotta, 1836).

[73] Diepgen.

Studie über Autenrieth diesen Brief aus dem Familienbesitz veröffentlicht.[74] Er zeigt nur Ablehnung; nirgends ist ein positiver Einfluß Johann Peter Franks, des berühmten Begründers des medizinischen Polizei, auf den jungen Arzt zu sehen. Es bleibt also dabei, J. H. F. Autenrieth war Carlsschüler und er hat Zeit seines Lebens an dem in der Carlsschule vermittelten Bildungsgut festgehalten.[75]

Im Juni 1797 wurde Autenrieth als Nachfolger des verstorbenen Clossius vom Tübinger Senat gewählt. Am 13. Mai 1805 konnte er mit dem klinischen Unterricht an dem von ihm in der ehemaligen Burse (jetzt Zahnklinik) mit vielen Schwierigkeiten eingerichteten *Institutum clinicum*, welches 15 Betten hatte, beginnen. Er nahm in diesem von Anfang an auch Geisteskranke auf, welche dann oft die übrigen Kranken störten und sich selbst gefährdeten, sodaß Autenrieth auf entsprechende Maßnahmen sinnen mußte, sie sicher und geräuschlos zu verwahren. Er kam so auf seine Maske und Birne, die den Kranken das Schreien unmöglich machen sollten, und auf die Einrichtung sogenannter „Palisadenzellen". Diese Zellen waren einfach Zimmer, in denen Fenster und Ofen mit einem Holzverschlag verwahrt waren. Leider sind diese heute museale anmutende Dinge, die doch nur ein Zeichen dafür sind, welch großes Interesse Autenrieth an den Geisteskranken hatte, daß er solche Unannehmlichkeiten auf sich nahm, um sie überhaupt im Clinicum haben zu können, fast das einzige, was wir von seiner irrenärztlichen Tätigkeit wissen. Auch R. Gaupp neigt zu der Ansicht, daß Autenrieth als Theoretiker geringen Einfluß auf die Entwicklung der Psychiatrie gehabt hatte, zumal es ihm auch an entsprechender Erfahrung gefehlt habe.[76] Wir werden im folgenden dieser Auffassung zu widersprechen haben. Es ist Autenrieth auf diesem Gebiet ebenso ergangen wie auf dem der allgemeinen Medizin. Man weiß von ihm bestenfalls noch, daß er auf die vertriebene Krätze viele Krankheiten glaubte zurückführen zu können und daß er geradezu einen wissenschaftlichen Feldzug gegen das Wegschmieren der Krätze mit Quecksilbersalbe führte.

Autenrieth war ein beherrschender Mann. Im Juni 1819 wurde er von König Friedrich I, dem straffen Organisator seines Landes zum Vizekanzler der Universität Tübingen ernannt. Es war dies eine aufsehenerregende Tatsache; war doch der Kanzler der Universität bisher immer ein evangelischer Theologe gewesen. Am 15. Mai 1822 wurde er Kanzler auf Lebzeiten. Er hatte die Universität durch schwere Zeiten zu führen, die revolutionären Burschenschaften zu dämpfen und gegen allen Widerstand die Universität in ein Staatsinstitut umzuwandeln. Beherrschend war er vor allem als Lehrer, verstand er doch seine Studenten trotz fehlender persönlicher Zuneigung auf Lebzeiten zu beeinflussen. Autenrieth wirkte schulbildend. Die von ihm gegründete Tübinger Medizinische Schule umfaßt Wilhelm Griesinger, C. A. Wunderlich, der dann später als Ordinarius für innere Medizin in Leipzig

[74] Stübler, 24–29.

[75] [Auslassung (ca. 90 Worte): Anmerkungen zu Autenrieths Persönlichkeit nach Robert v. Mohl, *Lebens-Erinnerungen von Robert von Mohl (1799–1875)* (Stuttgart: DVA, 1902)].

[76] Robert Gaupp, „Ferdinand Autenrieth (1772–1835)," in *Deutsche Irrenärzte: Einzelbilder ihres Lebens und Wirkens*, hg. von Theodor Kirchhoff (Berlin: J. Springer, 1921).

Lehrer so bedeutender Ärzte wie z. B. Strümpell wurde. Dieser von Autenrieth gegründeten Tübinger Schule gehört auch Albert Zeller an.

Autenrieth war Humoralpathologe im Sinne von Sydenham und von Franz de le Boë (Sylvius) (1614–1672). Vom Ersteren hatte er die Grundüberzeugung einer tiefen inneren Verwandtschaft der Krankheiten und der Möglichkeit des Übergangs der einen in die andere (*Transmotatio morborum*) übernommen; von Sylvius übernahm er die Lehre von den Krankheitschärfen, den *acrimoniae*. Diese Schärfen entstehen in bestimmten Organen und ergreifen metastatisch andere. Autenrieth unterscheidet akute und chronische und nennt unter den letzteren die Krätzschärfe, die Haemorrhoidalschärfe, die arthritische Schärfe. Die Regelmäßigkeit, welche er häufig bei der Metastasenbildung glaubte beobachten zu können, brachte ihn auf den inneren Zusammenhang der Organe, auf ihren Consensus. Die Lehre vom Consens der inneren Organe rückte somit immer mehr in den Mittelpunkt seines Denkens. Sein Nachdenken über diese Zusammenhänge führte zu bemerkenswerten Erkenntnissen. Autenrieth spricht unter anderem von einem Zusammenhang der Organe durch Gewohnheit, und wir glauben daß er dabei als erster im Auge hatte, was später Pawlow (1859–1936) als bedingte Reflexe beschrieb.

Die wesentliche therapeutische Aufgabe bestand darin, die Schärfen nach außen am besten auf den Darm abzuleiten. Dieser Gedanke ist ja wohl allen Humoralpathologien eigen. Das Haarseil im Nacken zur Erzeugung eines künstlichen Nackenkarbunkels, das Wiedereröffnen eines Unterschenkelgeschwürs, dessen Schärfe nach innen geschlagen war, das Wieder-in-Gang-Bringen des Haemorrhoidal- oder Menstrualflusses sind allgemein anerkannte Maßnahmen, die ja dann auch von den somatisch eingestellten Psychiatern gerne gebraucht wurden, ganz zu schweigen von den Mitteln der Blutentziehung mit Hilfe des Aderlasses oder der Blutegel.

Will man sich von der wissenschaftlichen Einstellung eines Arztes aus der Zeit der Wende vom 18. zum 19. Jahrhundert ein Bild machen, so wird man stets die Frage prüfen müssen, wie er sich zum Problem der Lebenskraft und des Zusammenhanges der Seele mit dem Körper stellte. Der Durchschnittsmeinung des 18. Jahrhunderts über die Lebenskraft hatte die Schule von Montpellier den treffendsten Ausdruck verliehen, indem sie von einer *force hypermécanique* sprach. Auch Frankreich war von Descartes abgefallen, der bekanntlich die Lebensvorgänge nach Art einer Uhr oder eines Automaten hatte erklären wollen: „Selon les règles des mécaniques qui sont les mêmes que celles de la nature.“[77] Georg Ernst Stahl hatte dann die den Körper gegen Fäulnis schützende, belebende und ausbildende Kraft mit der Seele gleichgesetzt.[78] M. Dessoir, dem wir auch hier wieder folgen, weist mit Recht darauf hin, daß diese Annahme für uns etwas Befremdliches habe, da wir beim Wort „Seele“ lediglich an die Summe der Bewußtseinsvorgänge zu denken pflegen. Ursprünglich aber umfaßte der Begriff „Seele“ in einer seiner verbreitetsten Anwendungen außer den psychischen auch alle anderen Lebenserscheinungen.

---

[77] Oeuvres I, 184.

[78] Georgii Ernesti Stahl, *Theoria Medica Vera* (Hallae: Orphanotropheum, 1708).

Aus der aristotelischen *anima vegetativa* ist späterhin die Lebenskraft geworden. Auch Stahl lehrt, daß ohne dies Prinzip der Körper eine unselbstständige und schnell zerfallende Maschine sei. Aber er erweitert den Begriff des bildenden und belebenden Prinzips, indem er die animalische Seele hineinbezieht, die Stelle der Bewegung und Empfindung. Daß die Lebenskraft mit dieser Seele identisch sei, folgert er aus den Bewegungen, die ja aus scheinbar seelenlosen zu bewußten oder umgekehrt aus willkürlichen zu unwillkürlichen werden können. Schließlich läßt er das Leben sogar von der Existenz der Vernunft abhängen und verwandelt dadurch einen nur im Menschen vorhandenen Tatbestand in einen allgemeinen und ferner ein bloßes Nebeneinander, nämlich das Nebeneinander von Leben und Vernunft, in einen Kausalzusammenhang, als dessen bedingendes Glied die geistige Seele fungiert.

Ein Anhänger Stahls, Robert Whytt (1714–1766) hat dann das Lebendige auf die „bloß empfindende" Seele eingeschränkt. Seele ist für ihn die Station, in der Empfindungskraft in Bewegungskraft umgesetzt wird, da der ganze Körper empfindlich und beweglich ist, so muß die Seele ihn überall durchziehen. Er kommt so zu der Meinung, daß das Rückenmark mehr als eine unselbstständiger Leitungsapparat sei. Dessoir macht hierzu die interessante Bemerkung, daß E. Pflügers Jugendarbeit über die „Rückenmarksseele" an diese Meinung Whytts anknüpfe. Dessoir zitiert E. Pflüger: „Aber auch so glaube ich [...] nachgewiesen zu haben, daß das Sensorium durch das ganze Cerebrospinalorgan verbreitet ist."[79]

Wir sind in diesem Punkte so ausführlich gewesen, weil A. Zeller sich wiederholt auf Stahl beruft und auch für ihn das Rückenmark Beziehungen zum Seelenleben hat. August Unzer hatte Stahls Lehre so umgebildet, daß sie ihre Eigentümlichkeit verlor, indem er zwischen die Seele als Träger des Bewußtseins und die körperlichen Funktionen eine Nervenkraft einschaltete, sodaß die Abhängigkeit des Leibes von der Seele zu einer mittelbaren wurde. Wir werden sehen, daß diese Lehre von der Mittelkraft sowohl bei Schiller als auch bei Autenrieth wieder auftaucht. Bei Autenrieth verbindet sie sich dann allerdings mit der Lehre Friedrich Hoffmanns, der, wie schon erwähnt, auch Schiller nahestand.

[¶] Dessoir sieht den Unterschied zwischen Stahls psychischem Vitalismus und dem dynamischen Vitalismus Friedrich Hoffmanns in zwei Punkten.[80] Erstens erkennt Hoffmann an, daß einige Lebensfunktionen (wie der Kreislauf) auf rein mechanischen Gesetzen beruhen, womit er sich den sogenannten Iatromathematikern nähert, die alle vom Willen unabhängigen Vorgänge nach Gesetzen der Mechanik und Hydraulik zu erklären versuchten. Frei von solchen mechanischen Bedingungen soll sein die *vis vitalis solidi*, die in den festen Körperteilen, besonders in Muskeln und Nerven, eigene Form der Lebenskraft. Hoffmann meinte, in den Nervenröhrchen zirkuliere diese Kraft als Nervenäther, ähnlich so wie das Blut in den Gefäßen. Zweitens soll diese Kraft als Äther auch in der gesamten übrigen Natur sich finden, zum Teil auch von den organischen Körpern aus der Atmosphäre angezogen werden.

[79] So Eduard Friedrich Wilhelm Pflüger, *Die sensorischen Functionen des Rückenmarks der Wirbelthiere: Nebst einer neuen Lehre über die Leitungsgesetze der Reflexionen* (Berlin: Hirschwald, 1853) nach Dessoir, 503, Fußnote 2.

[80] [Vgl.] Dessoir, 505 f.

Dessoir vermutet mit Recht, daß Hoffmann diesen Gedanken von Franz Anton Mesmer (1733–1815) übernommen habe. Nach Mesmer ist das ganze Weltall von einem ätherischen Fluidum durchströmt, das feiner ist als der Lichtäther. Die Bewegung dieses Fluidums oder der „Flut“ – genauer: die nach Polaritätsgesetzen sich vollziehende Schwingung – erzeugt sowohl den Einfluß der Himmelskörper aufeinander und auf die Erde als auch den in den bekannten Erscheinungen sich bekundenden Einfluß eines tierischen Körpers auf den anderen. Das Fluidum universale kann sich nämlich in den einzelnen Wesen anhäufen oder in ihnen abnehmen, sodaß ein mikroskopisches Analogon von Ebbe und Flut entsteht. Wie man nun die magnetisch-elektrische Kraft, die jenem Fluidum nahe verwandt, vielleicht sogar mit ihm identisch ist, in Stahl und Eisen ansammeln kann, so meinte Mesmer, habe er auch ein Mittel gefunden, in bestimmten Individuen den Naturmagnetismus zu dem Grad zu verstärken, daß er Erscheinungen, welche denen des Magnets analog seien, hervorzubringen vermöchte. Der Magnetismus animalis, der also nur eine Spielart des Magnetismus naturalis, das heißt der Bewegung der Allflut, beruhe auf einer Empfänglichkeit aller organischen Körper für das *Fluidum universale*, welches zunächst auf die Nerven wirke. Als dann Galvani (1737–1798) entdeckt hatte, daß von belebten Tierkörpern bzw. von den nerven Elektrizität erzeugt wird, folgerten Gelehrte wie Alexander von Humboldt, das bisher unbekannte Nervenfluidum, die Muskelreizbarkeit, ja der ganze Lebensprozeß seien galvanische Vorgänge, und auch Autenrieth schreibt in § 200 seines Handbuchs: „Wenn also auch das galvanische Fluidum nicht selbst die Quelle der Lebenskraft sein sollte, so nähert es sich doch am meisten unter allen bekannten imponderabilen Materien derselben.“[81]

Was die „Verbindung der Seele mit dem organischen Körper“ betrifft, so hält Autenrieth an der wohl von Unzer begründeten Lehre einer Mittelkraft ebenso wie Schiller fest. Autenrieth meint in dem Aufsatz mit ebendemselben Titel: „Die Verbindung des Geistes mit dem Körper wird seiner konstanten eigenen Unräumlichkeit ungeachtet dadurch denkbar, daß die mit ihm in Verbindung stehende organische Lebenskraft zwei gleichsam einander gegenüberstehende Beziehungen ihres Seins hat. Soweit sie sich in organischen Stoff einkörpert und als dem Raum nach teilbar sich ausspricht, wird sie räumlich. Als unräumlich aber zeigt sie sich, sofern die Verhältnisse jeder individualisierten Lebenskraft zur gemeinschaftlichen Quelle alles Lebens durch keinen Raum bedingt sind. Von dieser Seite aus kann sie also auch mit wesentlich Unräumlichem zusammenhängen. Soweit nun die Seele zunächst nur vermittelst der organischen Lebenskraft mit unserem Körper in enge, doch, wie oben bemerkt wurde noch eines Schwankens fähige Verbindung tritt, ist sie von der unräumlichen Welt aus durch diese doppelseitige Lebenskraft an ihn gebunden.“[82]

Es ist merkwürdig, daß Friedrich Schiller in seiner „Philosophie der Physiologie“ dieselben Ansichten, allerdings klarer und eleganter, entwickelt: „Oder endlich muß

[81] Autenrieth, *Handbuch*, Bd. 1, §200, 124.

[82] Johann Heinrich Ferdinand v. Autenrieth, „Verbindung der Seele mit dem organischen Körper: Entwicklung des Charakters der Persönlichkeit in der Reihe der Wesen,“ in *Ansichten über Natur- und Seelenleben*, hg. von Hermann Friedrich Autenrieth (Stuttgart: Cotta, 1836), 358.

eine Kraft vorhanden sein, die zwischen den Geist und die Materie tritt und beide verbindet, eine Kraft, die von der Materie verändert werden und die den Geist verändern kann. Dies wäre also eine Kraft, die einesteils geistig, andernteils materiell, ein Wesen, daß einesteils durchdringlich, andern teils undurchdringlich wäre, und läßt sich ein solches denken? – Gewiß nicht! Dem sei, wie ihm wolle, es ist wirklich eine Kraft zwischen der Materie (dieser nämlich, deren Wirkungen vorgestellt werden sollen) und dem Geiste vorhanden. Diese Kraft ist ganz verschieden von der Welt und dem Geist. Ich entferne sie: dahin ist alle Wirkung der Welt auf ihn. Und dennoch ist der Geist noch da. Und dennoch ist der Gegenstand noch da. Ihr Verlust hat einen Riß zwischen Welt und Geist gemacht. Ihr Dasein lichtet, weckt, belebt Alles um ihn. – Ich nenne sie *Mittelkraft*."[83]

Bevor wir zu Autenrieths eigentlicher Krankheitslehre übergehen, wollen wir kurz auf die Frage eingehen, ob er denn wirklich ein Kind seiner Zeit war und nicht nur ein verspäteter Aufklärer. Nun, dem ist nicht so: einmal benützt auch er den romantischen Zauberstab der Analogie oft und gerne, zum andern bemüht er sich in echt Okenscher Weise um eine Theorie der Anatomie, das heißt um eine Lehre von den Bildungsgesetzen. In Autenrieths Theorie der Anatomie spielt der romantische Begriff der Polarität eine große Rolle: „Alle diese Erscheinungen führen notwendig zuletzt auf einen tief in der Natur liegenden Gegensatz, der ja auch sonst überall, selbst [im moralischen], sich zeigt."[84] [Andernorts] glaubt er den Bau des weiblichen Brustkorbs auf ein geringeres Sauerstoffbedürfnis der Frau zurückführen zu können und spricht so von einer negativen Polarität des Weibes.[85] Die positive Polarität des Mannes, so meint er, werde durch einen stärkeren Oxydationsprozeß bewirkt. Es genügen diese kleinen Proben, um Autenrieth als einen echten romantischen Arzt auszuweisen. Andererseits hat gerade seine Polaritätslehre ihn davon zurückgehalten, sich der Brownschen Reiztheorie anzuschließen, die doch sonst die romantischen Ärzte weitgehend beherrschte. Autenrieth tadelt an Brown, daß er eben keine Polarität, sondern nur ein Mehr oder Weniger kenne.

Wenden wir uns nun Autenrieths eigentlicher Krankheitslehre zu, [die in zwei Bänden als Kollegnachschrift vorliegt].[86] Der erste Band ist den akuten Krankheiten, der zweite den chronischen gewidmet. Im ersten Band werden die Infektionskrankheiten und unter diesen das Nervenfieber abgehandelt. Unter diesem Titel fällt auch der Typhus. Autenrieth unterscheidet dabei den sporadischen Typhus, unseren

[83] Friedrich Schiller, „Philosophie der Physiologie," in *Friedrich Schiller: Medizinische Schriften. Eine Buchausgabe der Deutschen Hoffmann-La Roche AG aus Anlaß des 200. Geburtstages des Dichters* (Miesbach: W. F. Mayr, 1959 [1779]), 41.

[84] Autenrieth, *Handbuch*, Bd. 3, § 917, 121. [Zeller hat Autenrieths Text hier falsch wiedergegeben: Statt „Menschen" steht im Original „moralischen"!].

[85] Vgl. Johann Heinrich Ferdinand v. Autenrieth, „Bemerkungen über die Verschiedenheit beider Geschlechter und ihrer Zeugungsorgane, als Beytrag zu einer Theorie der Anatomie," *Archiv für die Physiologie* 7.1 (1807): 1–139.

[86] Johann Heinrich Ferdinand v. Autenrieth, *Specielle Nosologie und Therapie. Nach dem Systeme eines berühmten deutschen Arztes und Professors*, hg. von Carl Ludwig Reinhard, 2 Bde. (Würzburg: Etlinger, 1834–1835).

heutigen Abdominaltyphus und den eigentlichen contagiösen Typhus, unser heutiges Fleckfieber. Von letzterem meint er, es entstehe nur, wo mehrere Menschen beisammen seien, unter denen ein großes öffentliches Unglück herrsche. Autenrieth unterscheidet durchaus die beiden Formen, aber es liegt ihm gänzlich fern, obgleich er die Darmgeschwüre des Abdominaltyphus kennt, eine Untersuchung nach der Lokalisation im Darm = Abdominaltyphus und nach der Lokalisation im Hirn = Flecktyphus zu treffen. Die Lokalisation des Krankheitsprozesses war für ihn eben kein Unterscheidungsmerkmal erster Ordnung. Dies ist ja auch durchaus verständlich, wenn man sich seine Metastasenlehre vergegenwärtigt. Darüberhinaus war das scharfe Trennen von Krankheiten überhaupt nicht sein Anliegen. Dies ist besonders deutlich am Beispiel der mit Hautausschlägen einhergehenden Krankheiten zu zeigen, welche für Autenrieth alle zusammen nur Glieder einer Kette waren. Was den Typhus betrifft, so war für ihn die Bewußtseinsveränderung, das „Typhöse" das wesentliche Einteilungsprinzip. Er meinte, jedes Fieber könne typhös werden und auch beim sporadischen Typhus (Abdominaltyphus) könne der Patient gleich vom Kopf aus befallen werden. Das komme vor allem bei Geschäftsleuten vor, welche den Abend am Spieltisch verbringen würden und, um nachts arbeiten zu können, Wein und Kaffee etc. zu sich nehmen würden. Es entstehe so das Bild des Typhus encephalicus. Wir sehen, daß es so keineswegs zutrifft, was man oft lesen kann, daß Autenrieth der erste gewesen sei, der in das bis dahin unklare Gebiet des Typhus Ordnung gebracht habe. Nur wenn man dies bedenkt, wird es verständlich, daß Carl August Wunderlich, Schüler und Patenkind Autenrieths und späterer Vorstand der Tübinger und Leipziger Medizischen Klinik, der Freund Wilhelm Griesingers und Rosers, 1839 in seiner Dissertation *Die Nosologie des Typhus* zu dem Ergebnis kommen konnte, es gäbe nur einen Typhus[87]; jeder Versuch der Unterscheidung sei fehlerhaft und rein spekulativ. Für unser Thema ist Wunderlichs Versuch sehr wichtig, wenn wir bedenken, daß die Schule Autenrieths uns somit sowohl den Einheitstyphus als auch die Einheitspsychose beschert hat.

Im zweiten Band wurden die chronischen Krankheiten abgehandelt. Nach Autenrieths Meinung sind die meisten chronischen Krankheiten Nervenkrankheiten. Er entwickelt über ihre Entstehung folgende Gedanken: „Vermittelst des Gefäßsystems wirkt das Nervens-System auf die Ernährung. Vornehmlich scheint die passive Congestion durch Aufhebung des Nerven-Einflusses erregt zu werden. Stocken auf diese Art die Säfte in einem Theile, so giebt dies Veranlassung zur Erzeugung von Schärfen. [... Die] Ausstoßung dieser Schärfen [ist] die unmittelbare Folge des Nerven-Leidens, bald aber geht es weiter, es entsteht veränderte Ernährung, Bildung von Desorganisationen. So ist Hypochondrie ursprünglich ein Nerven-Leiden, mit der Zeit kommen aber arthritische Ausstoßungen oder arthritische Desorganisationen und After-Organisationen im Innern des Körpers. So endigt öfters Gesichts-Schmerz mit einem herpetischen Ausschlage oder einem

[87] Carl August Wunderlich, *Die Nosologie des Typhus: Eine Beleuchtung der wichtigsten Ansichten über dieselbe* (Stuttgart: Rieger, 1839).

Krebse. Bloße Adynamie, wo Frauenzimmer ohne sonstige Krankheit jahrelang im Bette liegen, geht in Hämorrhoiden oder chronische Frieseln über."[88] Wir sehen aus diesem kleinen Beispiel, wie sich Autenrieth die wandelbare Natur der Krankheiten vorstellte. Wer in diesem Geist erzogen wurde, der konnte unmöglich auf das scharfe Herausarbeiten von Krankheitseinheiten besonderen Wert legen.

Was nun Autenrieths Ansichten über die eigentlichen Geisteskrankheiten oder, wie er es nennt, die Krankheiten des Sensorium commune betrifft, so hat man ihm immer den Vorwurf zu geringer persönlicher Erfahrung gemacht. Dies wird sowohl von Stübler als auch schon von Gaupp mit Autenrieths eigenen Worten begründet, daß er bis 1807, also in 10 Jahren, 28 Geisteskranke behandelt habe.[89] Unter diesen war übrigens Hölderlin, über dessen Krankheit Autenrieth allerdings nie etwas geschrieben hat. Es wurde allerdings immer übersehen, daß Autenrieth wirkliches Interesse an den Irren hatte und daß er überall seine Augen offen und seine mächtige Hand bereit hatte. Er kannte so die Zustände, die damals in Zwiefalten herrschten, gut. In das 1089 gegründete, 1669 neu gebaute und 1803 säkularisierte Benediktinerkloster in Zwiefalten waren im Juni 1812 die bisher im Zuchthaus in Ludwigsburg untergebrachten Irren verlegt worden. Es befanden sich zu Autenrieths Zeiten dort etwa 160 Kranke. Außerdem hatte Bad Teinach im Schwarzwald damals den Ruf, besonders heilsam bei Geisteskrankheiten zu sein. Autenrieth machte auch dort seine Beobachtungen. Er zeigt ein scharfes, kritisches, durchaus auf Erfahrung gegründetes Verständnis für das Anstaltswesen, indem er sagt: „In den Tabellen von Irrenanstalten werden immer mehr als geheilt aufgeführt, als es wirklich sind, weil man längere Intervalla lucida als Heilung ansieht. Namentlich ist aber in neuen Anstalten das Verhältnis besser, weil hier alle Verhältnisse begünstigt sind. In alten Irrenanstalten sinkt die Heilung zu Null herab. In jeder neuen Anstalt ist das Resultat günstiger; zuletzt wird sie bloße Versorgungsanstalt. Die Gründe liegen darin: Narrheit hat unter allen Nervenkrankheiten die größte Hartnäckigkeit durch Gewohnheit [....] Die meisten [Nervenkrankheiten] werden umso hartnäckiger, je öfter sie der Mensch gehabt hat [....] Wenn man zu diesem in dem Übel liegenden Gründe hinzurechnet, daß zwei Faktoren bei der Narrheit ihr Spiel treiben, einer von der Seele und einer vom Körper aus, so ist die Gewohnheit von der Seele aus nicht anders zu unterbrechen, als wenn man ihre Aufmerksamkeit auf andere Gegenstände hinrichtet. Damit ist der erste Schritt zur Freiheit der Seele geschehen. Dies ist aber nicht anders möglich, als daß man sich beständig mit den Narren beschäftigt. Es gehört also dazu, daß jeder nur so viel Narren behandelt, als er den ganzen Tag beschäftigen kann. Dies ist aber in keiner größeren Anstalt möglich, besonders bei Narren, wo der psychische Faktor vorherrscht. Nun gibt in jeder neuen Anstalt jeder neue Arzt sich viele Mühe. Aber es ist kein Mensch imstande, dieses mit Interesse jahrelang zu treiben. Jeder erlahmt früher oder später, und kommt in einen Schlendrian, und es heißt zuletzt von den Ärzten, wie Goethe sagt: durchstudiert die groß und kleine Welt und gehen lassen am Ende, wie es Gott

[88] Autenrieth, *Specielle Nosologie und Therapie*, Bd. 2, 2.

[89] Gaupp, „Ferdinand Autenrieth," 57; Stübler, 99.

gefällt. Darum ist es notwendig, wenn man Narren heilen will, daß man einen jeden einzeln behandelt. Man sollte bei einer jeden Anstalt neben dem alten Arzt einen jungen nachziehen, welcher nach 10 Jahren eintreten könnte, denn über 10 Jahre hält es kein Narrenarzt aus, ohne zu erlahmen. Ich habe bei der Ständeversammlung darauf angetragen, dies bei der Irrenanstalt, welche in Winnenthal errichtet werden soll, zu berücksichtigen. Wenn es nicht geschieht, so stehe ich dafür, daß sie nach einiger Zeit so gut bloße Detentionsanstalt wird, wie Zwiefalten."[90] Autenrieth ist somit dafür verantwortlich, daß in Winnenthal genau nach zehn Jahren eine zweite Arztstelle zu besetzen war und dieser erste Assistent war kein Geringerer als Wilhelm Griesinger.

Autenrieths Systematik entbehrt eines durchgehenden Kriteriums. Katalepsie und Ekstase werden unter den Krämpfen abgehandelt. Unter den Krankheiten des Sensorium commune zählt er auf: 1. Hypochondrie, 2. Geisteskrankheit oder Narrheit, welche er dann nach ihren Ursachen einzuteilen versucht. Er erwähnt so eine Narrheit aus Mißbrauch geistiger Getränke, Narrheit aus vertriebener Krätze, Narrheit aus verhaltener Sekretion des Venensystems. Als 3. Gruppe nennt er die Manien, die er dann wieder unterteilt in Nostalgie (Heimweh), Melancholie, religiösen Wahnsinn. Die 4. Gruppe wird von Blödsinn und Cretinismus gebildet.

Es ist alles ein rechter Wirrwarr, mit dem man schwer etwas anfangen kann, und Autenrieth selbst legte auch wenig Wert auf die Systematik. Er schreibt: „Die Modifikationen zwischen Narrheit, Epilepsie, Katalepsie und andere Nervenkrankheiten sind sehr gering, doch scheinen bei der Narrheit die Ursachen häufiger im Gehirn selbst zu liegen. Wenn die Narrheit aber auch in anderen Teilen des Nervensystems ihren Sitz hat, so wird sie doch zuletzt idiopathische Hirnkrankheit, und namentlich ist dies beim Blödsinn der Fall."[91]

Autenrieth stellt klar heraus, daß die eigentliche Geisteskrankheit erst mit der körperlichen Krankheit beginnt: „Hierbei ist nun aber merkwürdig, die Grenze, welche zwischen der Narrheit aus psychischen und der Narrheit aus körperlichen Ursachen liegt. Ein Leidenschaftsnarr wird nicht eher ein wirklicher Narr, bis das Gehirn körperlich ergriffen ist. Ehrgeiz und Hochmut macht Männer am leichtesten zu Narren. Eigentlich verrückt wird der Mensch erst dann, wenn wirkliche Zeichen von Kopfleiden kommen, Kopfweh und Blutkongestionen gegen den Kopf [....] Etwas ähnliches ist mit dem religiösem Wahnsinne, das körperliche Leiden fängt mit dem an, daß der Mensch sein Gehirn abstumpft; es kommt Melancholie. Dann kehrt sich das Gehirn um, er sieht den dritten Himmel und Engel, oder die Hölle und den Teufel, und jetzt nützen alle vernünftigen Gründe nichts mehr. Etwas ähnliches ist beim weiblichen Geschlecht die verliebte Narrheit. Wenn ein Mann einen Korb bekommt, so gibt es immer noch genug Weiber in der Welt. Bei den Mädchen ist aber noch die Überzahl vorhanden, es kann darum eine leicht in den Bruch des Überschusses fallen; dazu kommt das feinere Gefühl des Weibes und die verletzte Eitelkeit; denn ein jedes Frauenzimmer glaubt doch, die Männer halten es für einen

[90] Autenrieth, *Specielle Nosologie und Therapie*, Bd. 2, 124–126.

[91] [Ebenda, 117].

Engel. Die eigentliche Narrheit fängt aber doch erst mit dem körperlichen Leiden an. Anfangs äußert sich diese Krankheit durch Melancholie, es kann aber auch krankhafte einseitige Tätigkeit miteintreten, d. h. Narrheit."[92]

Versuchen wir zusammenzufassen, was der Student Albert Zeller von seinem Lehrer Autenrieth über Geisteskrankheiten und Geisteskranke lernen konnte:

a) Die Formen, in welchen die Geisteskrankheit auftritt, sind untereinander verwandt, sie verhalten sich oft wie Glieder einer Kette.
b) Das Leiden beginnt häufig mit Hypochondrie oder Melancholie und geht später in Narrheit und Blödsinn über. „Mit Blödsinn endigen die meisten Fälle von Wahnsinn, wenn das Gehirn ganz abgestumpft ist".
c) Diesem Verlauf entspricht anatomisch ein Übergang des Krankheitsprozesses vom weichen Nervensystem, dem Gangliensystem, auf das Gehirn.
d) Psychische und körperliche Ursachen müssen zusammentreffen, um Geisteskrankheit zu erzeugen. Erst wenn körperliche Krankheit hinzukommt, wird der reaktiv Verstimmte geisteskrank.
e) Deshalb müssen auch die körperliche und die psychische Kurmethoden miteinander verbunden werden.
f) Irrenheilanstalt und Irrenverwahranstalt müssen getrennt werden.
g) Das zur Geisteskrankheit führende körperliche Leiden entwickelt sich nach dem Gesetzen der Metastasenlehre, dem Metaschematismus der Krankheiten, das heißt nach der allgemeinen Krankheitslehre.

Dem sachkundigen Lesen dieser Zeilen wird jetzt schon die große Ähnlichkeit mit den später von Zeller systematischer und deutlicher dargetanen Lehren ins Auge springen. Aber auch ein anderer Zusammenhang wird deutlich, nämlich der zwischen Autenrieth und Reil.

Persönlichkeit und Lehre J. C. F. Reils

Johann Christian Friedrich Reil, geboren am 28.2.1759 als Sohn eines Pfarrers in Ostfriesland, ist am 23. November 1813 an Fleckfieber gestorben, welches er sich als Inspekteur der Lazarette während der Völkerschlacht bei Leipzig (16.-19. Oktober 1813) zugezogen hatte.[93] Ein Mensch voll Feuer und Genialität, der vor allem im Stil seiner Jugendarbeiten noch vorwiegend dem Sturm und Drang verbunden ist. Aber auch ein Mann von Mäßigkeit und Bildung, der es nach seinen eigenen Worten stets abgelehnt hat, sich öffentlich zu streiten, man denke, in einer Zeit, in welcher die wissenschaftliche Pamphletistik blühte und in welcher das wissenschaftliche Publikum selbst so widerwärtige und bösartige Fehden wie die

[92] [Ebenda, 116].
[93] [Zu Reil, vgl. auch Gerhart Zeller (Hg.), *Albert Zellers medizinisches Tagebuch*, Bd. 2, 11–13].

zwischen Schelling und Paulus nicht nur duldete.[94] 1782 war Reil Doktor der Medizin in Halle geworden, 1787 Professor der inneren Klinik in Halle, 1789 Stadtphysikus in Halle, 1810 Professor der inneren Medizin in Berlin. Reil war fast zu allen Gebieten in der Medizin schöpferisch gewesen, aber wir müssen uns auf seine psychiatrische Wirksamkeit beschränken.[95] Reil war im Grunde ein Anhänger der analytischen Methode des Condillac (1714–1780) und Pinel (1745–1826): „Ich habe alle die Lehrgebäude älterer und neuerer Ärzte geprüft und bin bald ein Anhänger dieses, bald jenes Systems gewesen. Allein bei keinem, ich gestehe es aufrichtig, habe ich Beruhigung gefunden, die ich suchte."[96] Reil empfahl daher, alle Hypothesen zu verlassen und die Empirie einzuführen. Allein man könnte mit Kierkegaard sagen: Die Zeit des Unterscheidens war vorbei, das System hatte sie überwunden. Reil konnte sich diesen Einflüssen des Zeitgeistes nicht entziehen und so wurde auch er, wenigstens in vielen Punkten, spekulativer Systematiker.

Reils ganzes Denken kreist um den Begriff des Stoffwechsels, vor allem des intermediären. Ab 1796 erscheint sein *Archiv für die Physiologie*. Im ersten Band dieses Archivs druckte er seine mit Recht so berühmte Abhandlung „Über die Lebenskraft" ab.[97] In dieser unterscheidet er eine physische Kraft, die eine allgemeine Erscheinung der Materie sowohl in der toten als in der belebten Natur sei, und die Lebenskraft. Die Lebenskraft sei nur in der belebten Natur bei Pflanzen und Tieren anzutreffen, sie deute das Verhältnis mehr individualisierter Erscheinungen zu einer besonderen Art von Materie an. Das allgemeinste Attribut dieser eigentümlichen Art von Materie sei eine besondere Art von Kristallisierung, wobei der Begriff der Kristallisierung für alle chemischen Umsetzungen bei Pflanze und Tier dienen muß. Reil war kein Anhänger des Stahlschen Animismus, sondern eher ein Stoffwechselforscher ohne Forschungsmöglichkeit. So klingt auch der letzte Absatz der Abhandlung wie das Vorwort auf eine noch zu schreibende pathologische Physiologie: „Krankheit hat also immer ihre nächste Ursache in einer Veränderung der innern Kräfte des Körpers, und nie kann sein Verhältnis zu den Dingen außer ihm direkt und zunächst eine Krankheit hervorbringen. Krankheitszufälle sind tierische Wirkungen, und tierische Wirkungen können nie anderes als durch tierische Kräfte tierische[r] Organe wirklich werden. Die regelmäßigen Erscheinungen sind Wirkungen regelmäßiger Kräfte, und die anomalischen Erscheinungen Wirkungen kranker Kräfte [....] Alle Krankheiten des tierischen Körpers haben also ihre nächste Ursache entweder in einer widernatürlichen Organisation oder Mischung der tierischen Materie."[98] Da ja auch die Humoralpathologen im Grunde die Ursachen der Krankheit in einer unnatürlichen Mischung (Dyscrasie) gesehen hatten, so

[94] [Gemeint ist der Theologe und Rationalist H. E. G. Paulus (1761–1851). Vgl. Gerhart Zeller (Hg.), *Albert Zellers medizinisches Tagebuch*, Bd. 2, 19–21 und 26–28].

[95] Adalbert Gregor, „Johann Christian Reil (1759–1813)," in *Deutsche Irrenärzte: Einzelbilder ihres Lebens und Wirkens*, hg. von Theodor Kirchhoff (Berlin: J. Springer, 1921), 28–42.

[96] Johann Christian Reil, *Über die Erkenntnis und Kur der Fieber*, Bd. 4, 2. Aufl. (Halle: Curtschen Buchhandlung, 1805), iii.

[97] Johann Christian Reil, *Von der Lebenskraft* (Leipzig: Johann Ambrosius Barth, 1910 [1795]).

[98] Ebenda, 91.

bestand auch kein prinzipieller Widerspruch zu Autenrieth, mit welchem Reil schon in Halle ab 1804 freundschaftliche Beziehungen aufgenommen hatte und der dann auch später mit ihm zusammen das *Archiv für Physiologie* herausgab.

Reil hat mehr durch seine Hypothesen gewirkt als durch seine Analysen. Er war es, der den romantischen Anthropologen das Bild des Nervensystems entwarf: „Wir können uns unsern Körper als eine hohle Kugel denken, die eine innere und äußere reizbare Fläche hat. Jene ist gleichsam die nächste Werkstätte der Seele, wo sich die willkürlichen Bewegungen entwickeln, und die Imagination ihre gesetzmäßigen Spiele treibt. Diese ist der Welt zugekehrt, die sich gleichsam in ihr spiegelt. Zwischen beiden Flächen sind Nerven als Seile ausgespannt, mit zwei reizbaren Extremitäten versehen, deren eine, die peripherische, für die Welt und unseren Körper, die andere, die Centralendigung, für die Operationen der Seele reizbar sind.“[99] Die geflechtartige Formation ohne Zentrum, wie sie das Gangliensystem darstelle, so meint Reil, gäbe Richtungslosigkeit, sie gleiche der republikanischen Verfassung, in welcher kein einziges Glied sich zum König aufwerfen dürfe. Das Cerebralsystem sei dagegen dem Königtum zu vergleichen, dessen Thron unerschütterlich durch innere Souveränitat gesichert sei. Im Gangliensystem liege der somatische Pol des Ichs, es sei die Hauptquelle der Leidenschaften. Der pneumatische Pol sei das Gehirn. Ohne dieses würden die Empfindungen bewußtlos bleiben. Erst im Gehirn werde aus der Mannigfaltigkeit der Organempfindungen Einheit des Gefühls, das heißt: „Wahrnehmung des Körperlichen in uns, vermittelst eines Sinnes, den ich Gemeingefühl genannt habe.“[100] Reil hatte schon früher den Begriff des Gemeingefühls auf folgende Weise bestimmt: „Durch den äußeren Sinn schaun wir die Dinge außer uns, die Welt und unsern Körper, und diese im Raume, und unsern Körper, als den unsrigen, durch das Gemeingefühl an. Das Gemeingefühl ist gleichsam ein Mittelding zwischen dem äußern und innern Sinne, welches den Körper zwar als etwas Äußeres, aber ihn auch als unseren Körper, und seine Zustände, als die unsrigen vorstellt.“[101]

Reil mußte kein echtes Kind seiner Zeit gewesen sein, wenn er sich mit der Zweiteilung auch als Polarität begnügt und nicht letztlich Einheit als Steigerung oder als Ausgleich gesucht hätte. Seine Vermutungen hierüber spricht er im 4. Band der Kur der Fieber folgendermaßen aus: „daß die reale und ideale Seite des Menschen Äußerungen *eines* Wesens im Organismus sind, das sich nach zwei Richtungen entwickelt und dadurch die innige Abhängigkeit der einen Seite von der anderen begründet. In diesem Falle würde es eine höhere Naturlehre geben, der die

[99] Reil, *Über die Erkenntnis*, §18, 41. Diese Polarität hat er später noch eingehender dargestellt. Vgl. Johann Christian Reil, „Über die Eigenschaften des Ganglien-Systems und sein Verhältniss zum Cerebral-System,“ *Archiv für die Physiologie* 7.2 (1807): 189–254.

[100] Ebenda, 240.

[101] Johann Christian Reil, *Rhapsodieen über die Anwendung der psychischen Curmethode auf Geisteszerrüttungen* (Halle: Curt, 1803; reprint, Amsterdam, Bonset, 1968), 162–163. Vgl. auch die Rezension von Arthur Kronfeld, „Einige Bemerkungen über die ersten psychotherapeutischen Veröffentlichungen insbesondere J. C. Reil,“ *Allgemeine Zeitschrift für Psychotherapie* 1 (1928): 46–51.

Physiologie und Psychologie untergeordnet sind, sofern jene die objektive, diese die subjektive Seite jenes [Einen Urgrundes der Natur entwickelt].“[102]

Es wäre merkwürdig, wenn in Reils Auffassung von den psychischen Krankheiten diese Grundanschauung von Polarität und Einheit nicht wiederzufinden wäre. Man kann sich allerdings von seinen Ansichten auf diesem Gebiet nicht leicht eine Meinung bilden. Kahlbaum rechnet ihn unter die Forscher, welche „wenigerstellige“ Systeme geschaffen haben.[103] Die Kategorie der „vielstelligen“ Systeme mit ihrer großen Zahl von Einzelformen wird bei Kahlbaum durch Plater und Guislain sowie Flemming repräsentiert. Die wenigerstelligen Systeme mit einer beschränkten Zahl von Krankheitsformen findet Kahlbaum vor allem bei Esquirol, Reil und Pinel. Die 3. Gruppe der ‚Non-Systeme‘ wird durch Heinrich Neumann, J. B. Friedreich und Maximilian Jacobi repräsentiert. Kahlbaum führt als Reils System folgende schematische Unterteilung an: 1. Fixer Wahn, 2. Wut, 3. Narrheit, 4. Blödsinn. Dies ist im Grunde wohl nicht ganz richtig. Wir müssen allerdings etwas weiter ausholen, um dies deutlich zu machen.

Reil stand ursprünglich Johann Christian Hoffbauer sehr nahe.[104] Reil charakterisiert Hoffbauers Einteilung in dem wichtigen §20 seiner Rhapsodien auf folgende Weise: „Er will [seine Einteilung] nach den einzelnen Vermögen der Seele, die verletzt sind, deren abnormes Verhältnis gegen einander und nach der gestörten Gemeinschaft der Seele mit dem Körper ordnen und darnach als Geschlechter Geisteszerrüttungen, Verrückungen und Seelenkrankheiten im engeren Sinne festsetzen.“[105] Reil schließt sofort seine Kritik an: „Allein, wird diese Einteilung in das ganze System aller Krankheiten eingreifen? Ist sie nicht auf Symptome gegründet, sofern die Verletzungen der Seelenvermögen nicht Krankheiten sondern Produkte derselben sind? Sind die Seelenvermögen in Beziehung ihres zureichenden Grundes so heterogen, als sie es nach ihren Äußerungen zu sein scheinen?“[106] Reil möchte dann Hoffbauers Ansichten nur als Einleitung in das Studium der Arten gelten lassen. Aus allem, was Reil hier schreibt, wird noch das Suchen nach einem natürlichen System der Krankheiten entsprechend dem Linnéschen System deutlich. Reil ist jedoch viel zu überlegen, als daß er sich eng an eine solches Vorbild halten müßte. „Was sind wesentliche, was zufällige Differenzen? Wie unterscheiden sich Arten und Varietäten? Arten beziehen sich auf verletzte Qualitäten, die einer Tierart überhaupt eigen sind, Varietäten auf Modifikationen derselben durch

---

[102] Reil, *Über die Erkenntnis*, viii-ix.

[103] K[arl] Kahlbaum, *Die Gruppierung der psychischen Krankheiten und die Einteilung der Seelenstörungen* (Danzig: A. W. Kafemann, 1863).

[104] Johann Christian Hoffbauer (1766–1827) war Professor der Philosophie in Halle. Mit Reil zusammen gab er heraus *Beyträge zur Beförderung einer Kurmethode auf psychischem Wege*, 2 Bde. (Halle: Curt, 1808–1812). Hoffbauers Hauptwerke waren: Johann Christoph Hoffbauer, *Untersuchungen über die Krankheiten der Seele und die verwandten Zustände* (Halle: Hahn, 1802); ders., *Psychologische Untersuchungen über den Wahnsinn, die übrigen Arten der Verrückung und die Behandlung derselben* (Halle: Hahn, 1807).

[105] Reil, *Rhapsodieen*, 300–301.

[106] Ebenda, 301.

Individuen der gegebenen Tierart. Arten der Geisteszerrüttungen sind spezifisch-eigentümliche Verletzungen der Dynamik des Gehirns, in Beziehung auf seine Funktion als Seelenorgan, die sich daher durch einen Inbegriff steter Symptome zu erkennen geben müssen. Die Symptome dieser Krankheiten müssen als gestörte Geschäfte der Seele erscheinen, sofern das Gehirn nach seinen verschiedenen Zuständen zur Hervorbringung dieser Geschäfte mitwirkt. Varietäten entstehen durch das Verhältnis der Verrücktheit zu ihren mannigfaltigen entfernten Ursachen, durch die Verschiedenheit ihrer Stärke und Dauer, durch ihre Zusammensetzung mit anderen Seelen- oder Körperkrankheiten und endlich durch die Modifikation, welche die abstrakt gedachte Krankheit erleidet, wenn sie als wirklich in einem Individuum gesetzt wird."[107]

[¶] Wir sehen aus diesen Stellen, daß Reil weit eher wie schon Gregor ausführte,[108] zur Annahme nur einer Geisteskrankheit neigte und daß man ihn nicht, wie Kahlbaum dies tat, als Schöpfer eines wenigstelligen Systems charakterisieren darf. Was Reil von der Systematik im Ganzen hält, geht aus folgendem Abschnitt hervor: „Bei diesen absoluten Mängeln unserer Erkenntnis begnüge ich mich damit, zum praktischen Gebrauch für Ärzte vorerst nur einige feste Punkte in das Chaos der Geisteszerrüttungen zu stellen. Ich will nämlich solche spezifisch eigentümlichen Zustände derselben aufsuchen, die in sich selbst soviel Charakter haben, daß sie als Arten in jedes System passen müssen, und sie durch Merkmale bezeichnen, durch welche sie überall von jedermann erkannt werden können [....] Als Arten der Verrücktheit setze ich vorerst den fixen Wahn, die Wut, die Narrheit und den Blödsinn."[109] Ähnlich der hier von Reil in seinen Rhapsodien gegebenen Einteilung, jedoch losgelöster von starrer Systematik, ist die Einteilung andernorts,[110] wo Reil aufzählt]: 1. die Krankheiten des Gemeingefühls (Schmerz, Rheumatismus, Prosopalgie, Gicht, Taubheit der Glieder), 2. Krankheiten des äußeren Sinnes (Lichtscheu, nervöses Doppelsehen, schwarzer Star, Taubheit), 3. die Krankheiten des inneren Sinnes (Krankheit der Fantasie, des Gedächtnisses, der Aufmerksamkeit, des Bewußtseins) und endlich die Verrücktheiten, in welchen mehrere Vermögen der Seele zu gleicher Zeit ergriffen sind.

Weit wichtiger allerdings als diese eigentlich als Syndromlehre gedachte Einteilung und des durch sie hindurchschimmernden Abstractums der einen Krankheit „Verrücktheit" war für die Entwicklung der Zellerschen Lehre der von Reil anhand der Polarität von Gangliensystem und Cerebralsystem erdachte Entstehungsmechanismus der Verrücktheit, nach welchem das Gangliensystem primär und das Gehirn sekundär erkranke.[111] Reil sagt allerdings hierüber nichts dogmatisch aus. Er führt aber oft genug Beispiele dieser Art an: „Kurz, in allen den Geisteszerrüttungen,

[107] Ebenda, 299.

[108] Vgl. Gregor.

[109] Reil, *Rhapsodieen*, 302, 305.

[110] Reil, *Über die Erkenntnis*, xiii-xiv.

[111] Am deutlichsten ist die Lehre von der sekundären Erkrankung des Gehirns artikuliert in Reil, „Über die Eigenschaften".

die sich auf eine falsche Idee von dem Zustand des Körpers beziehen, scheint das Gemeingefühl eine Hauptrolle zu spielen, und als Reiz das Gehirn krank zu machen. Fast alle auf diesem Weg entstandenen Verrücktheiten führen eine Art von Melancholie bei sich.“[112] [Ferner]: „So hat die Tollheit ihren Zunder im Sonnengeflecht, erregt daselbst Brennen, Klopfen und Angst, bis die angehäufte Erregbarkeit in der Gestalt einer Aura zum Gehirn überschlägt, den Kranken aller Sinne beraubt, und zu gewaltsamen Handlungen treibt.“[113]

Auch zur Erklärung der Phänomene des tierischen Magnetismus wurde das Modell von der Polarität des Cerebral- und Gangliensystems mit Erfolg angewandt. Im magnetischen Schlaf, meinte Reil, sei die gesamte Lebenskraft vom Gehirn abgezogen und dem Gangliensystem zugeleitet, welches dadurch die Führung übernehme und in diesem Zustand auch als Erkenntnisvermögen funktioniere.

Wir möchten diesen Abschnitt, welcher der Bedeutung Reils für die Geschichte der Einheitspsychose gewidmet ist, nicht abschließen, ohne nocheinmal darauf hinzuweisen, daß Reil der eigentliche Begründer der psychischen Kurmethode ist. Er tritt daher auch entschieden für die Trennung von Heil- und Detentionsanstalt ein. Er macht sich gleichermaßen Gedanken über die Organisation der Heilanstalten wie über die Einrichtung der Versorgungsanstalten für unheilbar Geisteskranke. Der deutschen Übersetzung von Dr. Josef Mason Cox „Praktische Bemerkungen über Geisteszerrüttung“ fügte Reil einen Anhang über „Die Organisation der Versorgungsanstalten für unheilbar Irrende“ an.[114] Wir sehen hier eine klare geschichtliche Entwicklungslinie, die mit Reil beginnt, über Autenrieth zu Albert Zeller führt, und die darauf abzielte, getrennte Heil- und Pflegeanstalten anzulegen. Leider endet diese Entwicklung mit Albert Zeller. Damerow (1798–1866) hatte 1840 ein kleines Büchlein mit dem Titel „Relative Verbindung der Irrenheil- und Pflegeanstalt“ in Leipzig erscheinen lassen.[115] Dieses Büchlein machte Schule. In der Folge wurden alle Anstaltsneubauten nach Damerows Vorschlag errichtet.

Wir wollen nun versuchen, kurz stichwortartig zusammenzustellen, welche Ideen Reils besonders auf Albert Zeller und damit auf die Entwicklung des Gedanken von der Einheitspsychose gewirkt haben:

1. Es gibt nur eine Geisteskrankheit.
2. Das Nervensystem hat zwei Pole, das Cerebralsystem und das Gangliensystem. In der Geisteskrankheit wird der cerebrale Pol häufig sekundär befallen.
3. Im magnetischen Schlaf übernimmt das Gangliensystem die Führung von dem im Wachszustand herrschenden Cerebralsystem.

---

[112] Reil, *Über die Erkenntnis*, 302.

[113] Reil, „Über die Eigenschaften,“ 248.

[114] Johann Christian Reil, „Anhang über die Organisation der Versorgungsanstalten für unheilbare Irrende,“ in *Joseph Mason Cox: Praktische Bemerkungen über Geisteszerrüttungen* (Halle: Renger, 1811).

[115] Heinrich Damerow, *Über die relative Verbindung der Irren-Heil- und Pflege-Anstalten in historisch-kritischer, so wie in moralischer, wissenschaftlicher und administrativer Beziehung. Eine staatsarzneiwissenschaftliche Abhandlung* (Leipzig: Otto Wigand, 1840).

4. Die psychische Kurmethode ist notwendig trotz der vorwiegend somatischen Verursachung der Geisteskrankheiten.
5. Heil- und Pflegeanstalt müssen getrennt errichtet werden.

Nach diesem wichtigen Rückblick auf Reil wollen wir unsere Aufmerksamkeit nun wieder Albert Zellers geistigem Werdegang widmen. Wir haben ihn als Studenten in Tübingen verlassen, und zwar bei der Abfassung seines handschriftlichen Versuchs über den Consens der verschieden Organe im Sommersemester 1824. Wir wissen weiter von ihm, und zwar aus dem vernichteten Briefwechsel mit Jacobi, daß er 1825 den Sonnenstein bei Pirna besuchte. Er schrieb später: „Die erste teutsche Heilanstalt, die dieses Namens würdig war und die von Frankreich erhaltenen Impulse in sicherer und gründlicher und vollkommener Weise fortpflanzte, entstand auf dem Sonnenstein im Königreiche Sachsen unter der Leitung des trefflichen Dr. Pienitz und seiner Gattin, und der speziellsten und rühmlichsten Obsorge des edlen Ministers von Nostiz und Jänkendorf, der sich damit unsterbliche Verdienste um die leidende Menschheit erwarb; besonders da er in Colditz, neben der Heilanstalt auf dem Sonnenstein, ein wahres Ideal von Pflegeanstalt unter der Leitung des an Geist und Gemüth gleich ausgezeichneten Dr. Hayner erschuf.“[116]

Wir müssen diesem Hinweis folgen und prüfen, ob auch vom Sonnenstein sich wesentliche Einflüsse auf Albert Zellers Entwicklung herleiten. Pienitz (1772–1853), der erste Direktor der 1811 eröffneten Anstalt Sonnenstein, war Schüler von Esquirol und Pinel. Christian August Fürchtegott Hayner (1775–1837) war ebenfalls unter Pinel und Esquirol zum Psychiater gebildet worden.[117] Von den beiden großen Franzosen gehen allerdings wenig Anregungen auf Zeller aus, wie wir später anhand des Tagebuchs der psychiatrischen Reise sehen werden. Größeren Einfluß hatte indessen der Geist und die Art der Irrenbehandlung, wie sie auf dem Sonnenstein und in Colditz gepflegt wurde, auf den jungen, für Psychiatrie interessierten Mann.[118] Hayner hatte 1817 in Form eines Katechismus die Grundsätze einer menschlichen Behandlung der Irren eindringlich abgehandelt. Er ließ, wie später Zeller, von den mechanischen Beschränkungsmitteln nur die Zwangsjacke gelten. Obwohl Reil noch durchaus an die heilsame Wirkung einer körperlichen Züchtigung im richtigen Augenblick geglaubt hatte, schrieb Hayner in seinem Büchlein: „Verflucht sei also von nun an jeder Schlag, der einen Elenden trifft aus dieser bejammernswürdigsten Klasse der Leidenden!“[119] Von B. Gudden (1824–1886), dem Schwiegersohn von Maximilian Jacobi, einem Schüler Rollers

[116] A[lbert] Zeller, „Irrenanstalten, Irrenhäuser,“ in *Allgemeine Encyclopädie der Wissenschaften und Künste*, hg. von J. S. Ersch und J. G. Gruber (Leipzig: Brockhaus, 1845), 138.

[117] [Zu Hayner, vgl. Gerhart Zeller (Hg.), *Albert Zellers medizinisches Tagebuch*, Bd. 2, 17–18].

[118] [Zu Sonnenstein und Colditz, vgl. Gerhart Zeller (Hg.), *Albert Zellers medizinisches Tagebuch*, Bd. 1, 195–205, 209 und Bd. 2, 170 f. Um den Einfluß von Sonnenstein und seinem ersten Direktor Pienitz zu unterstreichen, beschreibt G. Zeller die Winnenthaler Anstalt als „Ableger des Sonnensteins“. Ebenda, Bd. 2, 171].

[119] Christian August Fürchtegott Hayner, *Aufforderung an Regierungen, Obrigkeiten und Vorsteher der Irrenhäuser zur Abstellung einiger schweren Gebrechen in der Behandlung der Irren* (Leipzig: Göschen, 1817), 35.

und einem aufrichtigen Verehrer Albert Zellers wissen wir, daß er in seinen Vorlesungen in jedem Jahr das Büchlein von Hayner vorwies und dabei den Verfasser als den ersten deutschen Irrenarzt ehrte, der eine menschliche Behandlung der Geisteskranken begründet und durchgeführt hatte.

1826 verfaßte Albert Zeller dann in Tübingen seine Doktorarbeit, und zwar bei dem Botaniker G. Schübler (1737–1834). Das Thema der Arbeit lautet: „Untersuchungen über die Einwirkung verschiedener Stoffe des organischen und anorganischen Reiches auf das Leben der Pflanzen."[120] Hätte es noch eines Beweises bedurft, welch großen Einfluß Autenrieth auf Albert Zeller hatte, so wäre er mit dieser Arbeit leicht zu erbringen. Zeller untersucht die Wachstumsverhältnisse verschiedener Pflanzen nach Zuführung von giftigen und ungiftigen Stoffen. Von den Ergebnissen dieser zahlreichen Experimente war ihm selbst wohl dies am wichtigsten, daß Giftpflanzen durch ihr eigenes Gift geschädigt werden. Das Fontanasche Gesetz, nach welchem giftige Tiere immun gegen ihr eigenes Gift sein sollen, wurde so, wenigstens für die Pflanzen, widerlegt. Albert Zeller vergleicht die Giftstoffe der Pflanzen mit den Auswurfstoffen der tierischen Körper, welche schädlich wirken, wenn sie daran gehindert werden, nach außen abzugehen. Wie wir wissen, ist dies ein Grundproblem der Autenriethschen Pathologie.

Georg Andreas Reimer und sein Kreis

1827 tritt Albert Zeller dann nach abgeschlossenem Studium in Tübingen seine zweite wissenschaftliche Reise an; sie führt ihn nach Berlin. Durch Zufall wurde er auf der Reise nach Berlin mit der Frau des Berliner Verlegers Georg Andreas Reimer bekannt. Reimers Haus öffnete sich ihm. Was war das aber für ein Haus! Schon äußerlich imponierend – hatte doch Reimer 1815 das stattliche Sackensche Palais in der Wilhelmstraße Nr. 73, in welchem sich später das Reichspräsidentenpalais befand, erworben. Reimers Haus und Verlag wurden zum Brennpunkt der Berliner Spätromantik. Schleiermacher wohnte die letzten 17 Jahre seines Lebens im Hause Reimers. Ernst Moritz Arndt fand während seiner Verfolgung durch Napoleon I als Deutschlehrer Alemand bei Reimer Unterschlupf. Fichte, Steffens, Tieck, Novalis, Kleist, Arndt, Fouqué, Jean Paul, die Gebrüder Grimm, Humboldt, Ritter ließen Teile ihrer Werke durch Reimer verlegen. 1801 erschienen die berühmten Schleiermacherschen Monologe im Reimerschen Verlag. Georg Andreas Reimer, der 1776 in Greifswald als Sohn eine Schiffers und Bierbrauers geboren wurde, war dazu voll echten Kunstsinnes. Er brachte eine Sammlung von 2000 Gemälden zusammen, die nach seinem Tode 1842 versteigert wurden und die seither einen wesentlichen Bestandteil der Berliner Museen bilden. Mit Peter Cornelius war er befreundet. Er verlegte dessen Illustrationen zu den Nibelungen und zum Faust. Die

[120] A[lbert] Zeller, „Untersuchungen über die Einwirkung verschiedener Stoffe des organischen und unorganischen Reichs auf das Leben der Pflanzen" (Medizinische Dissertation, Universität Tübingen, 1826).

Handzeichnungen zu den Nibelungen gingen aus Reimers Besitz in das Städelsche Kunstinstitut in Frankfurt am Main über. Caspar David Friedrichs „Klosterfriedhof im Schnee" (1819) befand sich länger im Besitz der Familie. Dies alles mag wohl nur ungefähr die Fülle der Bildungseindrücke charakterisieren, welche auf den jungen Arzt Albert Zeller einströmten, vor allem, wenn man die Persönlichkeit Georg Andreas Reimers hinzunimmt. Fouqué und Arndt schilderten ihn als einen rührigen und erfolgreichen Geschäftsmann, als einen aufrichtigen tapferen Patrioten im Krieg und Frieden, der seinen Verlag, einen der größten der damaligen Zeit, ebenso mit patriarchalischer Festigkeit und Würde regierte, wie seine große Familie.

Zeller ließ sich kräftig von diesen Eindrücken berühren. Ein Tagebuch, im Dezember 1827 begonnen, zeigt uns den Bildungsprozeß von innen und gibt Rechenschaft über die Lektüre dieses Zeitabschnitts.[121] Wir finden vor allem erwähnt Bichats Werk über Tod und Leben, Schleiermachers Dogmen, Friedrich Heinrich Jacobis Werke. Daneben machte Zeller, der an der Universität immatrikuliert war, galvanische Experimente an Tier und Pflanzen, und zwar ausdrücklich nach Ritter (Johann Wilhelm Ritter, 1776–1810). Ritter war wohl der unglücklichste unter den romantischen Naturwissenschaftlern, genial und trunksüchtig zugleich. Auf ihn geht die Theorie zurück, daß ein beständiger Galvanismus den Lebensprozeß im Tierreich begleitet und daß die Lebenskraft wahrscheinlich mit diesem Galvanismus identisch sei. Wie wir hörten, stand auch Autenrieth dieser Lehre nahe.

In dieser fruchtbaren Berliner Zeit entstanden Zellers erste Gedichte, charakteristischerweise in der Form des Sinngedichts nach Art des Angelus Silesius (1624–1672). Dies weist auf den Einfluß Schleiermacher hin. Zeller wohnt mit Schleiermacher zusammen im Reimerschen Haus. Seine Werke hatte er schon früher und auch während der Berliner Zeit gelesen. Von Schleiermacher wurde er in der Dreifaltigkeitskirche in Berlin mit Reimers Tochter Marie getraut.

Albert Zeller und die Seherin von Prevorst

Der 25 Jahre alte Doktor der Medizin ließ sich nach seiner Heirat in Stuttgart nieder, wo damals auf 35000 Einwohner bereits 50 Ärzte kamen. Es war dies für die damalige Zeit viel und die Konkurrenz war entsprechend groß. Der Sohn von Johann Peter Frank beklagt bereits die Jatromanie, welche die jungen Leute erfaßt habe, und verlangt eine staatliche Regelung. Zellers Praxis ließ sich dennoch gut an. Im Tagebuch der psychiatrischen Reise im Jahre 1832 spricht er selbst von der unbegreiflich gesegneten Praxis in Stuttgart. Das wichtigste Ereignis dieser Stuttgarter Zeit lag allerdings nicht auf praktisch-medizinischem Gebiet, sondern auf wissenschaftlich-publizistischem.

[121] Albert Zeller, Studientagebücher.

Im Jahre 1830 ließ der erst 26 Jahre alte junge Arzt ein kleines blaues Büchlein von wenig mehr als 100 Seiten, anonym erscheinen über die Seherin von Prevorst.[122] Zeller mußte seine Kritik an Justinus Kerner, welche dieses blaue Büchlein enthält, sehr rasch zu Papier gebracht haben, da Kerners Seherin von Prevorst im selben Jahre – 1830 – erschienen war. Kritiken, die so rasch nach dem Erscheinen eines Buches in die Öffentlichkeit gehen, sind immer feurig und Ausdruck dafür, daß beim Lesen Überzeugungen verletzt wurden. Zeller war in Berlin ein anderer geworden. Schleiermachers Geist und der große Zug der Berliner Romantik, wie er sich im Hause Wilhelmstraße 73 konzentrierte, hatten ihn aus schwäbischer Enge herausgeführt. Der Zusammenstoß mit den schwäbischen Theosophen und Spiritisten konnte nicht ausbleiben.

Wir haben hier kurz auf Schleiermachers Religionsphilosophie einzugehen, um das Entsetzen Zellers verstehen zu können, angesichts der naiv-ernsthaften und kritiklosen Schilderung der Geistererscheinungen, welche Frau Hauffe, die „Seherin von Prevorst" angeblich hatte.[123] Frau Hauffes Geister waren mit vielen Merkmalen und Attributen ausgestattet, die sie aus dem Leben in das Mittelreich der Geister mitgebracht hatten. Sie trugen altfränkische Tracht, merkwürdige Hüte, Werkzeuge oder Gegenstände, die mit ihren Verbrechen zu tun hatten. Den einen erkannte Frau Hauffe stets daran, daß er schielte.

Daß gerade Schleiermacher so stark auf Albert Zeller wirken konnte, wird einmal verständlich, wenn man den beiden gemeinsamen Wurzelgrund überdenkt. Schleiermacher war als Pietist erzogen worden, und zwar in der Brüdergemeinde in Barby. Zellers tiefe Beziehung zum Pietismus haben wir geschildert. Es kann nicht unsere Aufgabe sein, die Schleiermachersche Religionsphilosophie hier ausführlich darzustellen; wir wollen uns auf die wesentlichen Grundzügen beschränken. Schleiermacher ist erklärter Antirationalist, er vertritt die absolute Selbstständigkeit des religiösen Bereichs von Moral und gelehrter philologischer Theologie. Durchaus pietistisch und mystisch zugleich, rückt er das religiöse Erleben in den Mittelpunkt seiner Betrachtungen. Seine Religionsphilosophie ist so überhaupt nicht Lehre von Gott, den er für absolut unerkennbar hält, sondern Lehre vom religiösen Gefühl. Religion ist Sache des Herzens, das „fromme Gefühl" läßt das Absolute unmittelbar inne werden. Das Verhältnis der endlichen Natur zum Unendlichen ist das der Abhängigkeit, eine Abhängigkeit die gleichbedeutend ist mit Umschlossensein, Geborgensein und Aufgehen im Absoluten. Dies ist es, was Schleiermacher „das Gefühl schlechthinniger Abhängigkeit" nennt. In ihm besteht das religiöse Gefühl, in ihm und nicht anderem das Wesen der Religion selbst. Nicolai Hartmann weist

[122] [Albert v. Zeller], *Das verschleierte Bild zu Sais oder die Wunder des Magnetismus von einem Freunde der Wahrheit* (Leipzig: Weidmann, 1830). [Vgl. hierzu ausführlicher Gerhart Zeller (Hg.), *Albert Zellers medizinisches Tagebuch*, Bd. 2, 24–57. Dort beschreibt Gerhart Zeller die Seherin von Prevorst als eine „Genie der Empathie". Ebenda, 25. Er vermutet ferner, daß es bei der Abfassung dieser Schrift „Absprachen" mit dem Theologen H. E. G. Paulus gegeben haben könnten. Ebenda, 28 und 31].

[123] [Über Zellers enge Beziehung zu Schleiermacher, vgl. auch Gerhart Zeller (Hg.), *Albert Zellers medizinisches Tagebuch*, Bd. 2, 56–62].

mit Recht darauf hin, daß in diesem Gefühl nun doch ein gewisses Wissen um das Wesen Gottes ist, wenn es sich auch in den Grenzen der allgemeinsten Bestimmungen hält. Der amor dei intellectualis Spinozas und das Allgefühl der deutschen Mystik klingen so durch Schleiermachers Lehren hindurch, wenn er Gott als das Unendliche charakterisiert, welches alle Dinge durchdringt und mit ihrer Totalität identisch ist. Schleiermachers Religionsphilosophie geht so in die pantheistische Metaphysik über, die fast alle philosophischen Systeme seiner Zeit beherrscht. Die Einheit des Lebensgefühls der Romantik drängt sich für Schleiermacher in der Religion zusammen. Schleiermacher hat so viele Berührungspunkte mit Novalis. Paul Kluckhohn zitiert Novalis ("Gott ist die Liebe. Die Liebe ist das höchste Reale – der Urgrund") und führt dazu aus: „Der Welt- und Lebensgrund, das Absolute, die letzte Einheit, die alles Leben als Entzweiung und Individualisierung aus sich entlassen hat und in letzter Synthese wieder in sich vereinigen wird – so könnte man die Gottes- und Weltauffassung des Novalis und der Romantik überhaupt formulieren. Damit" – so fährt Kluckhohn fort – „wäre zugleich die religiöse Begründung des romantischen Synthesestrebens gegeben als der Synthese von Allheit und Individualität (Schleiermacher), von Einheit und Fülle (Fr[iedrich] Schlegel), von Natur und Geist (Schelling und Novalis), von Menschheit und Gottheit und Leben und Tod (Novalis), von Naturalismus und Spiritualismus (Baader) usw."[124]

Wir können es jedenfalls als erwiesen hinnehmen, daß das starke Einheitsstreben, welches das Denken Albert Zellers beherrschte, im religiösen Bereich wurzelt, so wie es ihm von Schleiermacher erschlossen wurde. Wir legen Wert auf diese Ausführung, da es uns letztlich darum geht, die Zeller-Griesingersche Einheitspsychose vom Einheitsstreben der Romantik als die „romantische Einheitspsychose" abzuleiten.

Schleiermachers Denken hat aber noch weiter prägend auf Zellers Weltanschauung und Anthropologie gewirkt. Schleiermacher scheute sich nicht, den traditionellen Begriff einer göttlichen Kausalität wieder aufzunehmen. Wir fühlen uns abhängig von Gott, indem wir ihn als Weltgrund fühlen, das ist als letzte Ursache aller Dinge außer uns wie aller Akte in uns. Bindet so das religiöse Gefühl den Menschen an das Universum, so läßt ihn doch diese Teilhabe an ihm nicht verschwinden, sondern bedeutet als Hineinwachsen des voll entfalteten Individuums ins Absolute Steigerung. Schleiermachers Individualismus drängt ihn vom eigentlichen Pantheismus fort, welcher für die Individuen als solche keinen rechten Platz hat. Wir glauben mit Nicolai Hartmann, daß die Wurzel des Schleiermacherschen Individualismus nicht Leibnizens Monadengedanke, sondern vielmehr die altchristliche Vorstellung vom absoluten Wert der Einzelseele, welcher das Erlösungswerk gilt, hat. Daß dieses Hineinwachsen des Endlichen ins Absolute, wie es auf Erden schon als Gefühl des Einsseins mit Gott erlebt werden kann und das nach dem Tode vollendet wird, die Lehre von der persönlichen Unsterblichkeit aller Naivität und Kleinlichkeit entkleiden mußte, leuchtet ein.

[124] Paul Kluckhohn, *Das Ideengut der deutschen Romantik* (Tübingen: Niemeyer, 1953), 142.

Wer sich so stark in Schleiermachers Lehren, vor allem in seine Lehre von der Unsterblichkeit hineingelebt hatte, dem mußte die Hauffesche Geisterwelt ein rechtes Ärgernis sein. Albert Zeller konnte nicht anders, er mußte entgegnen, und schon der Titel seiner Schrift „Das verschleierte Bild zu Sais“ zeigte, aus welchem Gedankenkreis die Kritik kam, nämlich aus dem des Novalis und der Berliner Romantik.[125]

Nach dieser Klärung des Motivs und der weltanschaulichen Wurzel des blauen Büchleins ist der Inhalt selbst für unser gegenwärtiges Thema nicht von allzu großer Bedeutung. Zeller beginnt mit einem Abriß der normalen Psychologie: „Nur wer die *gerade* Linie kennt, kann die Abweichung der *schiefen* bestimmen, nur wer das *gesunde* Leben kennt, das *kranke* beurteilen, nur wer das *kranke* erkannt hat in seiner Gesetzmäßigkeit, erkennen, wo das *kranke* heraustritt aus seinem *Charakter*, aus seiner gesetzmäßigen *Eigentümlichkeit*.“[126] Daß diese Psychologie getragen sein mußte vom Geiste der Einheit und der Vorstellung von Gott als dem Urgrund alles Seins, ist nach dem Vorstehenden nicht anders zu erwarten. Stahls Gedanken von der Seele als dem belebenden Prinzip werden von Zeller in echt romantischer Weise gesteigert. Gott ist für Albert Zeller das belebende Prinzip und der Urgrund der Einheit. „Die Kraft des Geistes und des Lebens [sind] Eins, die Seele [baut] ihren Leib.“[127] Wer spürte nicht die Nähe zu Schleiermacher, wenn wir lesen: „daß ein Wesen voll unendlicher Kraft und Weisheit und Liebe aus eigener Machtvollkommenheit Alles geschaffen hat, was da ist, daß wir mit Allem, was da ist, nur in ihm leben, weben und sind.“[128] Wie Gott in seiner Schöpfung allgegenwärtig ist und überall ganz ist, so ist auch die schöpferische Kraft in uns in allen Teilen ganz und unzertrennt, nur in jedem Teile auf eine besondere Weise wirksam. Zeller bedarf so auch keines Vermittlers zwischen Geist und Körper, keiner Mittelkraft, keines Nervenäthers, der im Denken der Seherin eine solche überragende Rolle gespielt hatte und der zur Erklärung aller Absurditäten willig dienen mußte. „Bedürfen wir denn solcher Mittelglieder zur Erklärung des eigentlichen Wesens des Lebens, bedarf das Leben selbst derselben, um den Leib zu bauen, zu erhalten, zu regieren? Ist denn der Geist und der Stoff einander so ganz fremd, oder sind nicht beide von Einer Kraft, von Einem höchsten Willen für einander bestimmt und geschaffen, also dem Ursprung nach eins. Wollen wir mit Rätseln Rätsel lösen? Ist denn der Nervengeist[129] Vater, oder Sohn oder Bruder der Nerven? Ist nicht der Geist, ehe die Nerven da sind? Elektrische und magnetische Kräfte stehen im Dienste des Lebens, wer will, wer kann das leugnen? Aber die gesteigertste Elektrizität, der innigste kräftigste Magnetismus bringt noch lange kein Leben, nicht einmal das einfachste zustande. Sie erklären so wenig als die zu unserem Leben

[125] Albert Zeller, *Das verschleierte Bild zu Sais*.

[126] Ebenda, 1.

[127] Ebenda, 20.

[128] Ebenda, 3.

[129] [Schiller verwendet den Begriff *Nervengeist* in seiner Dissertation. Vgl. Schiller, „Philosophie der Physiologie“].

notwendige Luft das Leben selbst. Wieviele Kräfte auch zusammenwirken mögen in dem Einen Menschenleben, so sind sie doch alle zusammen dieses nicht, es geht bei ihnen zu Gaste, sie bei ihm, sie dienen ihm freundlich, und hüten wir uns, sie nicht aus ihrer Dienstbarkeit zu entlassen."[130] Auch die herrschende Vermögenspsychologie mit ihrer geläufigen Einteilung in Gefühl, Vorstellung und Begehren wird zu einer Einheit zusammengefaßt, Albert Zeller kennt keine getrennten Vermögen, sondern Grundtätigkeiten des einen Geistes. Zeller folgt Reil, wenn er den Grundrichtungen und Tätigkeiten gewisse Gebiete des Leibes zuweist, „sodaß dem geistigen scheinbaren Auseinandertreten der *Einen* Seelenkraft wirklich eine leibliche Scheidung und Begrenzung entspräche, ohne daß darum der Geist zu etwas Räumlichem, zu einem Nebeneinander würde, was nie der Fall sein kann, da er dann aufhörte, er selbst zu sein."[131] Ebenso sind die fünf Sinne nur Äußerungen einer wahrnehmenden Kraft, der Sinnenkraft des Geistes. Reils Cerebralsystem finden wir wieder, „wir fühlen es, daß die Sonne unseres freien denkenden Lebens in dem Gehirn leuchtet."[132] Das dem Gefühlsvermögen entsprechende Nervensystem ist das Ganglien- oder Knotensystem mit seinem Mittelpunkt, dem sympathischen Nervensystem. Das Gefühlsvermögen selbst wird unterteilt in eines für den eigenen leiblichen und unseren geistigen Gesamtzustand. Wir treffen so Reils Gemeingefühl wieder an. Dem Begehrungsvermögen wird Brust und Unterleib zugeordnet. Im Zustand des magnetischen Schlafes scheint das ganze Gehirn von der Lebenskraft verlassen und alles Leben in die Herzgrube gegangen zu sein. In der folge prägt Zeller dann den Begriff des „somnambulen Wahnsinns", an welchem Kerners Patientin, Frau Hauffe, die Seherin von Prevorst, leide. Zeller leitet diesen Begriff des somnambulen Wahnsinns so sorgfältig und interessant ab, und man hat sich später über Charcots hysterische Hypnosepatienten so ähnliche Gedanken gemacht, daß es uns erlaubt sein möge, den entscheidenden Abschnitt hier anzuführen. Zeller schreibt: „Das ganze Streben der Heilkraft geht zwar dahin, das *magnetische* Leben wieder zu einem *gewöhnlichen* wachen zurückzuführen, allein wie eine andere Krankheit in den verschiedenen Graden ihrer Entwicklung aufgehalten und unterbrochen werden kann, so kann es auch hier geschehen, wiewohl es etwas Seltenes ist, daß sich der magnetische Zustand ungewöhnlich und gegen sein inneres Entwicklungsgesetz in die Länge zieht, daß er seinen Charakter des Periodischen fast gänzlich verliert, die einzelnen Anfälle kaum mehr sich erkennen lassen, sondern ineinanderfließen unter sich und mit gewöhnlichem Schlafen und Wachen."[133] Zeller führt dann weiter aus, das geistige Bild einer solchen Kranken werde so mehr oder weniger zu einer Fratze. Durch magnetisches Schlafen und Wachen verwirrt, müsse die Somnambüle zuletzt eine Wahnsinnige werden. „Eine solche Unglückliche weiß dann nicht mehr, ob sie wacht, schläft oder träumt. Dazu gesellt sich dann leicht eine absichtliche, willkürliche Verlängerung dieses

[130] Ebenda, 24–25.

[131] Ebenda, 26.

[132] Ebenda, 32.

[133] Ebenda, 82.

Zustandes, wobei denn die Somnambüle gar nicht mehr somnambül ist; hieraus ist es denn auch zu erklären, daß gemeiniglich am Ende eines somnambülen Lebens so viel verschuldeter und unverschuldeter Wahn sich findet, wenn auch die erste Zeit des magnetischen Lebens dem ursprünglichen Charakter treu bleib. Zieht sich nun die magnetische Krankheit durch das ganze Leben eines Menschen hindurch auf diese Weise, wird gewöhnliches Wachen und somnambüles Wachen immer auf neue durcheinander geworfen, so muß Leib und Seele miteinander zu Grunde gehen und zum gänzlichen Verderben ausschlagen, was eigentlich zum Heile führen sollte. Ein solches gänzlich zerrissenes somnambüles Leben nun finden wir in der vorliegenden Geschichte der unglücklichen Frau Hauffe, auf die neben so vielen Mißhandlungen auch alle Qualen des Magnetismus fallen mußten."[134] Albert Zeller schließt sein Büchlein mit der Hoffnung, daß er mit diesem dem Aberglauben eine große und tiefe Grube gegraben habe. „Der Schleier der Isis ist nicht gehoben, die Pforten des Geisterreiches sind nicht gesprengt [....] Was uns lähmt, freudig auf dieser Welt zu wirken, ist Sünde [....] Lasset uns wirken, solange es Tag ist, denn es kommt die Nacht, wo Niemand wirken kann."[135]

Das Büchlein wurde rasch bekannt. Noch im selben Jahre 1830 ließ C. A. Eschenmayer, welcher mit Kerner zusammen die Frau Hauffe bis zu ihrem Tode am 5. August 1829 insgesamt 3 Jahre lang beobachtet hatte, eine Rechtfertigung erscheinen.[136] Das Buch mußte sich vorwiegend mit dem verschleierten Bild beschäftigen, dessen Verfasser in der Zwischenzeit bekannt geworden war. Eschenmayer schreibt über Zellers Büchlein: „Diese Broschüre scheint viel Glück gemacht zu haben, und der junge Verfasser scheint schon so im Stillen den Siegerkranz *gegen die Seherin von Prevorst* in Rechnung nehmen zu wollen! Denn sonst würde die neue Ankündigung im Intelligenzblatt des Morgenblattes kein so lautes Rühmen machen, ‚daß diese Schrift die unparteiischte und wahrste Beurteilung der Seherin sei, ohne welche sie gar nicht verstanden werden könne; wer diese lese, habe durchaus jene Beleuchtung nötig'."[137] Eschenmayer tadelt an Zeller in erster Linie dessen religiöse Grundansicht, von der er meint, daß sie zur absoluten Liebestheorie der heutigen Schule gehöre, welche alles, was die Evangelien an Vernunft und Moral in sich enthalten, in das eigene System hinübernehmen wolle. Er tadelt, daß Zeller den Nervenäther nicht anerkennen wolle und daß Zeller Seele und Geist nicht getrennt betrachte. Eschenmayer beruft sich dabei auf Heinroth. Zeller habe, so meint Eschenmayer, den Somnambulismus und Magnetismus in seiner tieferen Bedeutung nicht erkannt. Im selben Buche nimmt auch Kerner selbst zum verschleierten Bild zu Sais Stellung. Er macht kein Hehl daraus, daß er den Verfasser kennt und beginnt so seine Erwiderung echt Kernerisch: „Es ist eine gewisse Wahrheit, daß alle die Herren vom A bis zu Z, die jetzt die

[134] Ebenda, 82 f.

[135] Ebenda, 168 f.

[136] Carl A. Eschenmayer, *Mysterien des innern Lebens: erläutert aus der Geschichte der Seherin von Prevorst* (Tübingen: Zu-Guttenberg, 1830).

[137] Carl A. Eschenmayer, „Das verschleierte Bild zu Sais," in *Mysterien des innern Lebens: erläutert aus der Geschichte der Seherin von Prevorst* (Tübingen: Zu-Guttenberg, 1830), 159.

Geschichte der Frau H[auffe] aus der Ferne mit ihren vorgefaßten Meinungen zu beurteilen unternehmen, für mich nahe Gestandenen von ihr nicht anders sprechen können, als wie Blinde von der Farbe."[138] Kerner fährt dann weiter fort, es tue ihm leid, daß er von seinen Kritikern, vor allem auch von dem einen sehr lieben, den er nicht kenne, von dem er aber nur gutes höre, dem Verfasser jenes blauen Büchleins „Das verschleierte Bild zu Sais" mißverstanden worden sei. Er, Kerner, sei der Frau Hauffe nicht kritiklos verfallen gewesen. Hierüber werde sich der Verfasser des blauen Büchleins freuen und sein Büchlein rot werden, daß es sich ganz anders verhalten habe. Er spricht dann direkt davon, daß Herr Z. der Wahrheit das kleine Opfer hätte bringen sollen, nach Weinsberg zu fahren, um mit den Ärzten und der Familie der Frau Hauffe persönliche Bekanntschaft zu machen. Er hätte dabei seine Zweifel und seine Ansichten offen äußern können. Er wäre dadurch der Wahrheit näher gekommen.

Wir müssen an dieser Stelle Eschenmayers kurz gedenken. Er gehört zum Bild, und er war einer der akademischen Lehrer Albert Zellers.

Adolf Karl August Eschenmayer, geboren am 4. Juli 1768 zu Neuenbürg im Schwarzwald, gestorben am 17. November 1857 in Kirchheim/Teck, ist wohl die absonderlichste Gestalt, welche je dem Tübinger Lehrkörper angehört hat. Sein Vater war Oberamtspfleger in Neuenbürg. Er selbst sollte Kaufmann werden, entzog sich dieser Laufbahn jedoch und studierte Medizin an der Hohen Carlsschule in Stuttgart. Der Einfluß Kielmeyers[139] auf ihn war ein bedeutender. Bald schloß er sich auch an Schelling an. Wie Kuno Fischer hervorhebt, hatte er durch die Differenzen, welche sich zwischen ihm und Schelling ergaben, einen bewegenden Einfluß auf Schellings Lehre. Schelling dankte ihm dafür auf besondere Art. Im ersten Heft von Schellings Zeitschrift „Allgemeine Zeitschrift in Deutschland für Deutsche" (1813) führt er Eschenmayer auf eine Weise ab, die Kuno Fischer wohl mit Recht perfide nennt.[140] Es scheint überhaupt Eschenmayers Schicksal gewesen zu sein, Zielscheibe des Spottes zu werden. Die Ursache hierfür lag wohl in seiner durchaus unharmonischen Persönlichkeit, deren widerstrebende Komponenten sich zu keiner Einheit zusammenschließen konnten. Auf der einen Seite war er ein mathematisch begabter, exakter Mann, der, an Kants Philosophie geschult, an Schellings Naturphilosophie vor allem die fehlende mathematische Untermauerung tadelte. Auf der anderen Seite war er mystisch-spiritistisch und der Erforschung und Deutung des Magnetismus verfallen. Er blieb allerdings auch hierbei zunächst noch

138 [Justinus Kerner, „Zur Geschichte des Geistersehens der Seherin von Prevorst," in *Mysterien des innern Lebens: erläutert aus der Geschichte der Seherin von Prevorst*, hg. von Carl A. Eschenmayer (Tübingen: Zu-Guttenberg, 1830), 84].

139 [Gemeint ist der Biologe und Tübinger Professor sowie späterer Direktor der kgl. wissenschaftlichen Sammlungen in Stuttgart, Carl Friedrich Kielmeyer (1765–1844). Vgl. Gerhart Zeller (Hg.), *Albert Zellers medizinisches Tagebuch*, Bd. 2, 63–64.]

140 [Vgl. Kuno Fischer, *Schellings Leben, Werke und Lehre*, 4th ed. (Heidelberg: Winter, 1923), 162.]

kritisch und erkenntnistheoretisch.[141] Später in seinem mit Kieser gegründeten *Archiv für den tierischen Magnetismus* geriet er dann immer tiefer hinein in unbegrenzte Spekulationen. Auf diesem Wege traf er sich mit Kerner, welcher ihn zur Beobachtung und Deutung der Seherin nach Weinsberg bat. 1811 war Eschenmayer außerordentlicher Professor für Medizin und Philosophie in Tübingen geworden. Er verfaßte 1814 eine Abhandlung spekulativer Art über die Philosophie in ihrem Übergang zur Nichtphilosophie. 1815 trat er dafür mit einer medizinischen Schrift über die Epidemie des Krupps hervor, 1816 mit einer Arbeit über Allopathie und Homöopathie. 1816 erschien sein Lehrbuch der Psychologie, welches 1822 sogar eine zweite Auflage erlebte. 1836 schied er freiwillig aus dem Lehramte aus und zog sich nach Kirchheim an der Teck zurück. Er lebte dort einsam und eingezogen; die mystisch-spekulative Seite gewann ganz die Oberhand. 1836 erschien seine Charakteristik des Unglaubens, des Halbglaubens und Vollglaubens, 1841 seine Grundzüge einer christlichen Philosophie. Einen Einfluß auf Albert Zeller konnten wir nicht nachweisen, obgleich Eschenmayer in Tübingen auch Vorlesungen über Psychiatrie gehalten hatte, welche der junge Zeller sicher hörte und die sicherlich für ihn eine gewisse Versuchung bedeuteten. Wir möchten den Eintrag im Tagebuch „Vor dem Mystizismus habe ich mich sehr zu hüten" auch als Zeichen einer Auseinandersetzung des jungen Studenten mit Eschenmayer werten.

Es ist sicher dem Aufsehen, welches *Das verschleierte Bild zu Sais* gemacht hat, zu verdanken, daß Albert Zeller 1832 auf die Direktorenstelle der neu gegründeten Irrenheilanstalt im Schloß Winnenthal, nahe dem Städtchen Winnenden bei Stuttgart, berufen wurde.[142] Seinem eigenen Vorschlage und den Gepflogenheiten der Zeit entsprechend wurde dem erst 26 Jahre alten Doktor die Auflage gemacht, ein Jahr lang durch Europa zu reisen und die wichtigsten psychiatrischen Anstalten und Lehrer des Faches aufzusuchen.

Wir verdanken dieser Reise das umfangreiche, schon oben erwähnte Tagebuch, dessen Inhalt bisher so gut wie unbekannt war, und zwar aus den eingangs erwähnten Gründen. Dieses Tagebuch völlig auszuschöpfen, würde den Umfang der Arbeit sprengen und vieles nicht zum engeren Thema Gehörendes bringen. Es soll an dieser Stelle daher nur daraufhin durchgesehen werden, welche Einflüsse aus der zeitgenössischen Psychiatrie, vor allem aus der englischen und französischen, auf Albert Zeller nachweisbar gewirkt haben und damit die Entwicklung des Gedanken der Einheitspsychose beeinflußten.

---

[141] Vgl. Carl A. Eschenmayer, *Versuch die Geseze magnetischer Erscheinungen aus Säzen der Naturmetaphysik mithin a priori zu entwickeln* (Tübingen: Heerbrandt, 1798).

[142] [Vgl. Gerhart Zeller (Hg.), *Albert Zellers medizinisches Tagebuch*, Bd. 1, 23 f. Kreuser kommt zum gleichen Schluß. Vgl. [Heinrich] Kreuser, „Zu Albert Zellers Gedächtnis," *MCBlWÄV* 74.45 (1904): 936].

Psychiatrische Reise 1832–1833

Die Reise begann am 20.2.1832 und führte zunächst nach Heidelberg, wo 1826 an unglücklichem Ort eine Anstalt für 200 Kranke eingerichtet worden war.[143] Der Direktor dieser Anstalt war Hofrat Friedrich Groos (1768–1852), der schon 1814 Physikus am Pforzheimer Irren- und Siechenasyl gewesen war und der 1826 mit seinen Kranken nach Heidelberg umzog.[144] Auch Groos war Carlsschüler, und zwar zunächst Jurist. Er studierte später Medizin in Freiburg. Er war ein interessanter Mann, ein scharfer methodischer Denker, dessen Bedeutung für die theoretischen Grundlagen der Psychiatrie besonders von Gruhle gewürdigt wurde.[145] Albert Zeller vermerkt über ihn, den er schon von einer früheren Reise, wohl von der nach dem Sonnenstein, her kannte, er, Zeller, habe Groos frischer und lebenskräftiger gefunden als früher, er scheine allerdings für das Detail der Anstalt kein besonderes Interesse zu haben, so mächtig ihn die Wissenschaften interessierten. Umso tätiger und tüchtiger sei Dr. Roller, der so alles in allem sein müsse. Dieser Eintrag ist charakteristisch für die ganze Betrachtungsweise Albert Zellers. Nur der Irrenarzt hat seine volle Achtung, der sich unermüdlich und intensiv mit seinen Kranken beschäftigt. Die Wissenschaftler und Theoretiker beeindrucken ihn wenig. Zeller war und blieb in erster Linie Arzt, Systematik war ihm niemals ein tiefes inneres Anliegen.

Mit dem zweiten Arzt der Heidelberger Anstalt, C. F. W. Roller, geboren am 11.1.1802 und gestorben kurz nach Zeller, am 4.1.1878 – Zeller war an Weihnachten 1877 gestorben –, blieb Zeller zeitlebens verbunden.[146] Rollers Werk, die 1842 eröffnete Badische Anstalt Illenau, galt als Musterbeispiel einer relativ verbundenen Heil- und Pflegeanstalt. Da Zeller, wie wir wissen, zeitlebens für die Trennung der Anstalten war, gab es durchaus Differenzen zwischen den beiden Männern; trotz allem fühlte man sich verbunden, vor allem durch den gemeinsamen Freund Maximilian Jacobi, der Roller und Zeller viele Jahre hindurch besuchte und durch seinen Briefwechsel mit beiden Verbindung hielt.

Auch mit Heinrich Eberhard Gottlob Paulus traf Zeller in Heidelberg zusammen.[147] Merkwürdigerweise enthält das Tagebuch keinerlei Hinweise auf die gemeinsame Kritik an der Seherin von Prevorst. Zeller rühmt den Ernst und den Scharfsinn an Paulus, er tadelt aber: „Es gebricht ihm aber gänzlich eine philosophische Beschauung der Welt, sowenig er etwas von dem Geheimnis der Seele mit

[143] [Zu Heidelberg, vgl. Gerhart Zeller (Hg.), *Albert Zellers medizinisches Tagebuch*, Bd. 1, 34–40].

[144] [Zu Groos, vgl. ebenda, Bd. 2, 9–10].

[145] Vgl. Hans Walter Gruhle, „Geschichtliches," in *Handbuch der Geisteskrankheiten*, hg. von Oswald Bumke (Berlin: Springer, 1932), 4–5.

[146] [Zu Roller und Illenau, vgl. Gerhart Zeller (Hg.), *Albert Zellers medizinisches Tagebuch*, Bd. 2, 7–9].

[147] [Zu Paulus, vgl. ebenda, 19–21].

Gott weiß und dem Bunde Gottes mit der Natur [….][148] Sein eigentliches Leben ist auch nur eine dürre Heide, und er hat keine christlich schöne Gegenwart um sich geschaffen."[149]

In Frankfurt am Main gilt der Besuch dem Kastenhospital, das 1683 erstmals erwähnt und 1785 neu eröffnet worden war.[150] Es hatte damals 84 Kranke. Ein Nichtarzt, der Verwalter Antoni, leitete es. Professor Varrentrapp war Physikus der Anstalt. Er besuchte diese jedoch nur gelegentlich. Er ist übrigens der Vorgänger von Heinrich Hoffmann (1809–1894). Antonis Name hat die Geschichte nicht bewahrt, obwohl es schlechthin vorbildlich war, was er an seinen Kranken tat. Zeller schildert ein Musterbeispiel der familiaren Verpflegung. „Antoni lebt mit seiner Familie ganz unter den Irren, beständig sind einige auf seinem Zimmer, was ihnen als eine äußerst große Gunst erscheint, sowie ein Ausschluß davon, durch ein unartiges Betragen veranlaßt, ihnen fast die höchste Strafe scheint."[151] Bemerkenswert ist auch Antonis Ausspruch, den uns Zeller bewahrt, der Unterschied zwischen einer Irrenanstalt und einem Gefängnis bestehe darin, daß die Irren nach außen, die Sträflinge aber nach innen geführt werden müßten. Zeller trägt in Frankfurt in sein Tagebuch ein: „Autenrieths Bemerkung nicht bestätigt, daß alle Irren zu betrügen versuchen."[152]

Von Frankfurt ging die Reise nach Eberbach, wo 1815 in einem Teil der Abtei Eberbach eine Landesirrenanstalt mit 60 Pfleglingen geschaffen worden war.[153] Zeller rühmt an den Ärzten Dr. Windt, gestorben 1848, und Dr. Basting sowie dem Verwalter der Anstalt, einem Juristen namens Lindpaintner die milde moralische Behandlung, welche sich frei von allem Heinrothschen Terrorismus halte.

In Bonn wurde Ernst Moritz Arndt besucht, mit dem ja die Familie Reimer eng befreundet war. Zeller traf dann auch in Bonn mit Friedrich Nasse (1778–1821) in Gesellschaft zusammen.[154] „Nasse ist ein wahrhaft gebildeter, sublimer Geist, er philosophiert wie er nur spricht, und dichtet, wie er nur philosophiert, und eine Fülle historischen Wissens in allen Zweigen der Wissenschaft bis in die feinsten Gebiete der Theologie stehen ihm zu Gebote."[155] Die große Sympathie, welche aus diesen Zeilen spricht, war sicher die Frucht der persönlichen Begegnung. Allerdings bestand zwischen Zeller und Nasse, dem Begründer der somatischen Richtung der damaligen Psychiatrie, grundsätzliche Übereinstimmung. Reil war Nasses Gönner. Er schlug ihn 1810 für den Lehrstuhl der Geburtshilfe in Berlin vor, den Nasse allerdings nicht annahm. 1815 wurde er nach Halle berufen als Professor der

[148] [Gerhart Zeller überspringt an dieser Stelle folgenden Satz: „Er glaubt nicht an Gott und glaubt doch an einen Gott, aber keinen geoffenbarten, er ist darum noch ein Jude, der nicht einmal einen Messias erwartet, oder vielmehr ein Heide, der noch dem unbekannten Gott dient"].

[149] [Gerhart Zeller (Hg.), *Albert Zellers medizinisches Tagebuch*, Bd. 1, 39].

[150] [Zu Frankfurt, vgl. ebenda, 42–45].

[151] [Ebenda, 43].

[152] [Ebenda, 42].

[153] [Vgl. ebenda, 47 f].

[154] [Zu Nasse, vgl. ebenda, Bd. 2, 71–73].

[155] [Ebenda, Bd. 1, 49].

Heilkunde und Vorsteher des klinischen Krankenhauses. 1819 erfolgte sein Ruf nach Bonn. Nasse war Internist, und er hatte auf die Ärzte seiner Zeit einen großen Einfluß. Für die Psychiatrie wurde er als Gründer der ersten rein ärztlich geleiteten psychiatrischen Zeitschrift wirksam. Ab 1810 erschien sie als *Zeitschrift für psychische Ärzte*, ab 1820 als *Zeitschrift für psychische Ärzte mit besonderer Berücksichtigung des Magnetismus*, ab 1823 nannte sie sich *Zeitschrift für Anthropologie*, diese endete 1830. Nasses somatische Grundanschauung soll durch folgendes Zitat verdeutlicht werden: „Durch Krankheit des Körpers entsteht eine Verrückung des normalen Verhältnisses von Seele und Leib [...], Empfinden ist vom Körper bestimmt, Denken und Wollen von der Seele, bei Irren aber vom Körper."[156] Nasse hält sich an die alte Einteilung der hypokratischen Ärzte. Er teilt die Geisteskrankheiten ein in Amentia (Blödsinn), Tobsucht (Mania), Wahnsinn (Melancholia). Er hält noch ganz an der Reilschen Vorstellung vom Cerebral- und Gangliensystem, wie wir sie oben dargestellt haben fort.

Von Bonn führte der Weg nach Siegburg, wo im Januar 1825 eine Irrenheilanstalt in den Räumen der 1051 gestifteten Benediktinerabtei errichtet worden war. Als erster Direktor dieser Anstalt hatte man nach langem Hin und Her auf Grund eines Gutachtens von Langermann Karl Wigand Maximilian Jacobi (1775–1858) berufen.[157] Welche Bedeutung dieser Mann für Albert Zeller gewann, geht vielleicht am deutlichsten aus folgender Tagebuchnotiz hervor: „Den 10. April [1833] verließ ich Siegburg gerade am Geburtstag von Dr. Jacobi, wo die ganze treffliche Familie beisammen war. Ich schied mit bitteren Schmerzen von diesem Orte, wo mir so viel Liebe und Treue gezeigt worden war wie fast nirgends in der Welt. Wenn ich in Zukunft etwas leisten werde, so verdanke ich es hauptsächlich diesem Aufenthalt und dem vortrefflichen Jacobi."[158]

Maximilian Jacobi war und ist in der Tat eine der bemerkenswertesten Persönlichkeiten der deutschen und darüberhinaus der europäischen Psychiatrie. Schon wenige äußere Daten seines Lebens und ein flüchtig gezeichnetes Charakterbild vermögen diese Sonderstellung zu begründen. Wir verdanken die gründliche Kenntnis von Jacobis Leben und Denken in erster Linie Dr. Johannes Herting, dem verstorbenen Direktor der Anstalt Düsseldorf-Grafenberg.[159]

Maximilian Jacobis Vater war der als Philosoph und Freund Goethes bekannte Friedrich Heinroth Jacobi (1743–1819). F. H. Jacobi war in erster Linie Polemiker. Seine kritische Auseinandersetzung mit Kant und Spinoza haben befruchtend

---

[156] [[Franz] Sioli, „Friedrich Nasse, 1778–1851," in *Deutsche Irrenärzte: Einzelbilder ihres Lebens und Wirkens*, hg. von Theodor Kirchhoff (Berlin: Springer, 1921), 112].

[157] [Über Siegburg und Jacobi, vgl. Gerhart Zeller (Hg.), *Albert Zellers medizinisches Tagebuch*, Bd. 1, 50–69 und Bd. 2, 73–79].

[158] [Ebenda, Bd. 1, 68].

[159] [Vgl.] Johannes Herting, *Carl Wigand Maximilian Jacobi*; ders., „Die erste rheinische Irrenanstalt Siegburg: Eine geschichtliche Studie, unter Benutzung amtlicher Quellen zur 100-jährigen Wiederkehr ihres Eröffnungstages 1. Januar 1925," *Allgemeine Zeitschrift für Psychiatrie* (*AZP*) 81 (1925): 163–241; ders., „Maximilian Jacobi, 1775–1858," in *Deutsche Irrenärzte*, hg. von Theodor Kirchhoff, Bd. 1 (Berlin: Springer, 1921), 83–94.

gewirkt. Seine Briefe über „Die Lehre des Spinoza in Briefen an Moses Mendelsohn" (1785) haben eine Spinoza-Renaissance eingeleitet, obwohl Jacobi Spinozas Pantheismus als Atheismus mißverstand. Kants transzendentalen Idealismus verkannte er als Subjektivismus. In seiner Kritik an Kant stößt Jacobi dann zu den irrationalen Momenten der Erkenntnis vor. Wie in dem von der sinnlichen Anschauung unabtrennbaren Glauben die Realität der Welt, so wird in dem Glauben der Vernunft, der „intellektuellen Anschauung", der „inneren Offenbarung", Gottes Dasein erfaßt. Und diese innere Offenbarung Gottes, so meint F. H. Jacobi, mache das eigentliche Wesen des Menschen aus. In dieser religiösen Grundüberzeugung des von Jugend auf pietistisch-schwärmerisch veranlagten Mannes wurzelt die breite und äußerst heftige Polemik, die F. H. Jacobi in seinen späteren Schriften gegen Fichte und Schelling richtete, ebenso wie seine nahe und freundschaftliche Beziehung zu Schleiermacher. Im Vorwort zur 3. Auflage seiner „Reden über Religion" bedauert es Schleiermacher mit warmen Worten, daß er diese Auflage nicht mehr F. H. Jacobi habe vorlegen können; er, Schleiermacher, verdanke ihm vieles. Erinnern wir uns kurz, wie sehr sich Albert Zeller in Berlin mit dem Werk F. H. Jacobis beschäftigt hat, dann verstehen wir es, vor allem wenn wir noch erfahren, daß Ernst Moritz Arndt,[160] der Freund Georg Andreas Reimers, mit Maximilian Jacobi eng befreundet, mit welchen Erwartungen Albert Zeller nach Siegburg kam und daß die sofort geschlossene Freundschaft des viel älteren Maximilian Jacobi keinem Fremden zuteil wurde. Nur so ist die Schnelligkeit verständlich, mit welcher diese Freundschaft geschlossen wurde. Maximilian Jacobi war nämlich kein Mann, der auf Fremde spontan einen gewinnenden Eindruck machte. Er war dazu viel zu ernst, zu schweigsam und zu mühsam im sprachlichen und schriftlichen Ausdruck. Allerdings mußte seine tiefe und echte christliche Religiosität in Albert Zeller gleichgestimmte Saiten berühren. M. Jacobis Frau war eine Tochter von Mathias Claudius. Eine Schwester von Jacobis Frau hatte den Verleger Perthes, der mit G.A. Reimer gut bekannt, wenn nicht befreundet war, geheiratet. Die Freundschaft, welche der damals 55 Jahre alte Mann, der fast 30 Jahre lang nach einem wirklichen Beruf gesucht hatte und diesen erst mit der Ernennung zum Direktor in Siegburg mit 50 Jahren gefunden hatte, dem 26 Jahre alten Jüngling entgegenbrachte, war dauerhaft. Als sichtbares Zeichen dieser Freundschaft entstand ein Briefwechsel, dessen Umfang und Schriftwechsel wir oben angeführt haben. In diesen Briefen fehlte wirklich nichts von allem, was Jacobi erfüllte, bewegte, erschütterte und erfreute. All dies teilte er mit Zeller. Dazu kamen häufige Besuche Jacobis in Winnenthal (1834, 1838, 1843, 1846, 1847, 1850, 1851, 1852, 1854, 1856) und Besuche Zellers in Siegburg (1840, 1843, 1845, 1846, 1855) sowie gemeinsame Wanderungen. Es ist rührend, zu sehen, wie sehr sich M. Jacobi um den jüngeren Albert Zeller bemühte. Man muß den Eindruck gewinnen, als ob M. Jacobi in Zeller eine Art Ergänzung sah und suchte. Schon im ersten Briefe schreibt er: „Das Gefühl, wie wenig ich bin und vermag, verläßt mich überhaupt nie und ist mir zumal wieder in dieser letzten Zeit bei der Aufgabe, die mir gestellt ist,

[160] [Zu Arndt, vgl. Gerhart Zeller (Hg.), *Albert Zellers medizinisches Tagebuch*, Bd. 2, 70–71].

und den Pflichten, die ich zu erfüllen habe, äußerst qualvoll geworden."[161] Er bewunderte offen das gesellige Leben, das Zeller an seiner Anstalt in Winnenthal zu erwecken vermochte und schrieb einmal an ihn, er möchte am liebsten alle seine Kranken nach Winnenthal schicken, da sie es doch dort viel besser hätten und rascher genesen würden. Immer wieder mußte er Zeller mahnen, ihm zu antworten. Er wurde darüber nicht müde und nicht verstimmt. Man hat fast den Eindruck, daß Jacobi die im ganzen nicht unerheblichen Unterschiede in wissenschaftlichen Grundfragen zwischen ihm und Zeller einfach nicht sehen wollte.

Was Zeller in Siegburg so tief beeindruckte, war in erster Linie die patriarchalische Anstaltsführung durch M. Jacobi, der ein wohlwollender, strenger, gütiger und würdiger Vater seiner Kranken und seiner Hilfskräfte war und der sich unverdrossen um seine Kranken bemühte. Zeller schreibt im Tagebuch: „Ich habe hier oft Jacobi bewundert, mit welcher Aufrichtigkeit und Klugheit und Liebe er die Einwilligung der Kranken selbst für einen längeren Aufenthalt zu erhalten wußte, und dabei gesehen, welchen wohltätigen Einfluß gerade der dabei in den Kranken angefachte und siegreich bestandene Kampf in seinem Gemüt und in seinem Körper hervorbrachte, so daß das Beherrschen des ungestümen Verlangens nach Entlassung als das letzte Kriterium der Genesung angesehen werden könnte."[162] Man spürt aus diesen Zeilen unmittelbar etwas vom Geiste, der in Jacobis Anstalt herrschte, und man versteht, daß Siegburg die hohe Schule der deutschen Psychiatrie wurde.

Wissenschaftlich bestand von Anfang an zwischen Zeller und Jacobi keine Einheit, aber doch Übereinstimmung in vielen Punkten. Es ist allgemein bekannt, daß M. Jacobi entschiedener Somatiker war. Es gab für Jacobi keine Geisteskrankheit, sondern nur mit Tobsucht, Schwermut, Wahnsinn, Blödsinn, Delirium und Narrheit einhergehende körperliche Krankheiten. Die psychischen Krankheitsäußerungen waren für ihn nur Symptome. Er kannte nur symptomatische Geisteskrankheiten in unserm heutigen Sinne. Man hat von jeher vermutet, daß diese strenge Einseitigkeit weltanschaulich-religiöse Wurzeln habe. Maximilian Jacobi schrieb in seinem Hauptwerk[163]: „Der Umstand, daß die Anthropologie bei der Betrachtung der Seelenstörungen so lange entweder zu gar keiner Geltung gelangte, oder aber bei dieser Betrachtung, teils der Psychologie, Ethik und Theologie entlehnten Elementen, teils den Ergebnissen anatomisch-physiologischer Forschung von vorn herein untergeordnet und damit vermengt ward, [...] hat die Psychiatrie bis jetzt in ihren Fortschritten wesentlich aufgehalten."[164] – „In der Anthropologie, in ihrer nächsten Beziehung zum Seelenleben, lernen wir ihr psychisches Element im Verhältnisse zu ihrem somatischen Elemente nach Maßgabe ihrer gegenseitigen Durchdringung kennen."[165] – „Aus jenem organischen Vereine von anthropologisch-psychischen Eigenschaften und Tätigkeiten kann indessen nie allein ein

[161] [Herting, *Carl Wigand Maximilian Jacobi*, 149].

[162] [Gerhart Zeller (Hg.), *Albert Zellers medizinisches Tagebuch*, Bd. 1, 52].

[163] Maximilian Jacobi, *Die Hauptformen der Seelenstörungen in ihren Beziehungen zur Heilkunde* (Leipzig: Weidmann, 1844). Jacobi widmete das Buch seinen Freunden Albert Zeller und C. F. W. Roller.

[164] Ebenda, xxvi.

[165] Ebenda, xxvi.

humanes Seelenleben hervorgehen, sondern nur ein, dem thierischen analoges, psychisches. Zu jenem gehört der Seele göttliches Element, vermöge dessen sie, ein an sich einfaches, persönliches, selbstständiges, selbstbewußtes, mit angeschaffenen Ideen des Guten und Wahren begabtes Wesen erscheint, welches sein Leben, unter den anthropologischen Bedingungen, in die es sich versetzt findet, als ein zur Freiheit bestimmtes und zur Freiheit, zu Gott anstrebendes, selbst mächtig führt."[166] – „Der Organismus wird dabei in einer gewissen Weise seelisch, indem die Seele ihn in einer ähnlichen Weise beherrscht, wie der tondichtende Künstler sein Instrument, und der menschliche Geist steht zu demselben in einem analogen Verhältnisse wie jener zu diesem. Denn auch das Instrument – die Cremonageige, die Flöte – kann durch den Künstler in einem gewissen Sinne veredelt werden. Je länger und unausgesetzter er nur reine Töne und Harmonien auf demselben hervorruft, um so mehr steigert sich die Fähigkeit des Instruments für solche Hervorrufung. Das Instrument kann aber auch durch den Künstler vernachlässigt, oder, ohne seine Schuld zerstörenden Einflüssen unterliegend, verderben und verfallen, so daß der Tondichter dasselbe für die Darstellungen seiner Dichtungen nicht mehr gebrauchen kann aber der dichtende Geist lebt fort, auch wenn er sich seiner Umgebung durch die Töne seines Instruments nicht mehr kund geben kann, und was in reinen Harmonien aus ihm hervorging, gehört, verhallte es auch für diese Welt, bleibend dem ewigen Reiche des Schönen an."[167]

Wir sehen Maximilian Jacobi als entschiedenen Vertreter eines leib-seelischen Dualismus am Substanzbegriff der Seele festhalten. Substanz aber ist einfach selbstständig, unzerstörbar und damit auch nicht erkrankbar. Nur weil Maximilian Jacobi diesen Seelenbegriff hatte, mußte er Somatiker werden. Wilhelm Griesinger, der Scharfsinnige, Kühle, legt dann auch in seiner Kritik zu Maximilian Jacobis Hauptformen[168] alle Mängel dieser Auffassung schonungslos dar. Jacobi mußte der Gefahr einer somatischen Spekulation und Hypostasierung erliegen, zumal seine allgemein-pathologischen Grundsätze – ein aus Erregungstheorie und alter Humoralpathologie gemischter Eklektizismus, jedoch mit sichtlichem Bestreben der Berücksichtigung der pathologischen Anatomie – keineswegs geeignet waren, alle Fragen körperlicher Krankheit zu klären, wie Griesinger mit Recht ausführt. Jacobi mußte auch Gefahr laufen, psychische Einflüsse zu übersehen, er mußte eine scharfe Grenze zwischen psychischer Gesundheit und Krankheit ziehen, und Griesinger vermutet, daß er, um seine wirksame und gründliche psychische Behandlung durchführen zu können, eigentlich seine Grundsätze vergessen mußte. Griesinger weist mit Recht darauf hin – und er ist in diesem Punkte wohl ganz das Sprachrohr seines Lehrers Albert Zeller -, daß die meisten Schwierigkeiten in Jacobis System

---

[166] Ebenda, xxvii.

[167] Ebenda, xxvii-xxviii.

[168] [Wilhelm] Griesinger, „[Rezension von] M. Jacobi: *Die Hauptformen der Seelenstörungen, in ihren Beziehungen zur Heilkunde nach der Beobachtung geschildert.* Erster Band: Die Tobsucht," *Archiv für physiologische Heilkunde* 3 (1844): 278–296.

verschwinden würden, wenn man mit dem Satze der Einheit von Leib und Seele Ernst machen würde; zum Beispiel würde dann auch der Satz der somatischen Theorie, daß überall, wo Irresein vorhanden ist, das heißt abnorme psychische Erscheinungen stattfinden, auch ganz sicher eine Erkrankung stattfindet, sich für immer von selbst verstehen.

Griesinger hat, scharfsinnig wie er war, den springenden Punkt aufgedeckt. Jacobi ist Dualist, Zeller idealistischer pantheistischer Monist. Es ist wirklich ein unersetzlicher Verlust für die Geschichte der Psychiatrie, das Zeller-Jacobis Briefwechsel unveröffentlicht vernichtet wurde. Man hätte aus diesen Briefen der beiden Freunde tiefere Einsicht in die beidseitigen Grundsätze gewinnen können.

Wir folgen Zellers Reiseroute, die jetzt nach Berlin führt. Am 8. Juni trifft Zeller dort ein. Er besuchte dort vor allem die Irrenabteilung der Charité, welche damals noch sehr ungenügend untergebracht war. Geleitet wurde diese Abteilung von Dr. Karl Wilhelm Ideler (1795–1860).[169] Ideler gehörte bekanntlich der psychischen Richtung der damaligen Psychiatrie an, ja er war mit dem älteren Johann Christian August Heinroth (1773–1843) der Hauptexponent dieser Richtung. Da die Namen Ideler und Heinroth so oft in einem Atemzug genannt werde, glaubte man ein Lehrer-Schüler-Verhältnis zwischen den beiden als gegeben annehmen zu können. Der Sohn Idelers hat sich mit Recht widersetzt und darauf hingewiesen, daß Karl Wilhelm Ideler allein Schüler Langermanns gewesen sei.[170] Unser Tagebuch bestätigt diese Auffassung voll und ganz, und es ist überhaupt in diesem Teil so unmittelbar und frisch, daß wir es im Auszug wiedergeben wollen. „Dr. Ideler, der Übersetzer von E. Stahls *Theoria medica vera*,[171] ist seit einigen Jahren Dirigent dieser Station, ein Mann voll stumm glühenden Eifers, der aber auf eine zum Teil sehr beschränkte, einseitige Weise sein oberstes Prinzip, daß fast alle Geisteskrankheiten aus Leidenschaften hervorgehen und durch diese erhalten werden, geltend machen will und an ein körperliches Bedingtsein der Seelenstörungen zum Unterschied von bloß leidenschaftlichen Zuständen nicht glaubt. Er verwirft sogar eine Unterscheidung als krass und materiell, indem er zwar im Allgemeinen bei einigen Krankheiten der Seele auch körperliche Ursachen annimmt, aber durchaus ärztlich im Leben keine Anwendung dieser Erkenntnis macht – nur das Eine, das Leiden der Seele, immer im Auge haltend. Selten wendet er darum Medizin an, wo nicht eine besondere Indikation laut schreit. Sein Hauptmittel ist eine strenge Pädagogik, mit Angst und Zittern müssen die Kranken meist in der ersten Zeit zu sich gebracht werden, und eine Subordination aller ihrer Gedanken, Gefühle und Begehrungen wird von ihnen verlangt, wie sie glücklicherweise nicht in der Hand eines Menschen stehen kann. Der Kranke muß zur Erkenntnis seines Zustandes, zur Erkenntnis seiner in diesem durch seine Schuld herbeigeführten Zustande

[169] [Über Berlin und Ideler, vgl. Gerhart Zeller (Hg.), *Albert Zellers medizinisches Tagebuch*, Bd. 1, 69–71 und Bd. 2, 81–86].

[170] [Carl Ludwig Ideler, „Carl Wilhelm Ideler und seine Stellung in der Entwicklung der Psychiatrie," *AZP* 51 (1895): 851–883].

[171] Vgl. Georg Ernst Stahl, *Georg Ernst Stahl's Theorie der Heilkunde*, 3 Bde. (Berlin: Enslin, 1831–1832).

begangenen Torheiten, Laster gebracht werden, d. h. von der Erkenntnis zum Bekenntnis, das bei ihm häufig der ersteren vorausgeht, und von der Erkenntnis zur Bereuung, Umkehrung und Selbstbeherrschung. *Arbeit* und *Reinlichkeit* sind zwei Hauptmittel für ihn. Zur Arbeit gehört bei den Männern und Frauen Lesen, Schreiben, besonders *Memorieren* von einfachen Liedern von Gellert usw. und *Rechnen*. Die Aufmerksamkeit der Männer wird aber durch das *Korbflechten* geübt, das selbst ein routinierter Korbmacher nicht treiben kann, ohne daß er seine Gedanken auf sein Geschäft richtet. *Disziplinarstrafen* sind außer den Entbehrungen von allerlei Annehmlichkeiten, von Essen und Trinken, die gewöhnlichen Zwangsmittel wie Zwangsweste, Zwangsstuhl, Drehstuhl, besonders noch das *kalte Bad* und die *Moxa*, die er *sehr häufig* anwendet [...].[172] Ideler sagte aber nicht, oder will nicht sagen, daß das Böse oder der Böse die Quelle der Seelenstörungen sei, sondern nur die Affekte, in dem die größten Verbrecher sehr häufig, weil ihr Gehirn und Verstand fest genug sitzt, nicht wahnsinnig werden, wohl aber schwache Menschen, bei denen oft nicht viel dazu gehöre. Auch er macht – und wie sollte es bei einer konsequenten Methode, die den Menschen als eine sittliche Kraft auffaßt und festhält, nicht der Fall sein – sehr glückliche Kuren, wobei freilich immer das bedacht werden muß, daß erstes, solange er seine Kranke hat, keine weiteren ungünstigen körperlichen Einflüsse auf sie wirken können, wie es früher wohl der Fall war, oder daß seine strenge Diät und die Heilkunst der Natur indessen auch leibliche Störungen entfernt, und daß endlich die psychischen Mittel, da die ganze menschliche Organisation ein psychisches Organ ist, zugleich auch physisch schon nach Stahls Theorien sein müssen [....] Über die großen Gebrechen seiner Methode will ich jetzt nichts sagen. Der Stoff ist da zu den mannigfaltigsten Bemerkungen. Nur das noch zu Dr. Idelers Ehrenrettung, daß, ehe er seine psychisch Kranken so attackiert, wie es immer geschieht, wenn sie einmal attackiert werden, er monatelang nach der Genesis der Krankheit forscht, ehe er es unternimmt, sie so zu schütteln [....] Besonders merkwürdig und instruktiv war mir Dr. Idelers Bekanntschaft um der Vergleichung mit Jacobis trefflichen Verfahren, das bei mir von allem, was ich kennenlernte, bis jetzt immer noch am höchsten steht, so abweichend und auch in mancher Beziehung unsere Ansicht sind, außerdem um der Verbindung willen, in der Dr. Ideler mit Geheimrat Langermann steht, dessen Persönlichkeit mir so reich und bedeutend erschien wie die von wenigen Menschen, die ich kennenlernte. Er ist der verklärte Dr. Ideler, der eigentlich nur seine Ansichten ausführt, ihm auch von Zeit zu Zeit, wenn es mit einem Kranken keinen rechten Fortgang haben will, diesen ihm ins Haus schickt, das der alte treffliche Herr schon seit Jahren nicht mehr verläßt. Kraft, Weisheit, Würde, Wohlwollen liegt in Langermanns Äußerem, er sieht aus wie ein kommandierender General der Geister und ganz geschaffen zur psychischen Heilmethode, so daß man wohl sieht, warum er diese ergriff, festhielt und als oberstes Heilprinzip geltend machte. Die größten Geister folgen dem Gesetz der Natur [...] und dieser Kreis der Persönlichkeit, der bei Langermann ein wahrhaft genialer

[172] [Die Auslassung bezieht sich auf den moralischen Verfall in der Großstadt („Brandwein und Hurerei“) und seinen Einfluß auf Ideler].

ist, indem ihm wirklich eine Weltanschauung zugrunde liegt, die überall leuchtend einschlägt, wohin ihr Blick auch fällt, wird auch bei ihm nicht verlassen; darum schätzt und stellt er Jacobi hoch und scheut sich auf eine wahrhaft weise und das innerste Leben anderer achtende Art seine Kreise zu stören, indem er nicht einmal Worte in den Weg und in die Seele werfen mag, um den Gang dieses stillen, schaffenden, fast tastenden Geistes nicht zu stören. Gerade diese Achtung des Besten, was in einem anderen liegt, macht ihn in meinen Augen groß, so abweichend oft meine Ansichten sind von den seinigen, die mich aber dennoch sehr angezogen haben [....] Es scheint ihm ganz unmöglich zu sein, den Menschen anders als eine sittliche Natur aufzufassen, und seine Eingeständnisse über die Resultate Jacobis gehen nur auf die Annahme einer gewissen Nervengewöhnung in bestimmten Situationen. Der Mensch ist zwar nach ihm ein freies Wesen, aber nur die wenigsten sind wirklich frei, indem ein bloßes Leben der Willkür kein Leben der Freiheit sei und die größten kombiniertesten Verstandesaktionen, die größten Bestrebungen nach allerlei zeitlichen Gütern und Erwerb kaum mehr seien, als wenn ein Hund über seine Kräfte nach einem Stück Fleisch in die Höhe springt. Er stimmt in vielem sehr auffallend mit Spinozas ‚De affectibus' überein und datiert den Ursprung der meisten Geistesstörungen viel weiter zurück als bloß bis zum Ausbruch der Krankheit der Seele. Sein erstes Augenmerk wie sein letztes bleibt darum, die Irren auf jede Art und Weise, vorzüglich aber oder eigentlich nie ohne den Weg der Autorität und eines absoluten Einschreitens zur Selbstbeherrschung zu bringen, indem er doch das Böse als Quelle der Seelenstörung sowenig als Ideler annimmt, das eigentliche Wesen des Bösen nicht erkennend. Nach seinem Vorschlag müßte in Preußen in jedem Bezirke als Seiten- und integrierendes Stück eines Irrenhauses (neben den Instituten für sogenannte Unheilbare) eine Art Korrektionshaus gebaut werden, das die aufnimmt, die nur unter Zwangsverhältnissen vernünftig sind und sich selbst überlassen, wieder rezidiv werden. Für die neue Köpenicker Anstalt ist diese Einrichtung schon festgesetzt. So müssen auch die Säufer und Huren, die in die Charité gebracht werden, unterschreiben, daß sie bei etwaigen Rückfällen ins Zuchthaus müßten[, sobald sie geheilt würden]. Nach Langermann muß mit militärischer Strenge verfahren werden. Auch hält er Disziplinarstrafen wie Moxa (Brenneisen) für notwendig und kommt daher auf dieselben groben physischen Methoden zurück wie Horn und Heinroth."[173]

Wir finden diese Bemerkungen über Johann Gottfried Langermann (1768–1832), den Albert Zeller etwa ein Vierteljahr vor dessen Tode kennenlernte, bemerkenswert genug. Dieser bedeutende Mann ist ja der eigentliche Begründer der wissenschaftlichen Psychiatrie in Deutschland und der Gründer zwar durch Reorganisation der Irrenhäuser in St. Georgen bei Bayreuth 1805. Wie treffend Albert Zellers Bemerkungen sind, wird deutlich, wenn man sie mit Hans Laehrs Biografie über Langermann in Kirchhoffs deutschen Irrenärzten vergleicht.[174]

---

[173] [Gerhart Zeller (Hg.), *Albert Zellers medizinisches Tagebuch*, Bd. 1, 70–72].

[174] [Hans Laehr, „Johann Gottfried Langermann, 1768–1832," in *Deutsche Irrenärzte*, hg. von Theodor Kirchhoff (Berlin: Springer, 1921), 42–51].

Ernst Horn (1774–1848) war von 1806 bis 1818 zweiter leitender Arzt an der Nervenabteilung der Charité. Er war ein Praktiker von großer Wirksamkeit, dessen Methoden heute recht merkwürdig berühren, zum Beispiel der berüchtigte Hornsche Sack, ein großer Sack aus Leinwand, in welchen Widerstrebende gesteckt wurden und in welchem dann auch einmal ein Kranker starb, was zu heftigen Angriffen auf Horn führte, der daraufhin seinen Dienst quittierte. Horn wirkte damals noch in Berlin. Zeller schreibt über ihn: „Horn ist immer noch sehr beschäftigt als Irrenarzt. er hat 2 kleine Anstalten vor den Toren und ist in jedem Betracht der alte große Indirekte, der im Aufruhr aller Kräfte des Leibes und der Seele gegen seine Maßregeln die Heilung der Kranken gewöhnlich zu suchen und zu finden scheint. Sein Blick ist katzenartig, schießend und schielend, voll Einsicht, aber auch fast wie etwas wahnsinnig. Mit großer Strenge hält er auch seine Damen täglich zu schweren körperlichen Arbeiten an. Sein Verfahren ist höchst energisch. Er schüttelt seine Kranken. Mancher, der genas durch ihn, will es nicht durch ihn, sonder durch eine andere Kur geworden sein. In dieser indirekten Methode liegt mehr, als Horn gewiß selbst weiß, von echt wissenschaftlichem Wert. Auch ihm verdanke ich und die Psychiatrie sehr viel. Seine Methode ist eigentlich nur die des Contrastimulus oder die konvulsorische, und recht umfassend diese betrachtet fragt es sich, ob nicht ein großer, vielleicht der größte Teil aller wirklichen ärztlichen Heilungen, nur auf eine konvulsorische, das heißt allopathische Weise geschieht.“[175]

Nach einem Besuch in der Irrenabteilung des Allgemeinen Krankenhauses St. Georg in Hamburg, in welchem merkwürdigerweise die Geisteskranken möglichst wenig getrennt von den übrigen Kranken untergebracht waren, verließ Albert Zeller am 14. Juli 1832 mit dem Dampfschiff Hamburg. Er wurde seekrank und empfand, wie er schreibt, alle Qualen eines Irren auf dem Drehstuhl.

Was England auf dem Gebiet der Irrenheilkunde zu bieten hatte, war zunächst mehr abschreckend als belehrend.[176] Obwohl 1774 das Parlament erstmals auf die Zustände der Irrenanstalten, vor allem in den weit verbreiteten Privatanstalten, aufmerksam geworden war, herrschte im Londoner Bedlam-Hospital, das von Heinrich VIII 1546 zur Aufbewahrung von Irren bestimmt worden war und das man 1812 neu erbaut hatte, noch immer ein sehr ungünstiger Zustand.[177] Das Intérieur in der Mitte des 18. Jahrhunderts hat uns William Hogarth (1697–1764) in seiner berühmten Kupferstichfolge „Der Weg der Liederlichen“ geschildert. Albert Zeller fand das Hospital 1832 wenig besser als zu dieser Zeit, in der man die Patienten noch wie wilde Tiere für 6 Pence pro zugelassener Person zur Schau stellte. Der Besucher tadelte besonders die schlechten baulichen Verhältnisse, die mangelhafte ärztliche Aufsicht, da die Anstaltsärzte den größten Teil des Tages außerhalb des Hauses in ihrer eigenen Praxis beschäftigt waren. Er fand sowohl die körperliche als auch die moralische Behandlung unzureichend. Arbeitsmöglichkeiten für Kranke fehlten ganz. Zeller klagte darüber, daß damals kein Arzt in England Vorlesungen

[175] [Gerhart Zeller (Hg.), *Albert Zellers medizinisches Tagebuch*, Bd. 1, 73].

[176] [Ebenda, 76–100].

[177] [Zu Bethlem Hospital, vgl. ebenda, Bd. 1, 82–89 und Bd. 2, 103].

über Psychiatrie hielt und daß man häufig auf seine Frage, mit welchen speziellen Mitteln man die Irren von ihrem Wahn abbringen wolle, nur mit Gelächter geantwortet habe. In welche Erbitterung der Besucher geriet, geht aus folgendem Satz hervor: „Ich konnte niemals die universale und wirklich wissenschaftliche und philosophische Art und den Geist der Deutschen finden“,[178] – „da das innere und geistige Leben des englischen Volkes nicht so groß ist wie in Deutschland, so benötigt auch die Behandlung nicht so unbedingt einen geistigen Charakter.“[179] – „Aber es ist bemerkenswert, wie sehr die äußere Seite der Religion hier mehr geschätzt wird als die innere.“[180] Dieser schlechte Anfangseindruck besserte sich im Laufe der Reise durch England rasch. Bei der Besichtigung der Irrenanstalt der Quäker bei York, „Friends Retreat“, am 10. und 11. September 1832 führt bereits echte Begeisterung die Feder: „Ich muß offen gestehen, dass meine Erwartungen in Bezug auf diese Anstalt nicht gering waren, aber in jeder Beziehung übertroffen wurden. Bis zum heutigen Tage kenne ich keine Einrichtung, die für ein gemischtes, aber hauptsächlich zur höheren Klasse gehörendes Publikum besser geführt wird.“[181] William Tuke (1732–1822) entwarf 1792 die Pläne für die Anstalt. Er leitete sie 30 Jahre lang. W. Tuke gilt als der Reformator des englischen Irrenwesens. Unser Tagebuch allerdings schreibt dieses Verdienst dem ersten Superintendenten der Anstalt Georges Jepson, gestorben 1836, zu. Dieser habe bemerkt, daß die wilden Tiere am leichtesten durch freundliche Methoden zu zähmen seien und habe daraus den Schluß gezogen, daß die Menschen, die des Verstandes beraubt seien, mit denselben Mitteln beeinflußt werden könnten. Mit Mut und Gefühl habe er das bislang herrschende System des Schreckens aufgegeben und begonnen, seine Kranken mit Freundlichkeit und Verständnis zu beeinflussen. Trotz dieser sichtbaren Erfolge einer psychischen Beeinflussung blieb man auch in York dabei, daß die Geisteskrankheiten in erster Linie körperliche Ursachen hätten. Albert Zeller zitiert aus dem letzten Bericht der Anstalt: „Eine Geistesstörung ist wahrscheinlich in allen Fällen mit einer körperlichen Krankheit verbunden, und häufig ist sie die erste Ursache, doch ihr Ursprung ist auch in vielen Beispielen in einer mentalen Affektion (*mental affection*) zu suchen und es ist sicher, dass das angemessene Funktionieren des Geistes wesentlich dazu beiträgt, dass Krankheiten verhütet werden.“[182] Der Superintendent der Anstalt gab auf Zellers Fragen zu, daß das zurückgezogene Leben der Quäker, ihr ständig nach innen gerichteter Blick sowie ihre Weichheit des religiösen Gefühls den geistigen Widerstand gegen krankhafte Einflüsse zu verringern vermöge.

Die vielen Eindrücke und Meinungen verwirrten den jungen Reisenden. Er trug in sein Tagebuch ein: „Nun habe ich in allen Büchern, bei jedem anderen und an mir selbst gesucht, um eine Erleuchtung über die Natur der Geisteskrankheit zu erhalten,

178 [Ebenda, Bd. 1, 89].

179 [Ebenda]

180 [Ebenda, 91].

181 [Ebenda, 134].

182 [Ebenda, 137].

aber umsonst, bis ich heute, am 20. September 1832 eine Erklärung in Spurzheims Arbeit über die Geisteskrankheit fand,[183] von der ich sehr wenig erwartete. Frage auf Seite 71: ‚Worin besteht die Geisteskrankheit' und Antwort: ‚In Bezug auf die krankhaften Affektionen des Verstandes (affections of the sense) und die Irrtümer der intellektuellen Kräfte sind wir dann geisteskrank, wenn wir die erkrankten Funktionen nicht erkennen können und sie als geordnet betrachten, und bei der Störung irgendeiner Empfindung sind wir dann krank, wenn wir entweder die Störung nicht wahrnehmen können (also z. B. wirklich glauben, wir wären König, Kaiser usw.), oder wenn wir die gestörte Empfindung wahrnehmen, aber den Einfluß des Willens auf unsere Handlungen verloren haben, z. B. einen krankhaften Hang zum Zerstören empfinden. So ist die Geisteskrankheit eine Abweichung einer Empfindung oder einer intellektuellen Fähigkeit vom gesunden Zustand, ohne die Möglichkeit, dies als krankhaft wahrzunehmen oder ohne den Einfluß des Willens auf die Handlungen, die aus dem Gefühl heraus entstehen (actions of feeling). Mit anderen Worten: die Unfähigkeit, die kranken Funktionen des Geistes wahrzunehmen und unsere Handlungen zu beherrschen (the irreversibility of our actions) bilden die Geisteskrankheit. Der größte Irrtum wird dadurch begangen, dass man den Geist als eine einheitliche Kraft darstellt oder wenn man die Gefühle von intellektuellen Fähigkeiten ableitet. Der Geist (Gemüt) ist eine Aggregation – oder besser gesagt ein Organismus – von Kräften, die individuell handeln oder gestört sein können, so wie es der Fall ist mit den äußeren Sinnen und Willensbewegungen; aber nur das Fehlen der Fähigkeiten, welche die Freiheit bilden, bildet die Geisteskrankheit.'"[184]

Was in Zellers Tagebuch über die französischen Anstalten festgehalten ist, entspricht keineswegs unsere Vorstellungen von der Anstaltskultur in Frankreich zu Beginn des 19. Jahrhunderts.[185] Die Zustände in der Salpêtrière und in Bicêtre waren heillos. In der Salpêtrière mit ihren 6000 Insassen, davon 1000 Irre, hätten sich die Närrinnen in großen Scharen singend, deklamierend, sich putzend und lachend herumgetrieben. Die Kranken seien in 3 Abteilungen eingeteilt gewesen.[186] In der ersten Abteilung hätten sich die befunden, die am meisten Behandlungschancen gehabt hätten. Diese Abteilung sei von Dr. Étienne Pariset (1770–1842), der von 1833 bis 1839 Chefarzt der Salpêtrière war, geleitet worden, die zweite von Esquirols Neffen, Dr. Jean Étienne Mitivie (1796–1871). Sie habe die bereits mehrere Jahre umsonst Behandelten beherbergt. Der Leiter der dritten Abteilung sei Dr. Jean Pierre Falret (1794–1870) gewesen. Er habe diese Anstalt erst 1831 für Idioten geschaffen; sie habe somit die Unheilbaren aufgenommen. Zeller vermerkt lakonisch: „Dr. Pariset scheint nichts zu tun. Dr. Mitivie wenig. Dr. Falret [...] kann nichts tun. Kurz: dieses weltbekannte Hospital verdient fast in nichts Lob, aber den

[183] Johann Caspar Spurzheim, *Observations on the deranged manifestations of the mind, or Insanity* (London: Baldwin, Cradock and Joy, 1817).

[184] [Gerhart Zeller (Hg.), *Albert Zellers medizinisches Tagebuch*, Bd. 1, 145–146].

[185] [Zu Frankreich, vgl. ebenda, Bd. 1, 149–181 und Bd. 2, 126–129].

[186] [Zur Salpêtrière, vgl. ebenda, Bd. 1, 162–170 und 177–178].

bittersten Tadel.“[187] Bicêtre, das 6100 männliche Sieche und arme Irre beherbergte, fand Zeller nicht besser. Vor allem seien die Kranken so gut wie unbeschäftigt gewesen.

In Frankreich wurden damals 5153 Geisteskranke gezählt. 2000 von diesen waren in 3 großen Anstalten in Paris, in Salpétrière, Bicêtre und Charenton aufgenommen. Im übrigen verfügte Frankreich nur über 7 Spezialanstalten, in denen nicht alle Kranken aufgenommen werden konnten, die übrigen waren in Hospizen und Hospitälern untergebracht. Die Zustände dort ließen offenbar manches zu wünschen übrig. Zeller fand es besonders unangebracht, daß eigentlich überall unheilbar Kranke mit noch heilbaren, frisch Erkrankten zusammen waren.

Albert Zeller und Jean-Étienne Dominique Esquirol

Die geistig beherrschende Gestalt der damaligen Französischen Psychiatrie war ohne Zweifel Dr. J.-E. Dom. Esquirol (1772–1840).[188] E. war Schüler Pinels. 1810 trat er an dessen Stelle in der Salpétrière. 1817 eröffnetet er die erste Klinik, 1822 wurde er Direktor der Salpétrière als Nachfolger Pinels, 1826 übernahm er die Stelle des Chefarztes an der staatlichen Anstalt Charenton bei Paris, welche 300 Kranke beherbergte. Er blieb Leiter dieser Anstalt bis zu seinem Tode, obwohl er 1824 noch eine eigene Privatanstalt in Ivry-sur-Seine nach seinen eigenen Angaben im Pavillonstil für etwa 100 Kranke eröffnet hatte. Mitivie half ihm bei der Versorgung der Privatanstalt, obgleich dieser nebenher noch die große Abteilung an der Salpétrière hatte. Zeller meint, die Erfolge an der Privatanstalt in Ivry seien auch nicht besser gewesen als die an der Salpétrière. Am besten gefiel dem jungen Besucher die Privatanstalt in Vanves, eine halbe Stunde von Paris entfernt, die vom Lieblingsschüler Esquirols Voisin geleitet wurde. Aber auch dort, meinte Zeller, werde die somatische Seite vernachlässigt. Man bewege sich zu sehr in den Gedankengängen Ideler und Heinroths.

Zeller hatte mit Esquirol wiederholt Gespräche. Er konnte sich dem Einfluß des bedeutenden Mannes nicht entziehen. Die bestehenden Differenzen in wissenschaftlichen Grundsätzen waren jedoch nicht zu überbrücken. Esquirol war kein so strenger analytischer Denker wie Pinel, sondern Eklektiker, der ohne klare Grundsätze ergriff, was günstig zu sein schien. Wie alle bedeutenden Psychiater des damaligen Frankreich war er Anhänger von Galls Gehirnlehre. Geisteskrankheiten waren für ihn Gehirnkrankheiten. Esquirol war Phänomenologe. Es ging ihm in erster Linie um die Klärung der vorliegenden psychiatrischen Zustandsbilder, ein eigentliches System der Geisteskrankheiten hat er nicht geschaffen. Er unterschied zwar Monomanien, Manie, Demenz, Imbezillität, ohne allerdings in diesen Zuständen mehr zu sehen als Symptomkombinationen. Allerdings weist Kahlbaum

[187] [Ebenda, Bd. 1, 178].

[188] [Zu Esquirol, vgl. ebenda, Bd. 1, 151–154 und Bd. 2, 127–129, 131].

mit Recht darauf hin, daß Esquirol eine abschließende Bearbeitung seiner psychiatrischen Ansichten nicht gelungen sei. Sein 1838 erschienenes Werk *Des maladies mentales* war nur eine lose Zusammenfassung seiner früher erschienenen monografischen Arbeiten.[189] Kahlbaum macht so in seinem oben zitierten Werkchen den Versuch, Ordnung in Esquirols Aufzählung zu bringen.[190] Wir halten diesen Versuch für ganz glücklich. Nach Kahlbaum unterschied Esquirol so Geisteskrankheiten mit *partiellem Wahn* (*Folie avec délire partielle*), und zwar Lypemanie, das ist Melancholie, Dämonomanie und die eigentliche Monomanie und solche mit *universellem Wahn* (*Folie avec délire universelle*) wie Manie, Demenz und Idiotie. Unseres Erachtens zeigt sich jedoch daraus, daß ein so leidenschaftlicher Systematiker, wie Kahlbaum es war, erst Ordnung in Esquirols System bringen mußte, wie gleichgültig Esquirol selbst solchen Einteilungsversuchen im Grunde wohl gegenüber stand. Offenbar wurde auch in den Gesprächen mit Zeller das Problem der Einteilung der Geisteskrankheiten nicht erwähnt.

Wir dürfen in diesem Zusammenhang nicht vergessen, daß damals F. J. V. Broussais (1772–1838) noch in Paris Ärzte und Medizinstudenten beherrschte, ja er hatte erst nach der Juli-Revolution im Jahre 1830 einen Lehrstuhl an der Fakultät erhalten.[191] Seine Polemik gegen die als Entitäten gedachten Krankheitseinheiten, höhnisch Ontologien genannt, war noch immer ungebrochen. Esquirol war nicht der Mann, der unter den Augen des gefürchteten Redners und Polemikers eine neue Ontologie schaffen konnte.

Albert Zeller mußte bei Broussais viel Ansprechendes finden. Alle Schüler Autenrieths sympathisierten eine längere oder kürzere Zeit mit ihm. Karl August Wunderlichs Doktorarbeit über die *Nosologie des Typhus* war eine solche Streitschrift im Sinne Broussais gegen die Ontologien. Das positiv Verbindende war die Idee einer physiologischen Heilkunde, welche vor allem von den Autenrieth-Schülern Wunderlich und Griesinger leidenschaftlich aufgenommen wurde und zur Begründung des *Archiv für physiologische Heilkunde* 1842 führte. Gemeint ist unter diesem Stichwort der physiologischen Heilkunde eine Pathologie, welche sich weder auf ein natürliches System der Krankheit im Sinne Linnés noch auf die Sektionsbefunde allein, sondern auf eine tiefere Erkenntnis der Lebensprozesse in der Krankheit stützen sollte. Bedenkt man, daß erst heute mit allen speziellen Mitteln der modernen Naturwissenschaft sich die Geheimnisse der pathologischen Physiologie teilweise zu lichten beginnen, dann wird es klar, daß der heuristische Ansatz des Broussais zwar richtig, aber zu seiner Zeit nicht auswertbar war. Da wirklich pathologisch-physiologische Erkenntnisse noch nicht erreichbar waren, mußte Spekulation die Lücke füllen. Es bot sich dazu die Theorie des Schotten John Brown (1735–1788) an, der die ganze Pathologie auf das Verhältnis von Reiz und Erregbarkeit reduzierte und der je nach der Reaktion auf den Reiz sthenische oder

[189] Jean Étienne Dominique Esquirol, *Des maladies mentales: considérées sous les rapports médical, hygiénique et médico-légal* (Paris: Baillière, 1838).

[190] [Gemeint ist Kahlbaum, *Die Gruppierung*].

[191] [Zu Broussais, vgl. Gerhart Zeller (Hg.), *Albert Zellers medizinisches Tagebuch*, Bd. 2, 132 f].

asthenische Krankheiten unterschied. Browns starke Wirkung auf die Naturphilosophie der deutschen Romantik, vor allem auf Schelling und die Bamberger medizinische Schule mit Adalbert Markus (1753–1816) und Andreas Röschlaub (1768–1835) ist bekannt.[192] Autenrieth war, wie oben schon gestreift, kein Freund der Brownschen Lehre, obwohl er während seiner Amerikareise mit einem begeisterten Vertreter des Brownianismus nämlich mit Benjamin Rush (1745–1813) zusammengetroffen war. Broussais kam zu folgenden Anschauungen: Der Unterschied zwischen den einzelnen Erkrankungen wird allein durch den Grad der Reizung bewirkt. Die pathologisch-anatomischen Veränderungen sind sekundär, Folge von Entzündung, welche durch die Reizung hervorgerufen wird. Durch Sympathie ergreift die Reizung dann die verschiedensten Organsysteme, die von dem Ort der primären Reizung weit entfernt sein können, Die Entzündung des Magen-Darm-Kanals, die Gastroenteritis ist in der Regel die nächste Folge der primären Reizung und damit die Grundkrankheit überhaupt. Bei so stark vereinfachter pathologischer Grundanschauung mußte auch die Therapie sehr einfach und damit auch sehr unwirksam sein. Sie bestand allein aus Diät und Blutentziehung in Form von Aderlässen oder durch Blutegel.[193] Wir müssen so Karl August Wunderlich Recht geben, wenn er in seinen Vorlesungen über Geschichte der Medizin in Leipzig im Jahre 1858 ausführt, Broussais habe an Stelle der alten Ontologien letztlich doch nur eine neue von Irritation und Gastroenteritis gesetzt.[194]

Albert Zeller gibt in seinem Tagebuch einen Auszug aus Broussais Werk: *De l'irritation et de la folie*.[195] Wir wollen diesen Auszug wörtlich zitieren, da der Abschnitt zeigt, wie nahe die Auffassung Broussais hier den älteren, allerdings anders begründeten Ansichten Reils und Autenrieths kommen. „In der Tat ziehen sich sehr viele Personen durch ein zu aufreizendes Regime (*régime irritant*) chronische Magenleiden zu, die, nachdem sie mehrere Jahre hindurch den Patienten im Zustand der Hypochondrie und der Neuropathie erhalten haben, schließlich zur geistigen Erkrankung führen. Bei anderen, die den Verstand aus demselben Grund verlieren, geschieht dies nach einer viel kürzeren Zeit. Wenn sie besonders kurz und das Magenleiden besonders schwer ist, wird das Delirium nicht mehr Geisteskrankheit genannt, es gehört zur Tobsucht (phrénesie) und den fieberhaften Delirien (délir fébriles). Aber sehr bemerkenswert ist die Tatsache, daß oft die moralischen Ursachen selbst, die am unmittelbarsten auf das Gehirn wirken, die Geisteskrankheit erst hervorrufen, nachdem sie eine gewisse Zeit gastritische Entzündungen entwickelt und unterhalten haben, so als ob es bei gewissen Kranken einer Erkrankung der

---

192 [Vgl. Werner Leibbrand, *Romantische Medizin* (Hamburg: H. Goverts, 1937), 50–60].

193 Henry Sigerist teilt mit, daß [1827] in Frankreich 33 Millionen Blutegel verwendet worden seien. Vgl. Henry E. Sigerist, *Grosse Ärzte: Eine Geschichte der Heilkunde in Lebensbilder* (München: Lehmann, 1932), 214.

194 [Vgl. Wunderlich, *Geschichte der Medizin*, 304].

195 François Joseph Victor Broussais, *De l'irritation et de la folie: ouvrages dans lequel les rapports du physique et du moral sont établis sur les bases de la médicine physiologique* (Brüssel: Melle Delaunay, 1828). [Zu Broussais, vgl. Gerhart Zeller (Hg.), *Albert Zellers medizinisches Tagebuch*, Bd. 1, 156 f]/

Eingeweide bedürfte, um zu einem hohen Grad der Erregung zu gelangen. Man darf sich darüber nicht wundern, dass bei vielen Menschen die moralischen Erschütterungen, obwohl sie das Gehirn erfassen, wenig Effekt auf die Organisation desselben als auf diejenige des Herzens, der Lunge oder des Magens hervorrufen. Das Gehirn leidet nie allein."[196] Man könnte beim Lesen dieses Zitats auf die Idee kommen, Broussais habe auch die Idee einer Einheitspsychose gehabt; dies wäre allerdings falsch, denn Broussais lehnt ja den Begriff einzelner Krankheiten generell ab. Es gibt für ihn keine Wesensverschiedenheit der Krankheit. Auf jeden Fall müßte Autenrieths Satz, daß erst durch Krankheit der Leidenschaftsnarr zum Geisteskranken werde, durch die Lektüre von Broussais Werk erneut Bestätigung für Zeller finden. Auch Zellers Ablehnung der Gehirnlehre konnte durch Broussais nur bekräftigt werden. Geisteskrankheiten waren für Albert Zeller nie ausschließlich Gehirnkrankheiten. Er sah das Wesen der Geisteskrankheit in einem individuellen Zusammengreifen körperlicher und seelischer Bedingungen. Zeller blieb auch Zeit seines Lebens dem alten Reilschen Schema von Cerebral- und Abdominalsystem verhaftet. Er konnte so auch kein tiefes Verständnis für die in Frankreich sich lebhaft entwickelnde pathologische Anatomie des Gehirns haben. Allerdings bemühte er sich, in diese Forschungen einzudringen, jedoch waren ihm dabei die ins Auge springenden Widersprüche und Ungereimtheiten der jungen Wissenschaft wichtiger als ihre konkreten Ergebnisse. Er beanstandet so auch mit Recht die Art der Hirnsektion, wie er sie in der Salpétrière sah und die notwendig zur Artefakten führen mußte. Man öffnete damals offenbar den Schädel mit einem einzigen Beilhieb; die Art der Rückenmarksektion, wie sie dort ausgeführt wurde, fand er rüde. Daß William Davidsohn in seinem Beitrag zur Pathologie des Gehirns bei Geisteskrankheiten, bei allgemeiner Paralyse und Epilepsie Erweichungen der Hirnsubstanz gefunden haben wollte, während Dr. Louis Foville (1799–1878), den Zeller in seiner Anstalt in St. Yon in Rouen besuchte,[197] fast immer Verhärtungen fand, schienen ihm unvereinigbare Widersprüche zu sein.

Die Lektüre von Dr. Étienne Jean Georget (1725–1828) verhalf Zeller dann zu einer kritischen Klärung seiner eigenen Betrachtungsweise.[198] Er tadelt an Georget, daß dieser nur ein Gehirn, das denke, empfinde, voller Wünsche sei und leide, anerkenne und keine Seele. Die Gedanken seien für Georget Produkte des Gehirns wie der Urin ein Erzeugnis der Nieren. Georget habe so den Wert des Gehirns für das organische und intellektuelle Leben sehr übertrieben. Zeller fügt hin zu, Esquirol habe ihm im Gespräch mitgeteilt, daß der früh verstorbene Georget in den letzten

---

[196] [Ebenda, 156].

[197] [Ebenda, 154 f].

[198] Étienne Jean Georget, *De la physiologie du système nerveux et spécialement du cerveau: Recherches sur les maladies nerveuses en général et en particulier sur le siège, la nature et le traitement de l'hystérie, de l'hypochondrie, de l'épilepsie et de l'asthme convulsif* (Paris: Baillière, 1821). [Zu Georget, vgl. Gerhart Zeller (Hg.), *Albert Zellers medizinisches Tagebuch*, Bd. 1, 158–160 und Bd. 2, 134–135. In Albert Zellers Auseinandersetzung mit Georget sieht Gerhart Zeller etwas „eindringlich Bekenntnishaftes aber nicht völlig Geklärtes. Es drängt ihn in Richtung eines ins Christliche gewendeten Spinozismus ..." Ebenda, 135].

Jahren seines Lebens seine Gedanken darüber grundsätzlich geändert habe. Daß Georget die Unabhängigkeit des seelischen Lebens verwirft, findet Zeller richtig. Georget vergesse aber, für Zeller hinzu, daß das Leben und die Seele ihr Dasein aus der gleichen Quellen beziehen und nicht etwa nur eine doppelte Manifestation derselben menschlichen Natur seien. „Im allgemeinen trennen wir viel zu sehr in unseren Beobachtungen und Folgerungen – was in der Natur kombiniert und verbunden und somit dasselbe ist; und hauptsächlich in den Geisteskrankheiten fehlt uns jeder Leitfaden für die Forschung, wenn wir vergessen, daß der Mensch nicht nur aus Körper und Seele zusammengesetzt ist, sondern daß er Körper und Seele gemeinsam (*ensemble*) ist.“[199]

[¶] Zeller bringt dann erstmals in kurzer Form in diesem Abschnitt, in welchem er sich mit Georget auseinandersetzt, seine eigene Meinung über die Entstehung der Geisteskrankheiten prägnant zu Papier: „Wenn der Mensch nicht vor der geistigen Erkrankung darauf achtet, den Einfluß der Sinne und der Einbildungskraft zu beherrschen, so kann die Zerrüttung seines Körpers bei Gelegenheit oft dazu führen, schlechte Gewohnheiten anzunehmen, die zusammen mit den erregten Störungen des Körpers bei der geistigen Erkrankung (*aliénation mentales*) enden können und sehr oft besteht die größte Schwierigkeit für eine vollständige Heilung in der zeitweiligen bzw. endgültigen Korrektur der schlechten Gewohnheiten als Endprodukt der Krankheit des Körpers.“[200]

Der letzte Teil der Reise, der nach Leipzig, auf den Sonnenstein zu Pienitz und Colditz zu Hayner sowie nach Prag und Hildesheim führte, steht ganz unter dem Eindruck der Auseinandersetzung mit Heinroth.[201] Vom 14.1.1833 bis 31.1.1833 war Zeller bei diesem in Leipzig. Am 24. März kam er auf der Rückreise von Prag noch einmal zu ihm. Beide Male kam es zu heftigen, leidenschaftlichen Diskussionen. „Ich hatte noch eine mir äußerst merkwürdige Unterredung mit Heinroth [am 24. März 1833]. Nochmals versuchte er, alle seine alten Geschütze vom freien Prinzip, von dem freien, wahren, nämlich dem sittlichen Standpunkt, von der Freiheit, von der Sünde, von dem tief verborgenen Leben derselben in den meisten Menschenherzen usw. aufzufahren. Ich wich diesmal aber keine Linie, dagegen verlor er immer mehr Land und Grund und machte mir zuletzt (im Vertrauen, wie er mir dreimal wiederholte) Bekenntnisse, die ich ganz füglich mit wenigen Klauseln als die meinigen ebenfalls unterzeichnen konnte.“[202] Zeller schließt seinen Tagebucheintrag mit den Worten: „Aber immer werde ich diesem Manne dankbar bleiben, der einen für das Ganze der Psychiatrie gewiß höchst notwendigen Gang der Betrachtung der sich gewählt hat.“[203]

[199] [Ebenda, Bd. 1, 158].

[200] [Ebenda, 162].

[201] [Zu Heinroth, vgl. ebenda, Bd. 1, 183–188 und Bd. 2, 149–155. G. Zeller beschreibt die Begegnung mit Heinroth als der „gedankliche Höhepunkt“ von Zellers Reise. Ebenda, Bd. 2, 150].

[202] [Ebenda, Bd. 1, 210 f].

[203] [Ebenda, 211].

Liest man dieses Zeugnis einer leidenschaftlichen, mit existenziellem Einsatz geführten Auseinandersetzung, dann drängt sich einem die Frage auf, welches wohl der eigentliche Grund und Motor dieses wissenschaftlichen Prinzipienstreites gewesen sein mochte. Ackerknecht sieht in der Auseinandersetzung zwischen den Somatikern und Psychikern im Grunde dasselbe zeitbedingte spekulative Element am Werk.[204] Wolfgang de Boor glaubt, daß der alte Universalismusstreit, das heißt der Streit um die Gültigkeit der Allgemeinbegriffe, welchen die Scholastiker mit großem Einsatz geführt hatten, auf solche Weise wieder auferstanden sei.[205] Wir müssen allerdings beide Deutungen für verfehlt halten, und wir finden in Albert Zellers Tagebuch erstmals einen Schlüssel zum Verständnis dieser Auseinandersetzung. Albert Zeller schreibt „Bei dem einen bleiben die größten körperlichen Veränderungen ohne irgendeine Umänderung seines Gemütszustandes, wenngleich vielleicht seine allgemeine Empfindlichkeit auf einen hohen Grad entwickelt ist, einem anderen macht ein leichtes Fieber phantasieren, ein wenig Wein berauscht."[206] – „Dr. Jessen hat – wie Jacobi und Roller – an sich selbst andere Erfahrungen gemacht als Herr Heinroth, der mich gar nicht zu verstehen schien, wie ich ihm von solchen mächtigen Verstimmungen erzählte, weil er selbst eine solche Gesundheit genießt, wo Leib und Seele gleichsam nebeneinander hergehen und die Affektionen der einen keine der anderen hervorrufen. Ein solcher weiß auch nichts von den Kämpfen, die wir innerlich zu bestehen haben."[207] Zeller führt uns hier an den letzten Ursprung der sich so sehr widersprechenden Überzeugungen. Er liegt nicht im Bereich des Rationellen, sondern im Bereich der Selbsterfahrung.[208] Wer sich beim Blick nach innen als frei erlebt, wird stets für Freiheit eintreten; wer sich unfrei erlebt, für Unfreiheit. Man denke nur an den zeitlich nicht fernen Arthur Schopenhauer (1788–1860), der mit starken Worten und großer Heftigkeit, vor allem in seiner abgelehnten Preisaufgabe über die Freiheit des Willens, für Unfreiheit eintritt.[209] Mußte nicht ein so leidenschaftlicher, zornmütiger, ehrgeiziger Mensch, wie Schopenhauer es war, sich beim Blick nach innen als unfrei fühlen und mußte diese unmittelbare Selbsterfahrung nicht stärker sein, als jedes logische Argument? Erinnern wir uns, daß Albert Zeller noch zu den subjektivistischen Analytikern gehört und daß er früh bei der Beobachtung seiner eigenen Seelenzustände auf einen Wechsel der Stimmung ohne äußeren Anlaß stieß. Zeller mußte diese unverständlichen Verstimmungen für die Folge körperlicher Vorgänge halten. Es wurde ihm so die Abhängigkeit der Stimmung von der körperlichen Gesamtverfassung

---

[204] [Vgl. Ackerknecht, 58].

[205] [Vgl. de Boor, 3–4].

[206] [Gerhart Zeller (Hg.), *Albert Zellers medizinisches Tagebuch*, Bd. 1, 187].

[207] [Ebenda].

[208] [Vgl. ebenda, 185–187].

[209] Vgl. Arthur Schopenhauer, „Über die Freiheit des menschlichen Willens," in *Die beiden Grundprobleme der Ethik, behandelt in zwei akademischen Preisschriften* (Leipzig: Brockhaus, 1860 [1840]), 3–106. [Zu Schopenhauers Einfluß, vgl. Gerlof Verwey, *Psychiatry in an Anthropological and Biomedical Context: Philosophical Presuppositions and Implications of German Psychiatry, 1820–1870* (Dordrecht: Reidel, 1985), 76–85, 156–175].

eine durch Selbsterfahrung erhärtete Grundüberzeugung. Aus der Selbsterfahrung speiste sich somit die Entschiedenheit und die Leidenschaft, mit welcher er Heinroth widersprach. Albert Zeller wurde so zu einem Konstitutionsbegriff geführt, der modern anmutet, und wir wollen daher folgende Stelle wörtlich wiedergeben und nichts hinzusetzen: „Eine durchgreifende umfassende Zusammenstellung aller uns bekannten Erscheinungen in der Seele, wie sie aus dem Organismus hervorgehen, was Nationalität, Fortpflanzen von äußeren und inneren Familienähnlichkeiten, Temperament und Konstitution (zwei Begriffe, die sich correlieren wie Leib und Seele oder vielmehr umgekehrt wie Seele und Leib, Kraft und Organ) in der Psyche modifizieren, wie die Prognose der Krankheiten aus dem Charakter des Individuums gestellt werden kann, und die Entwicklungsperioden des Leibes und der Seele einander parallel laufen. Wie Essen und Trinken, Ruhen und Handeln, Schlafen, die Zustände des Gemüts verändert, müßte uns das beste Licht über die psychischen Krankheiten geben.[….] Nachdem man so das Naturleben der Seele auseinandergesetzt hätte, das im Wachen immerfort produziert und das Leben der meisten Menschen allein ausmacht, könnte man in die Nacht der Träume und Wünsche und des Wahnsinns hinabsteigen und sehen, wie auch in ihnen ein Höheres wirkt und schafft und unsere armseligen Anthropologien auf der Fläche der Tiefen hinspielten, in denen Zauberkräfte spielen und walten."[210]

Wir müssen hier das Tagebuch, das noch viel Interessantes enthält, verlassen, und wir möchten diesen Abschnitt mit folgendem kleinen Zitat, welches Zellers anthropologische Grundüberzeugung enthält, beschließen: „Immer trennen wir Menschen, was Gott verbunden hat, und was Gott verbunden hat, soll der Mensch nicht scheiden."[211]

Die Geburtsstunde der Lehre von der Einheitspsychose: Albert Zeller und Joseph Guislain

Der folgende Abschnitt hat sich vor allem mit der Beziehung zwischen Zeller und Guislain sowie zwischen Zeller und Griesinger zu beschäftigen. Eine besonders exakte zeitliche Korrelation der Arbeiten ist hier erforderlich.

Am 1.3.1834 war die königliche Heilanstalt Winnenthal eröffnet worden.[212] In Zellers Schilderung der Anstalt wurde die Trennung der Heilbaren von den Unheilbaren als Grundsatz herausgestellt. Der somatischen Grundüberzeugung verleiht Zeller Ausdruck. Nur durch leibliche Störungen könne die Psyche so gebunden werden, daß Irrtum und Wahn zum Wahnsinn, Traurigkeit und Angst zur Schwermut, Sünde und Leidenschaft zur Tollheit und Torheit zur Narrheit sich ausbilde. Eine

---

[210] [Gerhart Zeller (Hg.), *Albert Zellers medizinisches Tagebuch*, Bd. 1, 184 f].

[211] [Ebenda, 184].

[212] [Albert Zeller, „Mitteilungen über die neu errichtete Irrenheilanstalt Winnenthal," *MCblWÄV* 3.5/14 (1834): 34–36, 108].

psychische Behandlung sei notwendig. Sie müsse in einem stillen, festen, aber ununterbrochenen geistigen Einfluß, einer sittlichen und weisen Lebensordnung beruhen, ihr Zweck müsse eine Rückerziehung sein, die nach dem Individuellen des Falles zu modifizieren sei.

1837 erschien dann [der erste vollständige Anstaltsbericht.] In diesem Bericht wird von Zeller erstmals klar ausgesprochen, daß die Hauptformen der Seelenstörungen für Hauptstadien, welche diese Krankheit zu durchlaufen pflege, gehalten werden. Wie überall in allen Bereichen des Lebens, binde sich die Natur an keine starren Formen. Merkwürdig ist folgender Passus: „Die sittlichen und intellektuellen Schwächen und Fehler des Menschen (die wohl in vielen Fällen in entsprechenden angeborenen und erworbenen Schwächen und Einseitigkeiten des Organismus begründet sein mögen), geben gewöhnlich die nächste Handhabe für die Überwältigung des Geistes durch körperliche Krankheiten. Bei weitem in den meisten Geschichten der Geisteskrankheiten läßt sich ein tiefer, den ganzen Menschen durchdringender, entweder mit plötzlicher Gewalt über ihn stürzender, oder lang und tief an ihm nagender und seine Kräfte verzehrender Schmerz, als die Mutter aller kranken Erscheinungen erkennen. Er entspringt entweder aus dem Verlust eines wirklichen oder vermeintlichen Gutes, das die Welt eines Menschen ausmacht, sei es nun äußerer materieller Besitz, oder Ehre, Liebe, Freundschaft, Unschuld, Friede, gutes Gewissen, oder aus der Furcht es zu verlieren, oder der Verzweiflung darüber, daß man dieses Gut sich nie zu eigen machen kann, oder dem Versagen an Hilfe in irgendeinem Unglück. Dieser Grundton der meisten Seelenstörungen, diese schmerzliche Stimmung, in der unangenehme, peinigende leibliche Empfindungen zu allgemeiner Traurigkeit der Seele und damit zur Trübung der geistigen Klarheit führen, hallt auch in den meisten Fällen durch alle selige Trunkenheit eines Wahnsinnigen nach; ja es ist der Wahn von unendlichem Glück meist nur das Wiederspiel desselben, in das die Seele, nach dem ihr angeborenen Triebe glücklich zu sein, überspringt. Soll daher eine Genesung gründlich erfolgen, so müssen in der Regel nicht allein alle, die Seelenstörungen begleitenden oder mitbedingenden, körperlichen Störungen gehoben sein, sondern eben dieser schmerzliche Zwiespalt des Innern. An die Stelle der verlorenen Welt muß ein Gut gesetzt werden, das nicht geraubt werden kann.“[213]

In diesem Bericht aus dem Jahre 1837 werden somit zwei wesentliche Faktoren der Lehre von der Einheitspsychose erstmals klar und deutlich formuliert. Erstens, daß die Haupterscheinungsformen nur Stadien sind, welche die eine Krankheit ohne scharfe Übergänge zu durchlaufen pflegt und daß der Seelenschmerz die Mutter aller kranken Erscheinungen sei. Während wir die Lehre von der einen Geisteskrankheit, welche sich in den verschiedenen Stadien jeweils anders manifestiert, schon bei Reil und Autenrieth vorgebildet fanden, finden wir den Schmerz als psychische Grundstörung von Zeller erstmals in diesem Bericht anerkannt. Zeller war auch in diesem Punkte nicht unvorbereitet; fanden wir doch sowohl bei Reil als auch

[213] Albert Zeller, „[Erster] Bericht," 327. [Erwähnenswert ist der gleich anschließender Satz: „Man muss dem Unglücklichen Hülfe zeigen und Nichts kann sie mehr zeigen und geben, als eben die Religion"].

bei Autenrieth wiederholt die Bemerkung, daß die Geisteskrankheit mit Melancholie, also mit Irritation des Bauchgangliensystems beginne und später durch Irritation des Cerebralsystems in Irrsinn übergehe. Aber dennoch ist die Auffassung, daß der Schmerz über den Verlust subjektiv hoher Werte der Grundstörung der Geisteskrankheit sei, in dieser prägnanten Form ganz neu und auch im Tagebuch nicht vorgebildet.

Es kann kein Zweifel sein, daß Albert Zeller in der Zeit zwischen 1833 und 1837 sich mit Joseph Guislains (1797–1860) *Traité sur les phrénopathies*[214] auseinandergesetzt und daß der Inhalt dieses Werkes klärend auf seine eigenen Gedanken und die von seinen Lehrern überkommenen Vorstellungen gewirkt hat. Welche Bedeutung er diesem Werke Guislains zumaß, geht am deutlichsten daraus hervor, daß er es 1838 in einer deutschen Übersetzung durch Wunderlich herausgab.[215]

Wer war nun dieser Joseph Guislain? Kurz und schematisch gesagt, der Reorganisator des Irrenwesens in Belgien. Was Langermann für Deutschland, Georges Jepson und William Tuke für England und Pinel für Frankreich, das war Guislain für Belgien. Leider ist, soweit wir sehen, die Biografie dieses bedeutenden Mannes, dessen zweites Hauptwerk *Leçons orales sur les phrenophathies* übersetzt von Heinrich Laehr erschienen, bis heute noch nicht geschrieben.[216] Zwar hat Brierre de Boismont (1798–1881), Direktor einer Privatanstalt in Faubourg St. Antoine in Paris, der vor allem Esquirols Arbeiten über die Halluzinationen fortsetzte, eine Biografie und Ergografie Guislains verfaßt.[217] Leider enthält das Buch auf 155 Seiten nur wenig Biografisches. Wir erfahren zwar, daß Guislain kein Freund der französischen Psychiatrie war, bekommen aber keinen Aufschluß über seinen tatsächlichen Bildungsgang. Wir wissen so von ihm nur, daß er aus einer Malerfamilie stammt und zunächst auch Maler oder Architekt werden sollte. Er hat offenbar eine entsprechende Ausbildung begonnen, diese dann unterbrochen und Medizin studiert. 1819 wurde er zum Doktor der Medizin promoviert. 1828 wurde er Chefarzt der Irrenanstalt in Gent. Vorher hatte er sich durch eine Preisaufgabe *Traité sur l'alienation mentale* bekannt gemacht.[218] Die 1821 von der Commission de surveillance medicale der Provinz Nordholland ausgeschriebene Preisaufgabe

[214] Joseph Guislain, *Traité sur les phrénopathies, ou doctrine nouvelle des maladies mentales, basée sur des observations pratiques et statistiques, et l'étude des causes, de la nature, des symptomes, du pronostic, du diagnostic et du traitement de ces affections* (Brüssel: Établissment Encyclographique, 1833).

[215] Joseph Guislain, *Abhandlung ueber die Phrenopathien*. Die Frage, wer dieser Dr. Wunderlich, der Übersetzer des Werkes, war, konnte bis heute leider nicht geklärt werden. [Auslassung (ca. 330 Worte): Erörterung darüber, wer der Übersetzer hätte sein können und daß es nicht Carl August Wunderlich (1815–1872) war].

[216] Joseph Guislain, *Leçons orales sur les phrénopathies, ou Traité théorique et pratique des maladies mentales* (Ghent: L. Hebbelynck, 1852); ders., *Joseph Guislain's Klinische Vorträge über Geistes-Krankheiten* (Berlin: Hirschwald, 1854).

[217] Alexandre Jacques Francois Brierre de Boismont, *Joseph Guislain: sa vie et ses écrits*, Esquisses de médecine mentale (Paris: B. Baillière, 1867).

[218] Joseph Guislain, *Traité sur l'aliénation mentale et sur les hospices des aliénés*, 2 Bde. (Amsterdam: J. Van der Hey et fils, 1826).

lautete: „Welches sind die Mittel, sowohl psychologisch als physisch, die für die Heilung der Geisteskrankheiten vorgeschlagen worden sind? Bei welchen von diesen Mitteln hat die Erfahrung gezeigt, daß sie den Zustand dieser Unglücklichen gebessert oder geheilt haben? Welchen Einfluß haben die Mittel auf die Krankheiten gehabt, die, obgleich sie nicht von den Geisteskrankheiten abhängen, diese doch manchmal begleitet haben? Welches ist der Einfluß der Krankheiten auf die Geisteskrankheiten und auf welche Weise wirken sie umgekehrt auf diese Krankheiten?“[219] Guislains Antwort auf diese Fragen, die er im Jahre 1823 eingereicht hatte, drang zunächst nicht durch. Einer erweiterten Bearbeitung, die er 1825 einreichte, wurde dann doch der inzwischen verdoppelte Preis zuerkannt. Die Arbeit imponierte durch die großherzigen Gefühle und den revolutionären Geist. Sie enthält bereits Guislains Grundauffassung, wie sie später in seiner Abhandlung über die Phrenopathien sowie in den Vorlesungen breit ausgeführt wurde. Die Arbeit ist allerdings nur im therapeutischen Teil umfänglich, sie hält sich im übrigen an Esquirols Einteilung.

Das, was Guislain psychopathologisches Denken charakterisiert, ist sein Suchen nach einer *altération fondamentale*. Er sieht sie im Seelenschmerz, in der krankhaften Erregung der Sensibilität. Guislain gibt im ersten Kapitel der Abhandlung über die Phrenopathien in wenigen Zeilen seine Grundüberzeugung: „Jedes Gewebe, wenn seine Sensibilität angeregt wird, äußert die Empfindung durch eine Lebensverrichtung, welche ihm eigentümlich ist. Die Empfindung, die von einem allzu starken Reiz entsteht, zeigt durch einen Schmerz, einen mehr oder weniger ähnlichen Charakter in den verschiedenen Organen, in denen sie erscheint. Die Seele hat ihre Reize, sie hat auch ihren Schmerz, aber er offenbart sich auf andere Weise als im Physischen. Es ist Sorge, Ärger, Schrecken: es ist mit einem Wort ein Seelenleiden [....] [M]an beleidige ein Individuum, man lasse es irgendein Leiden erdulden, alsbald wird sich eine Reihe von Erscheinungen entwickeln: es wird Tränen des Verdrusses, oder, des Zornes vergießen, es wird den Drohungen Trotz bieten, den Beschimpfungen sich widersetzen; es wird unruhig werden; alle seine Bestrebungen werden dahin gehen, das Agens, welches ihm beschwerlich fällt, zu ertöten, zu entfernen oder zu zerstören. Dieses ist die psychische Reaktion, welche physische Reaktion nach sich zieht.“[220] Alle Erscheinungsformen der Seelenstörung sind somit für Guislain Reaktionen auf die *altération fondamentale*. Diese Reaktion, so meint Guislain, vollziehe sich gesetzmäßig. Sie führe zunächst 1.) zu einer gesteigerten organischen Tätigkeit, 2.) zu einer Teilnahme des Nervensystems an der Ausprägung der Symptome[221]; 3.) zu einer Schädigung und 4.) zu einer Vernichtung der Seelenkräfte. Die unter 1 und 2 aufgezählten Reaktionen nennt Guislain primäre Elemente, 2 und 3 sekundäre. Durch diese Reaktion entstehen dann 4 konstitutive Elemente der Seelenstörungen:

---

[219] [Brierre de Boismont, *Joseph Guislain*, 5 f].

[220] [Joseph Guislain, *Abhandlung ueber die Phrenopathien*, 37 f].

[221] Guislain bekennt sich dabei ausdrücklich zur Gehirnlehre Galls. Das Gehirn ist der Sitz der Seelenstörung.

1.) Aufregung (Exaltation der Gehirntätigkeit),
2.) Verirrung (Aberration der Gehirnverrichtungen),
3.) Unterdrückung (Oppression der Gehirnverrichtungen),
4.) Vernichtung (Exhaustion der Seelenkräfte).

Aus diesen psychischen Elementen oder aus der Teilnahme gewisser somatischer Verhältnisse entstehen nun folgende Grundformen der Seelenstörungen:

A. *Erscheinungen des Reizes* (Seelenschmerz, Phrenalgie)

 1.) *Lyperophrenie* (Melancholie, einfaches Leiden der Sensibilität).

B. *Erscheinungen der Reaktion*

 2.) *Hyperphrenie* (Manie, Steigerung der Geistestätigkeit)
 3.) *Paraphrenie* (Folie, Wahnsinn, Aberration der Geistestätigkeit)
 4.) *Hyperplexie* (Stupidité, Melancholia stupida)
 5.) *Hyperspasmie* (Epilepsie, Veitstanz)
 6.) *Idéosynchysie* (Delir, Illusionen, Halluzinationen, Wahnwitz, Aberration der Vorstellungen)
 7.) *Anacoluthie* (Verwirrtheit, Mangel an Zusammenhang der Vorstellungen)

C. *Noasthenie* (Demenz, Verstandesschwäche)

Auf Ziffer 5 und 7 verzichtet Guislain in seinen Vorlesungen im Jahre 1845. Er kam so auf 6 Grundformen. Jede dieser Grundformen kann nun einfach bleiben und bildet dann das, was Esquirol eine Monomanie nannte und was Guislain als Monopathie bezeichnet; oder aber es verbinden sich mehrere Grundformen miteinander zu einer Krankheit, und zwar entweder gleichzeitig oder nacheinander. Die Kombination ist der häufigere Fall und sie ist es, welche in ihren mannigfachen Variationen die eigentlichen Arten der Seelenstörung bildet. Guislain glaubt über 100 bestimmte Formen unterscheiden zu können.

In seinem Bericht vom Jahre 1837 hatte Zeller Guislains Lehre, welche klärend auf seine eigenen, in ähnlicher Richtung gehenden Vorstellungen wirken mußte, offenbar begeistert aufgenommen. Die Kritik konnte jedoch nicht lange ausbleiben. Auf 106 Seiten der deutschen Ausgabe von Guislains *Phrenopathien* hat Albert Zeller dann in Form eines Vorworts und in Form von Bemerkungen zu jedem einzelnen Kapitel seine kritischen Bedenken ausführlich dargestellt.[222] Sie mußten sich nach allem, was wir bisher von seinen Ansichten wissen, hauptsächlich gegen 2 Grundüberzeugungen Guislains richten, nämlich gegen die von Guislain ausschließlich vertretene Psychogenie der Geisteskrankheiten und gegen die von Gall übernommene These, daß Geisteskrankheiten Gehirnkrankheiten seien. In der Widerlegung dieser Thesen gelingt Albert Zeller dann erstmals eine klare Darstellung seiner psychopathologischen Ansichten.

Er geht davon aus, daß die Erforschungsweise der Seelenstörungen eine anthropologische sein müsse, welche den Menschen weder ausschließlich von seiner

[222] Joseph Guislain, *Abhandlung ueber die Phrenopathien*, 1–28, 440–518.

geistigen und seelischen noch ausschließlich von seiner leiblichen Seite betrachtet, sondern immer von der Einheit der Menschennatur ausgeht, ohne irgendwie die innere, dynamische und die äußere leibliche Gliederung zu verkennen. Das Band des Lebens aber wird vom Nervensystem geknüpft. Es ist fähig, von allen leiblichen Zuständen, von allen festen und flüssigen Gebilden des Leibes aus bestimmt zu werden. Zudem kann von jedem Punkte des Nervensystems aus das gesamte System in den stärksten Konflikt gezogen werden. Im Rahmen des Gesamtnervensystems kommt nun aber dem Gangliensystem die unmittelbare Erregbarkeit unserer leiblichen und geistigen Persönlichkeit und das unmittelbare Innewerden dieser Erregungen und Zustände (der *sens affectif* Guislains) zu. So wird durch den inneren Sinne Reils die menschliche Persönlichkeit erst wahrhaft subjektiv, sie bekommt ein Herz, aus einer Art Gedankending[223] wird ein wirkliches Individuum. Es ist aber mit der Natur dieser Sensibilität, mit dem Charakter des Gefühls, in welcher das Unwillkürliche vorherrscht gegeben, daß der Mensch in ihr dem Unfreien, dem durch ein Leiden und Leidenschaften verursachten Gebundensein viel näher steht, als in den mehr objektiven Empfindungen des übrigen Nervensystems. Da nun aber erst in dem gesunden Ineinandergreifen von Freiem und Unfreiem, von Geist und Natur die menschliche Persönlichkeit und jede ihrer Handlungen zustande kommt, so muß in einer Verschiebung und Vernichtung dieses Verhältnisses von Gehirn und Gangliensystem in der Regel der letzte Grund der Seelenstörung liegen. Wie man nun bei solchen Konstitutionen, wo Leib und Seele sichtbar ineinanderspielen, gewöhnlich ein bestimmtes Organ oder eine bestimmte Reihe von Organen regelmäßig nach starken und unangenehmen psychischen Eindrücken ergriffen sieht, so wird man umgekehrt gerade auch bei Störungen der Funktionen dieser Organe in diesen Individuen psychische Affektionen entstehen sehen. Die Organerkrankung aber entsteht nach den Gesetzen der Metastasenlehre entsprechend dem Consens der Organe.

Auf diesem Wege kommt das zustande, was Jacobi erstmals in der Psychiatrie klar erkannte und was wir seither „Organische Gestimmtheit" nennen.[224] Albert Zeller schildert uns dies auf Grund eigener Erfahrungen als „bittere, schmerzhafte, trübe Stimmungen, über die wir uns selbst und Andern keine Rechenschaft geben können, Zustände, in denen uns jeder Blick der Liebe, jeder Ton der Freude, das friedlichste und harmloseste Wort verletzen und betrüben, ärgern und zum heftigsten Zorn und bösartigem Spott reizen kann, wo jeder Trost uns ängstigt, Mißtrauen in Alles uns erfüllt, wo uns Alles zuwider ist, was uns sonst angenehm und lieblich

223 [Immanuel Kant, *Kritik der reinen Vernunft* (Hamburg: Meiner, 1956), A489/B517, 23–29: „Mögliche Erfahrung ist das, was unseren Begriffen allein Realität geben kann; ohne das ist aller Begriff nur Idee, ohne Wahrheit und Beziehung auf einen Gegenstand. Daher war der mögliche empirische Begriff das Richtmaß, wonach die Idee beurteilt werden mußte, ob sie bloße Idee und Gedankending sei, oder in der Welt ihren Gegenstand antreffe"].

224 Maximilian Jacobi (Hg.), *Sammlungen für die Heilkunde der Gemütskrankheiten*, Bd. 2 (Elberfeld: Schönian, 1825). [Jacobi deutete psychische Erscheinungen naturhistorisch; für ihn waren sie „durchgehend das Resultat bestimmter Zustände des tierischen Organismus." Ebenda, 343].

dünkt, wo uns das eine Centnerlast däucht, was wir sonst spielend bewegten." [225] Auf der anderen Seite, so betont Zeller, gehöre auch der tiefste Seelenschmerz noch dem gesunden und vernünftigen Leben des Menschen an, solange ihm ein zureichender vernünftiger Grund entspreche. Zeller teilt Guislains Ansicht, daß die leiblichen Entstehungsweisen der Seelenstörungen ungleich seltener als die auf psychischem Wege seien. Er weist aber wiederholt auf die Beschränkung dieser Behauptung durch den Umstand hin, daß eben nur unter besonderen leiblichen Zuständen aus schmerzhaften Gemütsbewegungen Seelenstörungen sich erzeugen, sodaß es nicht selten geschieht, daß ein solches geistiges Moment, das ohne Hinzutreten eines leiblichen schnell erloschen wäre, im Verlauf der Entwicklung so in den Hintergrund treten kann, daß, wenn das leibliche Leiden, welches seinen selbstständigen Gang fortgegangen ist, wenn es gleich durch dieses geistige hervorgerufen worden war, gehoben wird, der geistigen Ursache von dem Genesenden gar nicht oder kaum mehr gedacht wird.[226]

An Guislains Einteilung übt Albert Zeller wenig Kritik. Er tadelt nur die Einschiebung der Krampfleiden unter die Seelenstörungen, und Guislain hat diese dann auch in seinen Vorlesungen 1854 aus dem System genommen. Albert Zeller weist aber auch darauf hin, daß die Abläufe keineswegs schematisch seien, daß individuelle Abweichungen vorkommen, ja häufig sind. Er gibt Guislain auch darin Recht, daß die Melancholie und die Manie innerlich verwandte Zustände seien. Gegen allzu subtile Unterabteilungen wehrt er sich, der überall Übergänge und keine festen Grenzen sieht. Soweit die Auseinandersetzungen mit Guislain. Kehren wir zu den Berichten über die Wirksamkeit der Heilanstalt Winnenthal zurück.

[Albert Zellers Anstaltsberichte und Encyklopädie Aufsätze]

Der zweite Bericht umfaßt den Zeitraum vom 1.3.1837 bis 29.2.1840.[227] Er ist deshalb besonders wichtig, weil er der letzte vor dem Zusammentreffen Zellers mit Griesinger ist, welcher vom 20.2.1840 bis 27.12.1841 in Winnenthal Assistenzarzt war. Wenn C. A. Wunderlich mit seiner Behauptung, daß Griesinger diese Berichte wesentlich beeinflußt habe, im Recht wäre, dann müßte man dies beim Vergleich des zweiten mit dem dritten und vierten Bericht erkennen können.[228] Der zweite Bericht ist aber auch deshalb von großem Wert, weil Zeller in diesem erstmals seine

[225] [Joseph Guislain, *Abhandlung ueber die Phrenopathien*, 16–17].

[226] [Vgl. hierzu so gut wie wörtlich Joseph Guislain, *Abhandlung ueber die Phrenopathien*, 18–19].

[227] [Albert Zeller, „Zweiter Bericht"].

[228] [Vgl. Carl August Wunderlich, „Wilhelm Griesinger: Nekrolog," *Archiv für Heilkunde* 10 (1869): 148. Tatsächlich ist Griesingers Einfluß nicht am Wandel der in der *MCblWÄV* veröffentlichten Berichten abzulesen, sondern in dem stark überarbeiteten und erweiterten Version des dritten Berichts, die in der *AZP* veröffentlicht wurde. Vgl. Albert Zeller, „[Dritter] Dreijähriger Bericht" und [Albert v.] Zeller, „[Dritter] Bericht über die Wirksamkeit der Heilanstalt Winnenthal vom 1. März 1840 bis 28. Februar 1843," *AZP* 1.1 (1844): 1–79].

Systematik der Geisteskrankheiten gibt. Eingeleitet wird allerdings dieser Bericht mit einer Diskussion über die damals wie heute brennende Frage, ob Irrenheilanstalt von Irrenpflegeanstalt räumlich getrennt oder relativ verbunden werden soll. Zeller trat, wie wir bereits wissen, entschieden für die räumliche Trennung ein.[229] Es war für ihn ein schwerer Schlag, daß er noch zu Lebzeiten 1875, gleichzeitig mit der Eröffnung der Heil- und Pflegeanstalt Schussenried die Umwandlung Winnenthals in eine Heil- und Pflegeanstalt hinnehmen mußte. Die Partei Damerow und Roller hatte damit gegen Reil, Autenrieth, Jacobi, Zeller und Griesinger gesiegt. Aber, wie oft in der Geschichte, kamen auch hier die zunächst Besiegten zu einem späten Triumph. Man ist heute, soweit wir sehen, damit beschäftigt, spezielle Pflegeanstalten, räumlich getrennt von den ursprünglichen Anstalten, zur Entlastung der eigentlichen Heilinstitute zu bauen. Es gehört dies nicht hier zu unserm Thema, und wir müssen daher die eingehende Behandlung der historischen Probleme des deutschen Anstaltsbaues auf einen späteren Zeitpunkt verschieben.[230] Hier soll es nur illustrieren, daß alle praktischen Fragen der Irrenheilkunde Zeller viel mehr beschäftigten und innerlich ergriffen als die Probleme der Krankheitssystematik.

[¶] Wir dürfen daher auch von ihm keine leidenschaftlich und apodiktisch vorgetragene Theorie erwarten, und wir glauben, daß der Leser erstaunt sein wird über Zellers eigene Worte: „Weil wir aber die Form des Irreseins nach generellen Zügen für noch bedeutender und entscheidender als die Dauer desselben erkannt haben, so eracht en wir es für notwendig, diesmal Einiges über die von uns gewählte Classifikation der Seelenstörungen zu sagen, was uns umso dringender erscheint, als über diesen Punkt noch eine wahrhaft babylonische Sprachverwirrung unter den Laien und Gelehrten herrscht, und wenn wir auch weit entfernt sind, unsern Versuch für den vorzugsweise wahren und richtigen zu halten, doch wenigstens unsere Bezeichnungsweise klar und verständlich zu machen. Der Hauptsache nach haben wir die in dem ersten Bericht gewählte Einteilung gelassen, und dieselbe nur in einigen Punkten noch mehr vereinfacht. Wir glauben zwar unsere Einteilung aus der Natur selbst und den erfahrensten und einsichtvollsten Schriftstellern aller Zeiten geschöpft zu haben, wollen aber weder in Abrede stellen, daß sich die mannigfaltigsten Assoziationen der angegebenen Grundformen in Einem [sic!] Individuum finden können, noch darüber rechten, ob dieser oder jener Ausdruck der allein geeignete sei, zufrieden, wenn es uns gelungen wäre, zu charakterisieren und festzustellen, was wir für wesentlich verschieden in der Natur erkannten. Es handelt sich bei solchen Einteilungen nicht um Auffindung von allen möglichen Unterabteilungen, sondern vor allem um Grundzustände des ganzen psychischen Lebens, und noch mehr um Stadien als Formen des Irreseins. Die einzelnen Gruppierungen

---

229 [Vgl. Albert Zeller, „Irrenanstalten, Irrenhäuser," 139–140].

230 [Zu diesem Thema veröffentlichte Gerhart Zeller später zwei Aufsätze: Gerhart Zeller, „Von der Heilanstalt zur Heil- und Pflegeanstalt: Ein Beitrag zur Geschichte des psychiatrischen Krankenhauswesens," *Fortschritte der Neurologie und Psychiatrie* 49 (1981): 121–127; ders., „Hat das psychiatrische Reformprogramm Wilhelm Griesingers aus dem Jahr 1868 heute noch eine Bedeutung?," in *Rehabilitationspsychiatrie*, hg. von Jürgen-H[elmut] Mauthe (Stuttgart: Enke, 1998), 1–14].

und Wechsel in gegebenen Fällen ergeben sich nach unserer Bezeichnungsart sehr leicht. Demgemäß sind wir auch der alten Einteilungsweise sehr nahe geblieben, jedoch mit dem wesentlichen Unterschied, daß wir die Melancholie der älteren Ärzte in die zwei Grundformen auflösten, welche sie und nach ihnen noch viele Neuere bis auf unsere Tage in ihr zusammengeworfen haben, nämlich in die Schwermut und Verrücktheit. So sehr wir auch überzeugt sind, daß das Delirium nicht von der näheren Erkenntnis und Bestimmung des Irreseins getrennt werden darf, vielmehr den unmittelbaren Übergang von den gewöhnlichen Krankheiten zu Seelenstörungen bildet, und sehr häufig die wirkliche Seelenstörung rein aus dem Fieberdelirium entspringt, ebenso die leibliche Begründung des Irreseins durch seine Erforschung am deutlichsten erkannt werden kann, so ist doch die übrige Reihe von pathologischen Symptomen bei ihm zu vorherrschend, als daß es zunächst mit den übrigen ausgebildeten Formen von Seelenstörung in eine Reihe gestellt werden kann. Die einfache Einteilung, welche wir daher wählen zu müssen glaubten, gibt 4 Grundformen oder Stadien des Irreseins: 1.) die *Schwermut*, Melancholia, 2.) die *Tollheit*, Mania, 3.) die *Verrücktheit*, partiellen Wahnsinn, Wahnwitz, Paranoia und 4.) den *Blödsinn*, Amentia, Dementia mit seinen verschiedenen graduellen Abstufungen von der bloßen Albernheit bis zum Erlöschen aller bewußten Sensibilität.“[231]

Albert Zeller gibt dann sehr eindringliche Schilderungen der Zustände. Er erwähnt dabei noch einmal ausdrücklich, daß für ihn die Schwermut die eigentliche Grundform und das erste Stadium aller nur halbwegs sich merkbar entwickelnder und nicht ganz in ihrer Ausbildung überstürzter Seelenstörungen ist. Sie kann, aber sie muß nicht, in andere Krankheitsformen übergehen, sie hat ihre Entwicklungs- und Ablaufsgesetze in sich selbst. Er arbeitet dann recht exakt heraus, das sich Manie und Melancholie wie Positiv und Negativ verhalten, wie Frost und Fieberhitze. Er unterscheidet außerdem Gehirn- und Ganglienmanie, immer verworrener, traumartiger, unzusammenhängender, anhaltender und tobender äußere sich die Tollheit, je mehr das Leiden des Gehirns, des Geistes das des Ganglienlebens und Gemüts überwiege. Die dritte Hauptform des Irreseins, die Verrücktheit, partieller Wahnsinn, Wahnwitz, Paraphrenie, Paranoia tritt fast nie, wie Zeller wörtlich ausführt, als primäre Form auf, *wenigstens nach unseren Beobachtungen*, wenn nicht auf dem Wege der Eifersucht, Prozeßsucht und der für Wirklichkeit gehaltenen einzelnen Sinnestäuschungen.

Zeller hat seine Lehre somit so vorsichtig formuliert, wie es der großen Erfahrung dieses Autors entsprechen mußte. Wie groß seine Erfahrung auf diesem Gebiet war, geht gerade daraus hervor, daß er die beiden klassischen Beispiele von Paranoia, von „primärer Verrücktheit“, nämlich den Eifersuchtswahn und den Querulantenwahn, bereits als selbstständige Bilder erkannt hatte. Im Blödsinn enden dann alle nicht heilenden Krankheitsverläufe. Er hat viele Grade und Ursachen. Seine Prognose ist umso schlechter, je besser der Allgemeinzustand des Kranken ist.

[231] Albert Zeller, „Zweiter Bericht“, 132.

Im zweiten Teil des Berichtes, welcher sich in sehr anschaulicher Weise mit der systematisch betriebenen Gruppen- und Arbeitstherapie, mit der „Gymnastik der Seele und des Körpers“,[232] beschäftigt, findet sich dann ein Satz, der wieder einmal beweist, wie sehr Albert Zeller seinem Lehrer Autenrieth wissenschaftlich verbunden blieb: „Wie schon oft erwähnt wurde, ist keine pathologische Lehre von größerer Bedeutung für die Psychiatrie, als die von dem Metaschematismus, der Metamorphose der Krankheiten, welche aber häufig nur in einer krankhaften Assoziation, das heißt in einer widernatürlichen und die gesunde Statik aufhebenden Verkettung zweier oder mehrerer sonst disparater Organe oder Systeme besteht.“[233]

Der dritte Bericht, welcher den Zeitraum von 1.3.1840 bis zum 28.2.1843 umfaßt, wurde in Band 1 der *Allgemeinen Zeitschrift für Psychiatrie*, 1844, auf Seite 1–79 abgedruckt.[234] Man darf dies wohl als einen Beweis dafür sehen, welches Interesse die Fachwelt an Zellers Berichten genommen hatte. Für uns ist dieser Bericht deswegen von Wichtigkeit, weil wir in ihm nach Spuren von Griesingers Mitarbeit suchen müssen. Diese finden sich auch, allerdings an wenig bedeutsamer Stelle. So taucht erstmals das bisher nicht gebrauchte Wort „Reflex“ auf.[235] Der Begriff der Spinalirritation wird eingeführt. Im übrigen ist aber gerade dieser Bericht der von Zeller propagierten und auf eine glückliche Weise praktizierten individuellen Krankenbehandlung und Krankheitserfassung gewidmet. „Wir haben immer mehr die Überzeugung gewonnen, daß nicht leicht bei einer anderen Krankheit die Ursache so rein individuell ist und daß nur im Allgemeinsten darüber sichere Anhaltspunkte aufgestellt werden können.“[236] Bei seiner im letzten Bericht aufgezeigten Klassifizierung bleibt Zeller ausdrücklich. Die Hauptformen sind Verlaufsformen, die Schwermut die primäre Störung. Sonst ist gerade dieser aus der Zeit der Zusammenarbeit mit W. Griesinger stammende Bericht besonders kurz. Nur die Statistik ist wohl als Werk Griesingers etwas detaillierter, die Sektionsbefunde sind ausführlicher, aber nicht unbedingt überzeugender, zum Beispiel wenn als Befund in 2 Fällen Verengung der Gehirnventrikel eingetragen ist. Es gelingen Albert Zeller aber in diesem Bericht Formulierungen, vielleicht als Früchte eingehender Gespräche mit dem jungen begeisterten Mitarbeiter, die so treffend sind, daß wir sie zitieren müssen: „Daß aber das Irresein eine Krankheit und kein bloßer Irrtum ist, kann man am besten aus [dem] tödlichen Ausgang der Seelenstörungen sehen. An Irrtum und Unsittlichkeit stirbt niemand, so kolossal sie auch sein

[232] [Ebenda, 139].

[233] [Ebenda. Autenrieths Einfluß auf Zeller zeigt sich nicht nur in der Krankheitslehre, sondern auch in der Einrichtung von sog. Authenriet'schen Zellen und Masken in Winnenthal. Vgl. Ebenda, 129 und Zeller, „Irrenanstalten, Irrenhäuser“, 148. Zu den Zellen, vgl. auch Hayner, *Aufforderung*, 13 ff].

[234] [Vgl. Albert Zeller, „[Dritter] Dreijähriger Bericht“ und ders., „[Dritter] Bericht“. Die in der *AZP* veröffentlichte Fassung war stark überarbeitet und erweitert, wahrscheinlich durch Griesinger].

[235] [Albert Zeller, „[Dritter] Dreijähriger Bericht“, 301].

[236] [Ebenda, 300].

mögen."[237] – „Daß wir aber den ganzen leiblichen Organismus im weiteren Sinne als Seelenorgan und die Seele selbst in ihm als das kräftigste und lebendigste Prinzip, als das Leben des Lebens betrachten und wir, wie wir von ihm aus Verderben und Zerstörung ausgehen sehen, so auch Leben und Heilung erwarten, haben wir schon früher wiederholt ausgesprochen."[238] Vielleicht ist dieser Bericht auch deswegen so knapp ausgefallen, weil Zeller zur selben Zeit mit der Vorbereitung seiner encyklopädischen Arbeiten befaßt war.

In der Allgemeinen Encyklopädie der Wissenschaften und Künste ist von Zeller bearbeitet der Artikel „Irre, Irren, Irrereden, Irrwahn" und der Artikel „Irrenanstalten, Irrenhäuser".[239] Beides Artikel bringen für unser Thema nichts Neues, zumal der Abschnitt über die Einteilung der Seelenstörungen eine wörtliche Wiederholung des zitierten Passus aus dem zweiten Bericht ist.[240] Trotzdem wurden diese Artikel von der Fachwelt beachtet. Kein Geringerer als C. F. W. Roller hat sie kritisch besprochen.[241] Diese Kritik ist recht interessant. So beanstandet Roller, daß Zeller den Unterschied zwischen primären und sekundären Seelenstörungen nicht scharf herausgearbeitet habe. Roller legt also hier bereits die Fassung des Problems, wie sie Griesinger in seiner *Pathologie und Therapie der psychischen Krankheiten*[242] gab, als Maßstab an. Er beanstandet weiter, daß Zeller von Tollheit spreche und den Begriff der Tobsucht, den Jacobi so scharf herausgearbeitet habe, nicht benütze. Er findet es auch nicht richtig, daß Zeller die Tollheit mit der *monomanie des grandeurs* vermische. Roller beanstandet somit gerade das, was wir als entschiedenen Fortschritt empfinden müssen, nämlich daß sich Zellers Begriff der Melancholie und Manie sehr gereinigt hatte und sich sehr stark unserem heutigen Gebrauch näherte. Roller beanstandet außerdem, daß Zeller von Gemütsnerven spricht. Er findet die Aufstellung eines solchen Begriffes für gewagt. Aus der Formulierung seiner Kritik geht hervor, daß er bereits nicht mehr weiß, daß die Bestimmung des Gangliensystems als Gemütsorgan auf Reil zurückgeht. Bei der Besprechung des Artikels über Irrenanstalten hebt Roller hervor, was tatsächlich große Beachtung verdient, daß Zeller für die Errichtung von Mittelinstituten zwischen Arbeitshäusern und Irrenanstalten eintritt. Wir haben gesehen, daß Langermann in Berlin etwas ähnliches schon gefordert hatte. Daß man heute in England durch Errichtung von Psychopathenheimen darangeht, diesen Gedanken zu verwirklichen, zeigt, wie

[237] [Ebenda, 299].

[238] [Ebenda, 298].

[239] Zeller, „Irrenanstalten, Irrenhäuser"; A[lbert] Zeller, „Irre, Irren, Irrereden, Irrwahn," in *Allgemeine Encyklopädie der Wissenschaften und Künste*, hg. von J. S. Ersch und J. G. Gruber (Leipzig: Brockhaus, 1845).

[240] [Ein genauer Vergleich zeigt eine nur teilweise wörtliche Wiederholung].

[241] [An dieser Stelle irrte sich Gerhart Zeller, insofern er die Besprechung E. von Feuchtersleben zuschrieb. Doch tatsächlich stammte die Rezension vom einflußreichen Direktor der badischen Anstalt in Illenau, C. F. W. Roller. Vgl. [Christian Friedrich Wilhelm] R[oller], „Zeller's Aufsätze in Ersch und Gruber allgemeiner Encyclopädie," *AZP* 2.4 (1845): 736–738. Der Text ist dementsprechend korrigiert worden].

[242] Griesinger, *Die Pathologie und Therapie*.

richtig er wohl im Grunde ist. Sonst schreibt Roller: „Der absoluten Trennung von Heil- und Pflegeanstalt redet Zeller – bald allein – noch immer das Wort – *sed victa Cantoni.*“[243]

Auch der vierte Bericht, umfassend den Zeitraum vom 1.3. 1843 bis 28.2.1846 wurde in der Allgemeinen Zeitschrift für Psychiatrie[244] abgedruckt. Zellers Klage über Platzmangel und über die ungenügende Aufnahmemöglichkeiten in der Pflegeanstalt Zwiefalten wird immer dringlicher. Man spürt einen Ton der Bitterkeit aus allem heraus. An seinen Grundsätzen hält Zeller nach wie vor fest, und er wird nicht müde, sie neu zu formulieren: „Oft entspringt die Seelenstörung einfach aus einem Mißverhältnis der gesamten leiblichen und geistigen Kraft zur gerade vorhandenen oder zur gesamten Lebensaufgabe, und hier zeigt sich dann die Wahrheit, daß bis auf einen gewissen Grad und in gewisser Art die seelische und leibliche Macht ganz dieselbe ist. Ein einziger lichter und kräftiger Gedanke, ein Strahl der Hoffnung und Freude im dringendsten Augenblick vermag zuweilen die Seele vor Wahnsinn zu retten, so wie umgekehrt das Hinzutreten einer einzigen, an und für sich geringfügigen leiblichen oder geistigen Schädlichkeit das Maß der Bedrängnis voll machen und Geist und Gehirn überwältigen kann, und wie von jedem einzelnen Punkt aus convulsivische Zustände entstehen können, so kann auch eine Seelenstörung sich von jedem einzelnen Nerven aus erzeugen, um diesen letzten Anfängen des Irreseins immer näher zu kommen und in ihrer einfachsten physiologischen und anatomischen Gestalt, wie in ihrer genetischen Verzweigung und Ausstrahlung, da auch hier die Gliederung des ganzen Krankheitsprozesses ein Gegenstand von der höchsten Wichtigkeit ist, und sie wie andere somatische Störungen heben zu lernen, dahin geht gerade das allseitige Streben der neueren Psychiatrie. Ist aber die Funktion eines Organs schon bei der Pathologie und Therapie der gewöhnlichen somatischen Störungen so wichtig als die anatomische Berücksichtigung desselben, so ist dies in noch ganz anderer Weise bei dem Seelenorgane, diesem wunderbaren Durchgangspunkt der menschlichen Persönlichkeit der Fall, und die rechte psychiatrische Meisterschaft wird sich deshalb gleicherweise in der individuellsten Leitung der geistigen wie in der individuellsten Herstellung der physikalischen Norm des Seelenorgans zeigen, und allseitig die lebendige Wechsel- und Ineinanderwirkung beider ins Auge fassen. Jede Psychiatrie ist unwahr und lückenhaft, geist- und seelenlos, die aus der Menschennatur Geist und Gemüt, diese höchsten und im materiellen mit keiner andern Kraft und Erscheinung vergleichbaren Faktoren ausschießt, so gewiß als die, welche den größeren spontanen und physikalischen Anteil des Gehirns an den geistigen Prozessen oder die große sensorielle und ökonomische Bedeutung des übrigen Organismus für die Energie des Seelenorgans übersieht. Der Vorwurf der Geheimlehre, welcher der Psychiatrie noch immer von manchen Seiten gemacht

---

[243] [R[oller], „Zeller's Aufsätze,“ 738].

[244] [Vgl. Albert Zeller, „[Vierter] Dreijähriger Bericht“ und [Albert v.] Zeller, „[Vierter] Bericht über die Wirksamkeit der Heilanstalt Winnenthal, vom 1. März 1843 bis 28. Februar 1846,“ *AZP* 5 (1848): 163–209. Die in der *AZP* veröffentlichte Fassung war erneut stark überarbeitet und erweitert worden].

wird, kann sich deshalb auch nur darauf beziehen, daß, um in das Geheimnis einer kranken Seele einzudringen und eine leitende vernünftige Gewalt über sie zu bekommen, das schlechthin abstrakte wissenschaftliche Interesse nicht ausreicht, und eine Hingabe der eigenen Persönlichkeit erfordert wird, wie sie nur aus dem tiefsten Mitleiden mit diesen Unglücklichen hervorgehen kann.“[245] Über seine bisherige Klassifizierung sagt Zeller ausdrücklich folgendes: „In Beziehung auf die Hauptformen der Seelenstörung und ihre Einteilung konnten wir indessen keinen Grund finden, zu einer anderen Klassifikation und Benennung überzugehen, da sie uns trotz der allen solchen Einteilungen anklebenden Mängel doch in Beziehung auf Diagnose und Prognose noch immer die leichteste Übersicht und Handhabung zu gewähren scheint. Wenn wir auch in manchen Fällen die Tollheit als Primärform, z. B. bei der Entstehung der Seelenstörung aus gastrisch-nervösen Fiebern, Arthritis, Trunksucht, Sonnenstich, Schrecken, und besonders aus Apoplexie beobachten konnten, so zeigt doch auch diesmal wieder die tabellarische Übersicht die Schwermut als die vorherrschende Grundform des psychischen Leidens. Mögen auch andere Beobachter andere Resultate gefunden haben, wie denn auch diesmal bei uns die Schwermut die vorherrschende Form bei den Frauen bildete und in andern Anstalten die Tobsucht bei den weiblichen Kranken vorschlug.“[246]

Der fünfte Bericht, der nun einen Zeitraum von 8 Jahren (1.3.1846 bis 28.2.1854) referiert, wurde 1855 der Allgemeinen Zeitschrift für Psychiatrie in Auszug wiedergegeben.[247] Der Bericht zeigt uns einen wesentlich reiferen, ernsteren, jetzt 50 Jahre alten Arzt, der schon 20 Jahre in der praktischen Irrenheilkunde steht, und nichts zeigt uns das Wesen dieses Mannes deutlicher als folgendes Zitat: „Wie der Sehende dem Blinden sein Auge, der Hörende dem Tauben sein Ohr zu leihen vermag, so haben die Ärzte und Pfleger solcher Unglücklichen ihnen ihre Seele zu leihen, bis und damit sie wieder selbst sehen, hören, vernehmen, wollen und handeln können, wie es sich vernünftigen Menschen geziemt. Um dieses zu erreichen, muß man nicht, wie man zu sagen pflegt, in ihre kranken Ideen eingehen, sondern es ist nötig, wie sich einer unserer ersten Kranken einmal ausdrückte, vor allem auf den Sinn im Unsinn sich verstehen zu lernen, und in ihr innerstes Geistes- und Gemütsleben durch jede Spalte, die sich darbietet, einzudringen, sich in ihr gesundes, wie in ihr krankes Sein hinein einzufühlen und zu denken, und mit ihnen zu leben um ihnen vorleben zu können. Nur wer ihr Herz gewinnt, kann hoffen, ihren Verstand zu gewinnen.“[248] Wir sehen aber auch bei dem 50-Jährigen schon Zeichen von Verhärtung der Meinungen, ein gewisses Erstarren vor allem in der Paralyse-Frage. Durch A. L. J. Bayle (1799–1858) und L. F. Calmeil (1798–1895) waren die wesentlichsten Forschungsergebnisse über diese Krankheit bekannt geworden.

[245] Albert Zeller, „[Vierter] Dreijähriger Bericht“, 11. [Vgl. die abweichende Fassung bei Albert Zeller, „[Vierter] Bericht“, 175 ff.

[246] Albert Zeller, „[Vierter] Dreijähriger Bericht“, 11. [Vgl. die abweichende Fassung bei Albert Zeller, „[Vierter] Bericht“, 177 f.

[247] Vgl. Albert Zeller, „[Fünfter] Bericht“ (1854) und „Bericht über die Wirksamkeit Heilanstalt Winnenthal vom 1. März 1846 bis 28. Februar 1854,“ *AZP* 12.4 (1855): 693–700.

[248] Albert Zeller, „[Fünfter] Bericht“ (1854), 306.

Zeller stand ihnen fremd gegenüber.[249] Ein ausschließliches Gehirnleiden als Ursache von Geisteskrankheit wollte und konnte er nicht mehr anerkennen, hatte er doch die Gallsche Hirnlehre von Jugend auf abgelehnt. Der ganze Körper war ja Seelenorgan und krankhafte Verstimmungen waren Folgen von abnormer Funktion des Gangliensystems. Daß er allerdings die progressive Paralyse als Krankheitsbild bis ins Letzte kannte, das zeigt mit wenigen Sätzen eine fast klassische Symptomschilderung derselben.

In die Berichtszeit fallen die Revolutionswirren der Jahre 1848/49. Es ist medizinhistorisch von Bedeutung, daß Zeller dabei erstmals die Beobachtung machen konnte, daß solche Massenkatastrophen und Erregungen die Zahl der Geisteskranken nicht vermehren. „Es ist fast unglaublich, welche Summe von Irrtum, Torheit, Jammer, Leidenschaftlichkeit aller Art, Unsittlichkeit, Gottlosigkeit, das Seelenorgan ertragen kann, ohne zu erkranken, wie man dies in den Zeiten der epidemischen Aufregung und Verwirrung in den Jahren 1848 und 1849 im großartigsten Maßstab sehen konnte, welche Jahre wenigstens uns keinerlei namhaften Zuwachs von Kranken, und nicht Einen [sic!] Fall, in dem nicht zugleich andere bedeutende körperliche Schädlichkeiten mitgewirkt hätten, gebracht haben.“[250]

Es klingt wie ein Abschied und es ist auch einer, denn Albert Zeller hat von 1854 an keinen wissenschaftlichen Aufsatz mehr veröffentlicht. Das geplante Werk über die Unsterblichkeit der Seele hat er nicht mehr zustande gebracht, nur die *Lieder des Leids* erschienen bis zum Tode 1877 immer wieder vermehrt. Er schreibt: „Wie wir in pathologischer und ätiologischer Beziehung keine Ursache fanden, von unseren anfänglichen Prinzipien abzugehen, so hielten wir bis jetzt auch an unserer Klassifikation der Hauptformen der Seelenstörung fest, weil sie sich uns nicht allein als die verständlichste und am leichtesten zu handhabende erprobt hat, sondern noch weit mehr darum, weil sie uns mehr als andere Einteilungen die meisten genetischen, diagnostischen und prognostischen Momente darbietet, und bereits hatten wir die Genugtuung, daß auch einige auswärtige öffentliche Anstalten sie in ihren Berichten über ihre Wirksamkeit angenommen haben. Wie wünschenswert aber eine endliche Verständigung in dieser Beziehung, sowohl den Ärzten als dem Richterstand gegenüber sein muß, leuchtet von selbst ein, zumal wenn man einen Blick in die wahrhaft babylonische Sprachverwirrung in diesem Gebiet, namentlich in den verschiedenen Gesetzgebungen wirft. Daß jede auch die naturgemäßeste Einteilung der Geisteskrankheiten ihre mannigfachen und großen Mängel haben wird, und so auch die unsere, wissen wir selbst am besten. Das Leben in seinem ewig regen Fluß läßt sich nun einmal nicht fest in bestimmte Rahmen bannen, die Zustände der Kranken sind oft so wechselnd, zuweilen auch so amorph, daß es schwerfällt, für den einzelnen Augenblick im Laufe einer Seelenstörung die rechte Bezeichnung zu finden; glücklicherweise handelt es sich aber auch in den meisten Fällen nicht darum, was nur momentan erscheint, sondern um die Reihenfolge und Gruppierung der Hauptzustände und vor allem um die Grundstellung, die das kranke

[249] [Vgl. hierzu Gerhart Zeller (Hg.), *Albert Zellers medizinisches Tagebuch*, Bd. 2, 134].

[250] [Albert Zeller, „[Fünfter] Bericht“ (1854), 302].

Bewußtsein gegen das freigebliebene gesunde einnimmt. In Beziehung auf die Form der Melancholie haben wir in neuerer Zeit immer mehr die doppelte Art derselben in passiver und aktiver Gestalt unterscheiden gelernt und sahen uns mehr und mehr genötigt, die größte Anzahl von Maniakalischen in die letztern einzureihen, wie wir schon früher bei der Tollheit (Manie) die Unterabteilung der Raserei und Narrheit festsetzten, und in neuester Zeit immer mehr darauf geführt wurden, die aus der Verrücktheit, dem partiellen Wahnsinn, Paranoia entspringende Manie als eine ihrem ganzen Zusammenhang in ihrer ganzen Erscheinungsweise nach andre als die der primären Tollheit aufzufassen [...].“[251]

Es ist interessant zu sehen, wie es gerade die Manie, dieser Prüfstein für die psychiatrische Diagnostik, ist, die Zellers Systematik nicht zur Ruhe kommen läßt, allerdings ohne daß das System der Verlaufsformen der einen Geisteskrankheit aufgegeben würde.

TEIL 3.3

Albert Zeller und Wilhelm Griesinger

Wir haben damit unsere Aufgabe, eine möglichst vollständige Geschichte der geistigen Entwicklung des Vaters der Einheitspsychose zu geben, erfüllt. Wir sahen den Jüngling unter dem Einfluß einer noch in der „Empfindsamkeit“ verhafteten Mutter in einer dem schwäbischen Pietismus nahestehenden Geistigkeit zu einem feinen Beobachter seiner selbst und zum subjektiven Analytiker heranwachsen. In der Schule Autenrieths wurde er für die Metastasenlehre und für eine Grundüberzeugung gewonnen, die vielfach eine innere Verwandtschaft der unterschiedlichsten Krankheitszustände, welche damit Entwicklungsstufen eines Krankheitsprozesses wurden, sah. Über Autenrieth wurde er zudem mit Reils Lehre vom inneren Sinn und mit seiner Theorie vom Ganglien- und Cerebralsystem bekannt gemacht. 1824 gewann er Anschluß an den Kreis um Georg Andreas Reimer in Berlin und damit an die Berliner Spätromantik, welche vor allem in der Gestalt Schleiermachers tief auf ihn wirkte. Auf diese Weise wurde er vom Einheitsstreben des Zeitalters berührt, dem seine Anthropologie zeitlebens verhaftet blieb. Leib und Seele sind eins, Ausdruck der einen göttlichen Kraft. Dies zu lehren wurde er nicht müde. Die Frage der somatischen oder psychischen Genese der Geisteskrankheiten mußte so für ihn zu einem Problem zweiter Ordnung werden. Er blieb jedoch im wesentlichen Somatiker, und zwar, weil er bei der Beobachtung seiner eigenen Seelenzustände immer wieder auf psychisch unmotivierte Stimmungsschwankungen stieß. Eine Reise zu den wichtigsten psychiatrischen Einrichtungen und Lehrern des damaligen Europas festigte vor allem seine aus der Reilschen Lehre vom Cerebral- und Gangliensystem hergeleitete Ablehnung der Gallschen Hirnlehre und ließ ihn ein

[251] Albert Zeller, „[Fünfter] Bericht“ (1854), 304.

klares Bild von der Behandlung psychischer Krankheiten gewinnen.[252] Eine individuelle körperliche Behandlung, verbunden mit individueller psychischer Behandlung, war von da an sein Ziel, das er als Direktor der Heilanstalt Winnenthal von 1833 bis zu seinem Tode 1877 weitgehend verbunden mit einer geschickten Gruppentherapie zu verwirklichen wußte. 3600 Kranke gingen durch seine Hand, zwei Drittel von diesen konnte er als geheilt oder gebessert entlassen. In der Auseinandersetzung mit Joseph Guislain und dessen *Traité sur les phrénopathies* (1833) festigte sich seine Ansicht soweit, daß er 1840 seine psychiatrische Lehre von der Einheitspsychose geschlossen vortragen konnte. Wir glauben nach dieser Darstellung auf keinen Widerstand zu stoßen, wenn wir Zellers Lehre von der Einheitspsychose als romantische Einheitspsychose bezeichnen. Die Einheitspsychose im Sinne Zellers ist ein legitimes Kind des Einheitsstrebens, ja der Einheitssüchtigkeit der Romantik.

Zellers unmittelbare wissenschaftliche Wirksamkeit war nicht groß; eine breite indirekte Wirksamkeit wurde ihm erst durch Wilhelm Griesinger und dessen Werk zuteil. Wir haben uns somit nun diesem bedeutenden Manne zuzuwenden, wobei wir entsprechend unserm Ansatz zunächst die Frage zu erörtern haben, ob auch er noch zu den Romantikern zu rechnen sei.

Wilhelm Griesinger wurde am 29. Juli 1817 in Stuttgart geboren. Er starb am 26. Oktober 1868 in Berlin an Perityphlitis.[253] Griesinger stammt aus einer Stuttgarter Familie, er studierte noch bei Autenrieth in Tübingen Medizin. Von Anfang an stand er modernen Einflüssen, vor allem jenen aus Frankreich kommenden, weit offen. Sein Weg führte ihn mit Carl August Wunderlich und Roser zusammen und 1842 zur Gründung des *Archiv für physiologische Heilkunde*. Daß Broussais der geistige Vater dieser Richtung war, wird von niemand bezweifelt, so sehr auch die Entwicklung über ihn hinauswachsen sollte.

Was Griesinger eigentlich bewegt haben mag, am 20. Februar 1840 als Assistenzarzt bei Zeller in Winnenthal einzutreten, ist unbekannt. Wir wissen nur, daß auf Autenrieths Veranlassung gleich bei der Gründung der Anstalt Winnenthal bestimmt wurde, daß nach 10 Jahren ein zweiter Arzt angestellt werden solle. Mit Griesinger wurde diese Stelle dann erstmals besetzt. Wir haben schon oben zitiert, was Griesinger selbst über die Winnenthaler Zeit und seinen Lehrer Zeller im Vorwort zur ersten Auflage seiner *Pathologie und Therapie der psychischen Krankheiten* schrieb.[254] Westphal hat das Verhältnis wohl am lebendigsten geschildert:

---

[252] [Vgl. Gerhart Zeller (Hg.), *Albert Zellers medizinisches Tagebuch*, Bd. 2, 64 f].

[253] Theodor Kirchhoff, „Wilhelm Griesinger," in *Deutsche Irrenärzte*, hg. von Theodor Kirchhoff (Berlin: J. Springer, 1921), 1–14; Wunderlich, „Wilhelm Griesinger"; Carl Westphal, „Nekrolog. Nach einer Rede gehalten zur Gedenkfeier für Griesinger," *Archiv für Psychiatrie und Nervenkrankheiten* 1 (1868): 760–774; Georg Stickler, „Wunderlich, Roser, Griesinger: ‚Die drei Schwäbischen Reformatoren der Medizin'," *Sudhoffs Archiv* 32/33 (1939/40): 32: 217–274 und 33: 1–54. [Zu Griesinger, vgl. auch die spätere Veröffentlichung Gerhart Zeller, „Welcher psychiatrischen Schule hat Wilhelm Griesinger angehört?," *Deutsches Medizinisches Journal* 19 (1968): 328–334].

[254] Vgl. das Vorwort in Griesinger, *Die Pathologie und Therapie*.

„In Winnenthal eröffnete sich für ihn eine neue Welt, in die er sich mit voller Hingabe versenkte; mit dem Direktor der Anstalt, dem Hofrat Dr. Zeller, knüpfte er ein Freundschaftsverhältnis, das bis zuletzt gedauert hat, und oft gedachte er später der in Winnenthal verlebten Tage, als eines der glücklichsten Zeitabschnitte seines Lebens. [….] Das bis in die späteste Zeit freundschaftliche und herzliche Verhältnis zu Herrn Zeller und dessen Familie ist umso bemerkenswerter, als beide Männer außerordentlich verschiedenen Anschauungen – namentlich auf religiösem Gebiet – huldigten."[255] Schon am 27.12.1841 schied Griesinger aus Winnenthal, seinem tragischen und abenteuerlichen Fatum folgend. Es ist für das Verständnis von Griesingers psychiatrischen Arbeiten notwendig, sich recht deutlich zu machen, wie sehr ihn Zeller und seine Anstalt beeindruckten. Enthalten doch Griesingers psychiatrische Aufsätze bis zum Erscheinen der ersten Auflage seiner *Pathologie und Therapie der psychischen Krankheiten* 1845 nichts anders als eine Auseinandersetzung mit den Ansichten seines Lehrers Albert Zeller.

Griesingers Kritik mußte an dem Punkte ansetzen, wo Zeller am meisten den Ansichten seiner Zeit verhaftet war, nämlich an dem für Zeller unbedingt gültigen Reilschen Denkmodell von Cerebral- und Gangliensystem, dem Denkmodell, welches die Grundlage von Zellers Lehre von der Einheitspsychose bildet. Das primär erkrankende Gangliensystem erzeugt krankhafte Gefühle und Stimmungen. Geht die Krankheit nach den Gesetzen der Metastasenlehre auf das Gehirn über so entstehen sekundär krankhafte Vorstellungen. Dieser Kernpunkt romantischer Anthropologie war für Griesinger nicht mehr annehmbar. Er mußte sich ein neues Denkmodell der psychischen Krankheiten schaffen, allerdings ohne an der überkommenen Lehre von der primären Depression und der sekundären Störungen des Denkens und Vorstellens etwas zu ändern. Wie Zeller von den physiologischen Anschauungen seiner Zeit beeindruckt war, so mußte Griesinger nun die modernen Ergebnisse physiologischer Forschung heranziehen. Er tat es in zwei grundlegenden Arbeiten. In der ersten Arbeit[256] geht Griesinger davon aus, daß im Rückenmark, aus den zentripetalen Eindrücken der sensitiven Nerven, gleichsam in der Sonnenferne des Bewußtseins, eine Aktion entstehe, die der scheinbaren Ruhe, oder richtiger dem mittleren Tätigkeitsgrade des sensorischen und motorischen Systems entspreche, nämlich der Tonus der Muskeln, des Zellgewebes und der Gefäße. Geradeso, meint Griesinger, bilde sich im Gehirn aus der ganzen Masse der zuströmenden und im Organ zerstreuten Vorstellungen ein Zustand scheinbarer Ruhe, welcher die Kraft und die Richtung der psychischen Bewegung, daß heißt der Bestrebungen reguliere. Dies Verhältnis der Summe aller Vorstellungen als eines Ganzen zu der Kraft, Leichtigkeit und Richtung der möglichen Bestrebungen, dieser psychische Tonus – so meint Griesinger – werde zum großen Teil mit den Worten Gemüt und Charakter bezeichnet. Wie aber der zentripetale Reiz im Rückenmark nicht nur durch Zerstreuung auf den Gesamtzustand des Organs wirke, sondern

[255] [Westphal, 761].

[256] Wilhelm Griesinger, „Ueber psychische Reflexactionen. Mit einem Blick auf das Wesen der psychischen Krankheiten," *Archiv für physiologische Heilkunde* 2 (1843): 76–113.

auch in zentrifugale Aktion umgesetzt werde, so würden die dem Gehirn teils direkt von den Sinnesorganen, teils indirekt vom Rückenmark zugeleiteten Eindrücke nicht nur unbewußte Anregungen für den psychischen Tonus bleiben, sondern sie würden auch in bewußte Vorstellungen und dann in Bestrebungen übergehen. Vorstellungen regen Strebungen an und werden zu solchen, Strebungen regen wieder Bewegungen, Aktionen der Muskeln, an und werden zu solchen. Wie nun die Rückenmarksreflexe vom Gehirn aus gehemmt werden, so werde auch im Gehirn der Übergang der Vorstellungen in Bestrebungen gehemmt, und zwar durch das gemeinschaftliche Wirken aller übrigen Vorstellungen auf die im Fluß befindlichen. Dies ist nach Griesinger die Grundlage dessen, was man Besonnenheit nennt. Der Wahnsinn beruht nun auf Anomalien in der Zerstreuung der Vorstellungen und deren Übergang in Bestrebungen. Hemmungen im freien Fluß der Vorstellungen sowohl in ihrer Zerstreuung in das Gesamtorgan als in ihrem Übergang in Strebungen erzeugen psychische Unlust, Traurigkeit bis zur Verzweiflung, also Schwermut, Melancholie. Daß der Zustand der psychischen Depression in der unendlichen Mehrzahl der Fälle der Ausgangspunkt für die ganze Reihe weiterer Veränderungen, welche den Wahnsinn konstituieren, bilde, daß er der eigentlich primäre sei, dies, betont Griesinger, habe er selbst an einigen Hundert selbstbeoachteten Fällen in Winnenthal gesehen, es sei ihm unantastbares Gesetz geworden. Dieser Hemmungszustand könne nun von den verschiedensten äußeren Erlebnissen aus angeregt sich bilden, teils könne das Gehirn als Vorstellungs- und Strebungsorgan primär oder durch sympathische Reizung von anderen Organen (häufig von den Genitalien) aus in der Weise erkranken, daß die Zerstreuung der Vorstellungen und namentlich die Strebungen vermindert, gehemmt werden.

Griesinger setzt seine Bemühungen um ein neues Denkmodell als Grundlage der Einheitspsychose 1844 in den „Neuen Beiträgen zur Physiologie und Pathologie des Gehirns" fort. Der einleitende Abschnitt ist für seine wissenschaftsgeschichtliche Stellung so wichtig, daß wir ihn zitieren: „Wir nehmen die am Schlusse einer früheren Arbeit[257] zusammengeknüpften Fäden wieder auf, um sie weiter zu führen, indem wir die Vergleichung von Empfindungs- und Bewegungs- (im physiologischen Sinne Rückenmarks-) und von psychischen (Gehirn-) Phänomenen in kranken und gesunden Zuständen fortsetzen. Wie sich Goethes Idee und Okens Nachweis gemeinschaftlicher Bildungsgesetze für die Wirbel- und Kopfknochen höchst fruchtbar erwies für das Verständnis des Schädelbaues, so dürfen wir hoffen, daß auch aus der Vergleichung zwischen den Lebenstätigkeiten des Rückenmarks und des Gehirns sich gewisse fördernde Anhaltspunkte für die richtige Auffassung der psychischen Erscheinungen ergeben werden."[258]

Griesinger ist ein Mann des Übergangs, in allen weltanschaulichen Fragen von größter Zurückhaltung, alleine auf positives Wissen aus, schwenkt er hier den romantischen Zauberstab der Analogie, und zwar mit ausdrücklichem Bezug auf

---

[257] [Vgl. ebenda].

[258] Wilhelm Griesinger, „Neue Beiträge zur Physiologie und Pathologie des Gehirns," *Archiv für physiologische Heilkunde* 3 (1844): 69.

Oken! Wir sind sicher, daß sich viele Schwierigkeiten seines Wesens auf diesen inneren Zwiespalt an der Schwelle von romantischer Naturphilosophie und Positivismus zurückführen lassen.

Die Abhandlung beginnt mit einem Bekenntnis zu einer pathophysiologischen Betrachtung der Geisteskrankheiten und mit dem Hinweis auf die unbefriedigenden Resultate einer pathologischen Anatomie derselben. Auch Zeller hatte in seinem vierten Bericht über die Wirksamkeit der Heilanstalt Winnenthal auf das durchweg negative Ergebnis einer pathologischen Anatomie der Geisteskrankheiten hingewiesen.[259] Griesinger führt nun den Begriff der Spinalirritation ein und bestimmt diese als eine Krankheit ohne sichtbare Beeinträchtigung der Substanz. Den Begriff der Cerebralirritation bildet er analog. Die Schwermutszustände werden als Cerebralirritation mit dem vorstechenden Symptom des Schmerzes definiert und in Analogie gesetzt zu den Neuralgien. Wie der Neuralgie subjektiv Schmerz, objektiv Kontraktur, Zittern und Lähmung entspricht, so geht auch die Cerebralirritation subjektiv mit Schmerz einher, objektiv mit Hemmung oder Erregung. Die Manie wird von Griesinger als psychisch-convulsiver Zustand aufgefaßt. Die sekundären Formen (Wahnsinn, partielle Verrücktheit, Narrheit) werden der chronischen Spinalirritation gegenübergestellt. Wie bei dieser Rückenmarkskrankheit, steht auch hier die Schwäche im Vordergund. Es handelt sich somit um psychische Schwächezustände. Der Blödsinn endlich ist psychische Paralyse. Er entspricht der Lähmung, welch nach Spinalirritation zurückbleibt.

So hatte Griesinger nun in Analogie zu Spinalirritation und Neuralgie sein Denkmodell gefunden, das in der Lage war, den Verlauf der Geisteskrankheit von schmerzhafter Depression bis zur vollständigen Lähmung in der Demenz, entsprechend der Zellerschen Stadieneinteilung, zu erläutern.

[¶] Wie sehr sich Griesinger dadurch im Gegensatz zu seinem Lehrer Zeller gebracht hatte, wird deutlich, wenn man bedenkt, daß Zeller zeitlebens einen Kampf gegen die Gallsche Hirnlehre geführt hatte. Geisteskrankheiten waren für ihn nie eine Sache des Gehirns allein, der ganze Körper war Seelenorgan. Zeller hatte gerade an Guislain die Überbewertung des Gehirns für die Entstehung der Seelenstörungen beanstandet. Nun mußte er erleben, daß sein Schüler Griesinger die Geisteskrankheit kurzweg als Cerebralirritation bestimmte und in § 1 seiner *Pathologie und Therapie der psychischen Krankheiten* 1845 auf die rhetorische Frage: welches Organ muß als überall und immer notwendig erkrankt sein, wo Irresein vorhanden ist? die Antwort gab: „Zeigen uns physiologische und pathologische Tatsachen, daß dieses Organ nur das Gehirn sein kann, so haben wir vor allem in den psychischen Krankheiten jedesmal *Erkrankungen des Gehirns* zu erkennen."[260] Es wäre sicher zum Bruch zwischen den beiden Männern gekommen, wenn nicht Griesinger im übrigen, wenigstens zunächst, ein getreuer Schüler seines Lehrers geblieben wäre.

---

259 Vgl. Albert Zeller, „[Vierter] Dreijähriger Bericht", 14.

260 [Griesinger, *Die Pathologie und Therapie*, 1].

Als einen solchen getreuen Schüler, ja geradezu als ein Sprachrohr seines Lehrers, sehen wir ihn in seiner Rezension über Jacobis Hauptformen der Seelenstörungen. Er bekennt sich hierbei in erster Linie zu Zellers Anthropologie und der von ihm vertretenen Einheit von Leib und Seele. Griesinger schreibt: „Der dualistischen Hypothese stellt sich die nach den empirischen Daten weit wahrscheinlichere Hypothese einer unmittelbaren Einheit der leiblichen und Seelen-Erscheinungen entgegen. Diese Ansicht ist bis jetzt viel weniger bearbeitet und ausgebildet worden, als die dualistische, und zwar aus Gründen, unter denen die Scheu, die vor dem Worte ‚materialistisch' verbreitet ist, nicht zu den letzten gehört."[261] Auch im Folgenden ist er mit Albert Zeller, der immer wieder davon sprach, daß der Geist seine Physis, seine Physik habe und daß sein höchstes und freiestes Wirken an diese organische und dynamische Gesetzmäßigkeit gebunden sei, einig, wenn er schreibt: „Die Psychologie hat sich nach unserer Überzeugung gerade so zur Psychiatrie zu verhalten, wie die Physiologie zur Pathologie und Medizin. Beide haben die wichtigsten gegenseitigen Aufschlüsse von einander zu fordern. Daß wir aber unter Psychologie überhaupt nichts Anderes, als eine empirische, eine Beobachtungs-, eine Naturwissenschaft verstehen können, wird keiner weiteren Ausführung bedürfen. Für eine solche aber ist die Mechanik der Gehirnaktionen die erste Grundlage, welche dann auch der abstrakteste Spiritualismus anerkennen muß. Dort, auf diesem Gebiete, kann mit dem auch in der Psychiatrie so oft proklamierten, aber so selten konsequent festgehaltenen Satze der Einheit von Seele und Leib endlich Ernst gemacht werden."[262]

Wilhelm Griesinger und Johann Friedrich Herbart

Wir müssen annehmen, daß Griesinger sich intensiv um eine solche Psychologie als Grundlage der Psychopathologie bemühte, ja bemühen mußte. Bei Albert Zeller war sie nicht zu finden. Er bedurfte ihrer nicht. Was der ältere Lehrer auf dem Wege der Einfühlung und subjektivistischen Analyse an psychologischen Einsichten gewonnen hatte, war dem jüngeren naturwissenschaftlich ausgerichteten Schüler nicht mehr zugänglich. Die ganze Methode mußte auf ihn als vorwissenschaftlich wirken. Griesinger mußte aber, wollte er seiner Richtung der physiologischen Medizin, welcher er im Verein mit Roser, Carl August Wunderlich leidenschaftlich verbunden war, treu blieben, seine *Pathologie und Therapie der psychischen Krankheiten* auf eine Psychologie aufbauen. Griesinger hatte das Werk kurz nach seinem Weggang aus Winnenthal zu schreiben begonnen. Es erschien 1845 erstmals in Stuttgart. Er schreibt im Vorwort der ersten Auflage: „Die psychologische Analyse des Irreseins, mit deren bisheriger Behandlung ich in vielen Punkten nicht übereinstimmen konnte und deren eigene Darstellung deshalb eine Hauptaufgabe bildete,

[261] Griesinger, „[Rezension von] M. Jacobi," 296.

[262] [Ebenda].

machte es notwendig, Einiges über das gesunde Seelenleben vorauszuschicken. Es galt hier nicht eine Psychologie zu schreiben, sondern nur einige Hauptpunkte von unmittelbarer Anwendung auf die psychische Krankheit hervorzuheben. Ich befand mich hier an einigen Stellen in der besonderen Lage, eigene Ansichten über den Zusammenhang der psychischen Erscheinungen unterdrücken zu müssen, weil sie nicht ohne eine für die notwendige Kürze dieser Schrift allzu weitgreifende Auseinandersetzung hätten dargestellt werden können, und mich dafür der Formen und Termini einer anerkannten (der Herbartschen) Psychologie bedienen zu müssen. Ich werde mich für diese Resignation ein andermal entschädigen."[263]

Es ist wohl der Seltenheit dieser ersten Ausgabe von Griesingers Pathologie und Therapie zuzuschreiben, daß mancherorts übersehen wurde, daß die Benutzung der Herbartschen Psychologie für Griesinger ausdrücklich nur eine Notlösung bedeutete und daß daher der Versuch, Griesingers ganze Psychiatrie aus der Herbartschen Psychologie abzuleiten, wenig ergiebig sein mußte; auf jeden Fall weniger ergiebig, als wenn man Griesingers Herauswachsen aus der Lehre seines Lehrers Zeller aufmerksam verfolgte.

Allerdings war Herbarts Psychologie keineswegs ungeeignet und Griesinger mußte, wie wir sehen werden, manches in ihr finden, was seinen auf anderem Wege gefundenen Vorstellungen entsprach.

[Zwei von Herbart zwischen 1816 und 1825 veröffentlichte Werke gelten als die ersten Lehrbücher der Psychologie als eigenständige Wissenschaft.][264] Der Untertitel seines zweiten Werkes mußte Griesinger anziehen; er versprach eine „Psychologie als Wissenschaft, neu gegründet auf Erfahrungen, Metaphysik und Mathematik". Herbart war eigentlich noch ein Vertreter der Assoziationslehre, seine geistigen Einheiten waren Vorstellungen, nicht Vermögen. Wir sehen schon hier eine gewisse Beziehung zu Griesinger, in dessen Arbeit über die psychischen Reflexaktionen die Vorstellungen eine große Rolle gespielt hatten. Herbart allerdings hatte keine Verwendung für Physiologie, alle Erklärungen mit neurologischen Begriffen fehlen in seinem Werk. Umso reizvoller mußte für Griesinger der Gedanke sein, ihn in dieser Hinsicht zu ergänzen. Herbarts „Vorstellungen" waren jedoch von denen Griesingers grundverschieden. Sie waren dynamische Einheiten, die miteinander um einen Platz im Bewußtsein kämpften und gemäß bestimmter quantitativer Gesetzmäßigkeiten aufeinander wirkten. Die Vorstellungen, so meinte Herbart, können sich entweder zu einem harmonischen Ganzen verschmelzen oder aber gegenseitig verdrängen. Wenn sie von gleicher Kraft sind, ist die gegenseitige Hemmung vollkommen, sind zwei oder mehrere sich gegenseitig behindernde Vorstellungen von gleicher Stärke vorhanden, so geben sie die Resultate an das Bewußtsein weiter, dessen Inhalt nun jederzeit in dem wechselseitigen Spiel der konkurrierenden Vorstellungen ausgedrückt werden kann. Herbart hat bekanntlich

[263] [Griesinger, *Die Pathologie und Therapie*, iv-v].

[264] Johann Friedrich Herbart, *Lehrbuch der Psychologie* (Königsberg: 1816); ders., *Psychologie als Wissenschaft* (Königsberg: 1824/25). Wir folgen in der Darstellung von Herbarts Psychologie der deutschen Übersetzung von John Carl Fluegel, *Probleme und Ergebnisse der Psychologie: Hundert Jahre psychologischer Forschung* (Stuttgart: Klett, 1947).

den Versuch gemacht, diese Verhältnisse mathematisch zu erfassen. War somit das Bewußtsein durch Vorstellungen, die dem Bewußtsein nicht oder nicht vollständig gegenwärtig sind, zu erklären, dann mußte dem Unbewußten eine breite Bedeutung zukommen. Herbart unterscheidet drei Bewußtseinsstufen: erstens die im Blickfeld stehenden Vorstellungen, die klar wahrgenommen und begriffen werden, zweitens Randvorstellungen, die verschwommen und nur unklar gegenwärtig sind, und drittens jene, die ganz und gar aus dem Bewußtsein verdrängt wurden. Eine Vorstellung, die eine Verdrängung erfahren hat, hört nicht auf zu existieren; sie verbindet sich nur mit der großen Menge anderer aus dem Bewußtsein verdrängter Vorstellungen, die wiederkehren können, entweder bei Nachlassen der entgegenwirkenden Vorstellungen oder durch Verbindung mit einer ähnlichen, da kombinierte Kräfte solche Widerstände, die vorher zu stark waren, nun zu überwinden imstande sind. Wir müssen es dem Leser überlassen, die gedankliche Verbindung zwischen Griesingers Lehre vom psychischen Tonus und Herbarts Bewußtseinslehre zu ziehen. Wir sind jedoch ganz entschieden der Ansicht, daß nicht Herbart der Anreger Griesingers war, sondern daß Griesinger auf seiner Suche nach einem neuen Denkmodell der Geisteskrankheit und einer der Psychopathologie zu Grunde legbaren Psychologie, also in seinen Ablösungsbestrebungen von seinem Lehrer auf Herbart eigentlich mangels anderer Möglichkeit zurückkommen mußte.

Nachdem wir so die Grundprinzipien aufgezeigt haben, nach welchen Griesinger seine Pathologie und Therapie abgefaßt hat, dürfen wir sein übriges Werk als nicht zum Thema gehörig und den Rahmen der Arbeit sprengend beiseite lassen. Es kann nicht unsere Aufgaben sein, Griesingers Bedeutung für die Psychiatrie hier erschöpfend darzustellen. Was seine Systematik betrifft, so haben wir diese bereits eingangs nach der ersten Auflage der Pathologie und Therapie zitiert. Wir dürfen hinzufügen, daß sie sich unverändert in der vierten und letzten zu Lebzeiten erschienenen Auflage 1876, welche allerdings im wesentlichen ein Nachdruck der zweiten Auflage von 1861 ist, wiederfindet.

Es möchte uns scheinen, daß Griesingers Formulierung der Lehre von der Einheitspsychose nur darin von der Zellers abweicht, daß sie wesentlich apodiktischer ausgesprochen wird. Hatte Zeller noch geschrieben „Die dritte Hauptform der Irreseins, die Verrücktheit [...] tritt fast nie als primäre Form auf, wenigstens nach unserer Beobachtung, wenn nicht etwa auf dem Wege der Eifersucht, Prozeßsucht und der für Wahrheit gehaltenen einzelnen Sinnestäuschungen“,[265] so findet sich keine dieser Einschränkungen mehr bei Griesinger. Bei Griesinger ist die Unterteilung im einzelnen differenzierter; er unterscheidet als primäre Zustände die psychischen Depressionszustände und die psychischen Exaltationszustände, unter denen ersteren Hypochondrie, Melancholie, Melancholie mit Stumpfsinn, Melancholie mit Äußerung von Zerstörungstrieben, Melancholie mit anhaltender Willensaufregung; die psychischen Exaltationszustände umfassen die Tobsucht, den Wahnsinn. Die sekundären Zustände werden in Analogie mit Neuralgie und Spinalirritation als psychische Schwächezustände definiert; sie umfassen die

[265] [Albert Zeller, „Zweiter Bericht,“ 135].

partielle Verrücktheit, die Verwirrtheit, den apathischen Blödsinn. In den späteren Auflagen ist noch Idiotismus und Cretinismus angefügt.

Wilhelm Griesinger und Ludwig Snell

Bei der großen Verbreitung des Griesingerschen Lehrbuchs und einer zunächst fast allgemein anerkannten Gültigkeit seiner Lehre konnte die Kritik ganz im Sinne der von Zeller gemachten Vorbehalte und Einschränkungen nicht lange auf sich warten lassen.

Die Kritik kam von sehr berufener Seite. Dr. Ludwig Snell, geboren am 18. Oktober 1817, gestorben am 12. Juni 1892, aus einer alten Gelehrtenfamilie stammend, war 1849 Direktor der neuen Irrenanstalt zu Eichberg geworden. 1856 hatte man ihm die Direktion der damals größten Irrenanstalt Deutschlands in Hildesheim übertragen, welcher er 1873 die erste deutsche Ackerbaukolonie anfügte. Snell hielt auf der Naturforscherversammlung zu Hannover vom 18. bis 22. September 1865 einen Vortrag „Über Monomanie als primäre Form der Seelenstörung".[266] Er trug 8 Fälle vor, welche wir heute unschwer als paranoid-halluzinatorische Schizophrenie diagnostizieren. Er kam zu folgendem Ergebnis: 1.) Die Monomanie (oder der Wahnsinn) entwickelt sich in ihrer reinen Form als primäre Geistesstörung. 2.) Die aus Manie und Melancholie hervorgegangenen ähnlichen Krankeitszustände unterscheiden sich von der reinen Monomanie durch allgemeines Ergriffensein des Seelenlebens. 3.) Die Entwicklung der Monomanie ist zweifacher Art: in der Mehrzahl der Fälle entsteht sie allmählich, selten unter den mehr stürmischen Erscheinungen eines akuten Leidens. 4.) Die Verfolgungsideen mit gehobenem Selbstgefühl bilden den Grundcharakter dieser psychischen Krankheitsform. 5.) Die Überschätzungsideen sind gewöhnlich sekundär, können aber auch den Verfolgungsideen vorangehen oder sich gleichzeitig mit denselben entwickeln.

Mit Snells Kritik war der erste entscheidende Einbruch in die zur Herrschaft gekommene Zeller-Griesingersche Lehre gelungen. Sehen wir, wie Griesinger darauf antwortete. Er tat dies charakteristischerweise nicht in seinem Lehrbuch, das er nach diesem Einbruch grundsätzlich hätte überarbeiten müssen. Waren doch die sogenannten sekundären Zustände, von Griesinger als Schwächezustände gedeutet, fest und unverrückbar in Griesingers System eingebaut. Der Gedanke einer primären Schwäche war auch mit dem zu Grunde gelegten Denkmodell von der Neuralgie und der Spinalirritation nicht zu vereinheitlichen. Es war ein schwerer Schlag für Griesinger, und er sah sich gezwungen, die Grundlagen seine psychiatrischen Denkens zu überprüfen.

Griesinger brachte seine noch keineswegs geklärten und in einer tiefgreifenden Wandlung befindlichen Auffassungen in seinem Vortrag zur Eröffnung der

[266] Ludwig [Daniel Christian] Snell, „Über Monomanie als primäre Form der Seelenstörung," *AZP* 22 (1865): 368–381.

psychiatrischen Klinik in Berlin in die Öffentlichkeit. In ihm findet sich der programmatische Satz „Halten wir uns noch fern den sogenannten ‚Formen‘ der Psychiatrie; kehren wir zurück zu den Elementen, die wir eben betrachten, zu unsern Primordialdelirien."[267] Unter diesen Primordialdelirien, die er auch typische oder fundamentale Delirien nennt, möchte Griesinger immer wiederkehrende falsche Gedankenverbindungen verstehen, die von 10 Kranken mindestens 7 aussprechen und vielleicht bei 5 Kranken durch die ganze Dauer der Krankheit den Hauptinhalt des Deliriums bilden und die so häufig die ersten und letzten aller Wahnvorstellungen seien.

Griesinger glaubt mehrere Hauptgruppen solcher Primordialdelirien unterscheiden zu können. Bei der einen Gruppe hätten die Wahnvorstellungen den Inhalt eines Leidens, einer Beeinträchtigung, einer Unterdrückung. Die andere Gruppe trage aktiven, expansiven, gesteigerten Charakter. Daneben möchte Griesinger auch die körperlichen Wahnvorstellungen, die Sexualdelirien sowie die eigentümliche Gefühls- und Vorstellungsweise des allgemeinen Anderssein als Primordialdelirien ansehen. Die beiden erstgenannten hält er für Hauptarten. Sie können sich mit anderen verbinden. Griesinger meint, so würden dann durch Mischung von Größen- und Verfolgungsideen die Bilder entstehen, welche Snell beschrieb und die Griesinger mit einem neu eingeführten Ausdruck als „primäre Verrücktheit" bezeichnen möchte. In dieser Bezeichnung steckt noch das alte System, in welchem ja bekanntlich die psychisch anomalen Grundzustände, welche auf Affekten oder affektartigen Zuständen beruhten, als primär im Sinne des zeitlichen Ablaufs den Zuständen gegenübergestellt wurden, die ohne tiefere Gemütsbewegung mit falschem Denken und Wollen einhergingen. Aber Griesinger hatte 1867 das System bereits völlig gesprengt. Führt er doch in der Eröffnungsansprache vom Jahre 1867 aus: „Jetzt zweifle ich selbst, ob auch für die Fälle, wo die Erklärung ganz zu passen scheint, die Fassung, die Primordialdelirien *entstehen* aus der pathologischen Gemütsbewegung [...], der richtige Ausdruck ist [...]. Die Betrachtung in den letzten Jahren hat mir gezeigt, daß dies zum mindestens nicht so allgemein ist, als ich früher glaubte."[268]

Wir gebrauchten oben im Zusammenhang mit Griesingers Lebenslauf das Wort „tragisch", und wir sehen jetzt, wie richtig es angewandt war. Ein Jahr vor seinem Tode sehen wir ihn als Herausgeber der unveränderten dritten Auflage seiner *Pathologie und Therapie der psychischen Krankheiten,* in welcher er sein bisheriges System der Geisteskrankheiten unverändert wiedergab und gleichzeitig in seinem Vortrag zur Eröffnung der psychiatrischen Klinik zu Berlin als einen gründlichen Zerstörer derselben.

Wir können nur ahnen, wie Griesinger sich die weitere Entwicklung seiner Forschungen gedacht haben mag. Offenbar wollte er mit den Methoden der Statistik eine Reihe von Initialsyndromen herausarbeiten und diese dann während des

---

[267] W[ilhelm] Griesinger, „Vortrag zur Eröffnung der psychiatrischen Klinik zu Berlin am 2. Mai 1867," *Archiv für Psychiatrie und Nervenkrankheiten* 1 (1867): 148.

[268] [Ebenda, 150].

Verlaufes der Krankheit verfolgen. Daß dies ein methodisch richtiges Vorgehen gewesen wäre, das dann wohl auch zu ähnlichen Ergebnissen wie die Untersuchungen Kraepelins hätte führen müssen, kann wohl nicht bezweifelt werden. Griesingers unerwarteter Tod an einem perityphlitischen Abszeß schnitt die weitere Entwicklung ab. Da Griesinger aber in erster Linie durch sein Lehrbuch bekannt wurde, lebt er weiter als Vertreter der Einheitspsychose, obwohl er diese im letzten Jahr seines Lebens gründlich zerstört hatte. Schon aus diesem Grunde wäre es gut, wenn man in Zukunft nicht mehr von der Zeller-Griesingerschen Einheitspsychose reden würde, sondern von der romantischen Lehre von der Einheit der Psychosen (Albert Zeller). Ganz unvorbereitet war diese Entwicklung in Griesingers Denken allerdings nicht. Sehen wir ihn doch schon bei der Abfassung der ersten Auflage seines Lehrbuchs damit beschäftigt, durch Analyse der Erscheinungsbilder zu Elementarstörungen vorzustoßen. Es ist kein Zweifel, daß Joseph Guislain hier der Anreger war, welcher ja im Grunde nichts anderes suchte als solche Elementarstörungen, die für ihn typische Reaktionsformen waren und die dann untereinander beliebige Verbindungen eingehen konnten. Guislain war, so betrachtet, keineswegs auf der Suche nach der Einheit der Psychosen, sondern ein Vorläufer einer psychiatrischen Syndromlehre. Guislain steht somit am Anfang einer Entwicklung, die mit E. A. Hoches „Die Bedeutung der Symptomenkomplexe in der Psychiatrie“[269] endete, ohne ganz ausgeschöpft worden zu sein.

Um dieses Suchen nach letzten Elementarteilchen der Geisteskrankheit konsequent durchhalten zu können, hätte es eines kälteren analytischen Verstandes bedurft. Griesinger, der Mann des Übergangs, der innerlich seinem in Schleiermacherschem Denken gereiften Lehrer Albert Zeller stets verbunden blieb, dem die 2 Jahre in Winnenthal ein Höhepunkt seines Lebens blieben, der den Zauberstab der Analogie nach dem Vorbild Okens und Galls schwang und der dabei leidenschaftlich nach positivem Wissen strebte, mußte auf diesem Wege scheitern. Für uns liegt Griesingers Bedeutung für die Psychiatrie darin, daß er für eine wahrhaft anthropologische Psychiatrie eintrat, das heißt für eine Psychiatrie, welche der geistig-seelischen Seite des Menschen ebensoviel Aufmerksamkeit schenkt wie seiner körperlichen.

Friedrich Wilhelm Hagen

Wir begegnen auf diesem Wege wissenschaftlicher Entwicklung einem Manne, dessen Namen im ersten Kapitel der Arbeit erwähnt wurde, nämlich Friedrich Wilhelm Hagen (1814–1888). Hagen war Schüler Friedreichs. Er ging 1844 auf eine wissenschaftliche Reise, die ihn zu Jacobi nach Siegburg, zu Guislain nach Gent, zu Roller in der Illenau und zu Zeller in Winnenthal führte. Von 1860 bis 1887 war er

[269] Alfred Erich Hoche, „Die Bedeutung der Symptomenkomplexe in der Psychiatrie,“ *Zeitschrift für die gesamte Neurologie und Psychiatrie* 12 (1912): 540–551.

dann Direktor der Heil- und Pflegeanstalt und ex. ord. Professor für Psychiatrie an der Universität in Erlangen. In seiner akademischen Antrittsvorlesung vom Jahre 1860 wirbt er mit klugen und wohlabgewogenen Worten für eine Physio-Psychologie oder eine medizinische Psychologie als Sonderfach. Er sagte: „Die einseitige Betrachtung führt eben, wie überall, so ganz besonders bei diesem Gegenstande, zu nichts; es muß von beiden Standpunkten aus geforscht und dann versucht werden, die Ergebnisse dieser verschiedenen Untersuchungsweisen miteinander zu vereinigen."[270] Kraepelin weiß, daß Hagen die Zeller-Griesingersche Lehre übernommen hat. Wir können dies heute nicht mehr prüfen, da Hagen uns kein abschließendes Werk über psychiatrisch Systematik hinterlassen hat. Sie lag ihm wohl nicht so sehr am Herzen, wie seine große Arbeit über den goldenen Schnitt. Vielleicht war er aber auch der Meinung Neumanns, daß keine Systematik besser sei als eine falsche. Aber damit ist der genannt, der uns nunmehr beschäftigen wird: Heinrich Neumann.

TEIL 3.4

Heinrich Neumann und der Positivismus

Heinrich Neumann, geboren 1814, gestorben 1884, ist eine scharf profilierte wissenschaftliche Erscheinung. Er stammte aus einer jüdischen Gelehrtenfamilie. Sein Vater wirkte für die Judenemanzipation. Er wurde von einer englischen Missionsgesellschaft beauftragt, das Neue Testament ins Hebräische zu übersetzen. Dies führt dazu, daß er mit seiner ganzen Familie zum Christentum übertrat. Er lebte später in Breslau als Privatgelehrter. Heinrich Neumann war vielseitig gebildet. Seine Erscheinung war die eines Weltmannes. Schon mit 22 Jahren promovierte er *multa cum laude* zum Doktor der Medizin. Nachdem er einige Jahre Militärarzt gewesen, habilitierte er sich in Breslau für innere Medizin. Da er in allem ausgesprochen modern dachte und sich zur naturhistorischen Schule Schönleins bekannte, kam es innerhalb der Fakultät zu Unzuträglichkeiten. 1846 gab er seine Dozentur auf und ging als Assistenzarzt an die Provinzial-Irrenanstalt Leubus, welche damals von Dr. G. M. Martini (1830–1872), mütterlicherseits einem Nachkommen Melanchthons, geleitet wurde. Mit ihm, der vorwiegend statistischen und juristischen Fragen zugewandt war, harmonierte Neumann nicht. 1849 schied er aus Leubus und wurde wieder Militärarzt. Als solcher war er während des polnischen Aufstands und während der Choleraepidemie 1850 tätig. 1852 gründete er dann die erste Privat-Irrenanstalt Norddeutschlands in Pöpelwitz bei Breslau. In den fünfziger Jahren habilitierte er sich zum zweiten Male für Psychiatrie. 1862 wurde er

[270] [Friedrich Wilhelm Hagen, „Der Werth und die Bedeutung der Psychologie für die Psychiatrie," in *Studien auf dem Gebiete der ärztlichen Seelenkunde: gemeinfassliche Vorträge*, hg. von Friedrich Wilhelm Hagen (Erlangen: Besold, 1870), 8].

Professor extraordinarius für Psychiatrie und kam neben Griesinger und Dr. August von Solbrig (1809–1872), dem Direktor der Kreisirrenanstalt zu München, für die Besetzung des Berliner Lehrstuhls in Frage. 1867 wurde er Primärarzt der Irrenabteilung des Allerheiligen-Hospitals in Breslau. Diese Abteilung wurde 1874 in eine psychiatrische Klinik umgewandelt, deren erster Direktor Heinrich Neumann wurde. Ab 1881 begann er zu kränkeln. Eine Diagnose konnte nicht gestellt werden, weil er jede körperliche Untersuchung ablehnte. Erst als 1884 eine Karbunkulose auftrat, war die Diagnose Diabetes mellitus sicher. Am 10. Oktober 1884 starb er im Coma diabeticum.

Nimmt man Neumanns *Lehrbuch der Psychiatrie*[271] zur Hand, dann fühlt man, vor allem, wenn man vorher in Griesingers *Pathologie und Therapie* gelesen hat, einen ganz besonders analytischen, skeptischen, positivistischen Geist am Werke. Man kann sich die Kluft in Stil und Weltanschauung gegenüber Albert Zeller nicht tief genug vorstellen. Albert Zeller war romantisch, pantheistisch auf Synthese aus. Neumann kalt und klar, ganz moderner Naturwissenschaftler, unreligiös und in allen Seelenfragen auf das positiv Wißbare eingeschränkt. Neumann ist dadurch auch präzis in seinen Formulierungen und er steckt gleich auf den ersten Seiten seines Buches die Grenzen scharf ab: „Die Wissenschaft vom räumlichen Dasein des Menschen nennen wir die Anatomie, die vom zeitlichen Dasein die Physiologie; ein drittes Wissen, sofern es auf den Namen einer Naturwissenschaft Anspruch macht, vom Menschen gibt es nicht.“[272] Der Begriff der Seele erscheint nicht mehr in seinem Werk. „Ein lebendes Ganze, dessen Verrichtungen in ihm selbst ganz oder teilweise zum Bewußtsein kommen, heißt ein *beseeltes* Wesen […. Man sage nun] nicht mehr, der Mensch hat *eine Seele*, sondern: der Mensch ist *beseelt.*“[273] – „Der Weg der Naturwissenschaften führt weder zu Gott hin, noch von ihm hinweg; er berührt den Weg der Religion in keinem einzigen Punkt.“[274]

Wenn man bedenkt, daß diese Zeilen nur 5 Jahre nach Zellers letztem Bericht über die Wirksamkeit der Heilanstalt Winnenthal geschrieben wurden, dann gewinnt man einen lebendigen Eindruck von der ungeheuren weltanschaulichen Wandlung welche sich in der ersten Hälfte des 19. Jahrhunderts abspielte. Wir verstehen aber auch, warum Albert Zeller 1854 aufhörte, wissenschaftlich zu publizieren.

Einer der großen Anreger dieser Wandlung war Auguste Comte (1797–1858), und wir müssen in aller gebotenen Kürze uns ins Gedächtnis zurückrufen, was dessen „Positivismus“ eigentlich aussagt. Wir benützen der Prägnanz und Kürze wegen die *Geschichte der Philosophie* (1932) von Ernst von Aster. „Die Grundthese des Comteschen ‚Positivismus‘ ist der Gedanke, daß wir erstens, nur eine Kenntnis von *Phänomenen* besitzen und daß zweitens unsere Kenntnis von den Phänomenen eine *relative*, keine absolute ist. Es hat keinen Sinn, nach dem ‚Wesen‘ einer Tatsache oder nach ihrer wirklichen ‚Ursache‘ zu fragen, sondern nur nach ihrer Beziehung

---

271 Heinrich Neumann, *Lehrbuch der Psychiatrie* (Erlangen: Enke, 1859).

272 [Ebenda, §3, 4].

273 [Ebenda., §20, 9].

274 [Ebenda., §6, 5].

zu anderen Tatsachen in der Form der Aufeinanderfolge oder der Ähnlichkeit. Diese Beziehungen sind konstant, wir nennen sie, soweit es sich um die Beziehungen der Ähnlichkeit handelt, Begriffe, soweit es sich um solche der Abfolge handelt, Gesetze der Phänomene. Die Gesetze der Phänomene kennenzulernen, um dann mit ihrer Hilfe die kommenden Phänomene vorhersagen zu können [– *savoir pour prévoir* –] ist der Sinn aller wissenschaftlichen Erkenntnis."[275]

Wir verstehen jetzt Neumanns Bemühungen um die Klärung der psychologischen Phänomene besser. Die Methode, mit welcher er diese Erklärung zu erreichen sucht, ist die analytische, zu welcher er sich ausdrücklich in §1 seines Werkes bekennt und die er am Beispiel der analytischen Chemie erläutert. Er führt allerdings logisch fortschreitend aus, daß Analyse immer eine Einheit, ein Ganzes, voraussetze, was zerlegt werden könne. Die analytisch zu unterscheidende Einheit der Psychiatrie sei der Mensch, das heißt dessen Funktionen.

Eine der Grundfunktionen, deretwillen man ihm das Prädikat eines beseelten Wesens erteilt habe, sei die Metamorphose, das heißt diejenige Tätigkeit, kraft welcher der Mensch seine Sinneseindrücke in Bewußtseinszustände verwandle.[276] Derjenige Zustand, bei welchem die Tätigkeit der Metamorphose sich vorherrschend auf Kosten der anderen Seelentätigkeiten gelten mache, nennt Neumann Hypermetamorphose.[277] Sie wird von Neumann dadurch charakterisiert, daß die Aufmerksamkeit fortwährend für die Sinnenwelt in Anspruch genommen wird. Dieser Zustand ist gleichbedeutend mit Erethismus des Bewußtseins. Er ist ein exzessiver Wachzustand (Pervigilium). Aus der Erregung wird Gereiztheit, alle Sensationen werden als unangenehm und schmerzhaft erlebt. Die Hypermetamorphose artet in Tobsucht aus. Die Tobsucht ist allerdings für Neumann keine besondere Krankheit, sondern „nur eine Aufforderung zur Diagnose, d. h. eine Aufforderung zur Erforschung der Elemente, welche die Tobsucht bedingten und der Folgen, welche sie notwendigerweise mit sich bringen muß."[278] Die Hypermetamorphose ist aber auch der genetische Bereich für die Entstehung von Illusionen.

Der der Hypermetamorphose entgegengesetzte Zustand ist die Ametamorphose.[279] Wurde das Bewußtsein in der Hypermetamorphose von den Sinneseindrücken und damit von der Außenwelt beherrscht, so schließt sich in der Ametamorphose der Mensch zunehmend von der Außenwelt ab. Seine Tätigkeit nimmt die Richtung nach innen. Die geistigen Kräfte gehen zurück. Der Kranke empfindet nicht, will nicht, vernachlässigt sich, Halluzinationen und Wahnvorstellungen treten hinzu. Die Ametamorphose umfaßt sowohl die Melancholie als auch die Ekstase oder, wie wir heute sagen würden, die gehemmte Depression und den Stupor.

---

[275] [Ernst v. Aster, *Geschichte der Philosophie* (Leipzig: Kröner, 1932)].

[276] [Neumann, *Lehrbuch*, §91, 40].

[277] [Ebenda, §159, 71].

[278] [Ebenda, §162, 75].

[279] [Ebenda, §176, 91].

Wir sehen so, wie Neumann aus den beiden Grundzuständen der Hypermetamorphose und der Ametamorphose alles ableitet, was er Elemente nennt, Elemente, die noch keineswegs das Vorhandensein einer Krankheit beweisen. Krankheit ist erst da, wo aus einem Element fortschreitend andere sich entwickeln, also ein Krankheitsprozeß stattfindet.[280]

Wo nun solcher Prozeß stattfindet, da liegt Seelenstörung vor. Neumann betont: „[E]s gibt nur eine Art der Seelenstörung. Wir nennen sie *Irresein.*"[281] Irresein hat so nicht verschiedene Formen, wohl aber verschiedene Stadien. Sie heißen Wahnsinn, Verwirrtheit, Blödsinn. Hieraus folgt, daß ein Wahnsinniger, der nicht geheilt wird, sicherlich in Verwirrtheit und schließlich in Blödsinn verfallen wird.

Es wird auf den, der sich in das System Neumanns vertieft, ungemein befremdend wirken, daß er die ganze Gruppe der affektiven Psychosen, welche Griesinger, Zeller folgend, so sauber den nicht affektiven entgegengestellt hatte, gänzlich unter den Tisch fallen läßt, obwohl er in seinem Lehrbuch zugeben muß, daß die Schriftsteller, „welche behaupten, dem Wahnsinn gehe ein Stadium melancholicum voraus, *der Sache nach*, wenigstens für die große Mehrheit der Fälle, recht hatten."[282] Dennoch bleibt Neumann ausdrücklich dabei, daß die Melancholie als Krankheitsklasse unbrauchbar sei.[283] Die schwermütige Stimmung könne zu jeder Form und zu jedem Stadium der Geisteskrankheit hinzutreten.

Schließen wir mit der Ausführung dessen, was Neumann selbst für das Spezifische seiner Auffassung hält. Er betont in §266 seines Lehrbuchs, daß es 2 Punkte seien: Erstens habe er versuchst, die konkreten kranken Seelenzustände so lange zu analysieren, bis eine weitere Trennung unmöglich geschienen habe. Was er so fand, habe er Elemente genannt. So sei die Hypermetamorphose ein Element, so die Tobsucht, die Halluzination. Nach Elementen allerdings sei eine Klassifikation nicht zu machen. Der andere spezifische Punkt seiner Auffassung sei der, daß eine reelle Einteilung der Geisteskrankheiten sich nur auf die geistigen Verrichtungen stützen dürfe. Diese seien aber in Wirklichkeit nicht so leicht zu trennen wie in den psychologischen Systemen.

Es komme bloß auf den Mut an, es auszusprechen: besser gar keine Klassifikation als eine falsche. „Man mache sich einmal mit der Vorstellung vertraut, daß die *Krankheiten des Menschen* den Klassenbegriff abgeben, unter welchem die *Geisteskrankheiten* als *Genus* erscheinen, die einzelnen vorkommenden Fälle aber die *Spezies* repräsentieren [....] Es ist aber allen Spezies gemein, daß sie als Wahnsinn beginnen, in Verwirrtheit übergehen und als Blödsinn enden."[284] Nur eine Form wird von Neumann aus diesem Verlauf ausgenommen. Es ist der angeborene Blödsinn (Idiotie, Cretinismus).

---

280 [Ebenda, §155, 69].

281 [Ebenda, §247, 167].

282 Ebenda, §255, 170–171.

283 Ebenda, §267, 182–184.

284 Ebenda, §266, 182.

Die Romantische und die Positivistische Einheitspsychose

Haben wir bei der Besprechung der Zeller-Griesingerschen Lehre von der romantischen Einheitspsychose oder von der romantischen Auffassung von der Einheit der Psychosen gesprochen, so müssen wir Heinrich Neumanns Lehre als die positivistisch-skeptische Auffassung von der Einheit der Psychosen nennen. Trotz mancher gemeinsamer Grundgedanken, zum Beispiel der deutlichen Verwandtschaft von Neumanns Lehre von der Metamorphose mit der schon 1843 von Griesinger vorgetragenen Lehre von der psychischen Reflexaktion, müssen wir eine scharfe Trennung der romantischen und positivistischen Einheitspsychose vollziehen. Man sollte in Zukunft Zeller-Griesinger und Neumann nicht mehr in einem Atemzug nennen, vor allem auch der so ganz unterschiedlichen Wertung der Verstimmungszustände wegen. Liegt doch für Zeller auf ihnen der Hauptakzent, während sie bei Neumann nur unwesentliche Begleitumstände sind. Eigentlich kam Neumann zu seiner Einheit nur dadurch, daß er mit kühnem Strich Zellers Primärformen beseitigte.

Dieses ungewöhnliche und den Tatsachen Gewalt antuende Verfahren hat seine Ursache sicher in persönlichen Bedingtheiten. Zellers Temperament schwang harmonisch zwischen heiter und traurig. Neumanns Temperament scheint ganz nach der psychästhetischen Proportion gebaut gewesen zu sein.[285]

TEIL 3.5

Von der Einheitspsychose zur Vesania Typica *Kahlbaums*

Niemand hat wohl die große Einseitigkeit im Neumann-System klarer erfaßt als Karl Ludwig Kahlbaum (1828–1899). Kahlbaum stammte aus der Neumark, sein Vater war Fuhrunternehmer. Seine Neigung zog ihn zum Studium der Naturwissenschaften und der Mathematik. Aus praktischen Grunde studierte er jedoch Medizin in Königsberg, Würzburg, Leipzig und Berlin.1854 promovierte er. 1856 trat er in die ostpreußische Provinzial-Irrenanstalt Allenberg als zweiter Arzt und Stellvertreter des Direktors Bernhardi (1804–1872) ein. Von Allenberg aus erwarb er sich die *venia legendi* in Königsberg und verfaßte 1863 die bereits öfters erwähnte Arbeit *Die Gruppierung der psychischen Krankheiten und die Einteilung der Seelenstörungen*. Kahlbaum war finanziell sehr beschränkt, und er sah bald, daß sich seinem Plane, die Universitätslaufbahn einzuschlagen, unübersteigbare

---

[285] [G. Zeller greift hier auf Ernst Kretschmers Theorie der Temperamente zurück. Rückblickend diagnostiziert er Neumann als ‚schizothym', was durch eine ‚psychaesthetic proportion' von Überempfindlichkeit und Kühle gekennzeichnet ist, und Zeller als ‚cyclothym'. Vgl. Ernst Kretschmer, *Körperbau und Charakter: Untersuchungen zum Konstitutions-Problem und zur Lehre von den Temperamenten*, 11. und 12. Auflage (Berlin: Springer, 1936), 136–140].

Hindernisse entgegenstellten. Er nahm daher im Oktober 1866 das großzügige Angebot von Dr. Hermann Reimer (7.5.1825–8.6.1906) an, der ihm die Stelle des zweiten Arztes an seiner 1850 für Epileptische gebildeter Stände eröffnete Anstalt in Görlitz anbot.[286]

Kahlbaum war Heinrich Neumann hauptsächlich verpflichtet. Er spricht dies an vielen Stellen seines Buches über die *Gruppierung der psychischen Krankheiten* deutlich aus.[287] Kahlbaum hatte auch keinen Zweifel an der Richtigkeit von Neumanns Stadienlehre, ja er hält den von Neumann aufgezeigten Verlauf für typisch. Unter Berufung auf Zeller, Griesinger und Guislain bildet Kahlbaum aus ihm eine Klasse der Geisteskrankheiten, die er dann mit dem alten Namen *Vesania* belegt. Er definiert den Begriff der *Vesania* als idiopathische Seelenstörung mit deutlichem Ergriffensein des mehr oder weniger ganzen Umfangs des Seelenlebens.

Kahlbaum unterscheidet dann 3 Gattungen von *Vesania*:

1.) *Vesania acuta*, das ist fieberhaftes Irresein ohne ätiologische Begleitung extracerebraler Krankheiten.
2.) *Versania typica*, das ist idiopathische Seelenstörungen in bestimmten regelmäßigen Stadien verlaufend. Diese Stadien sind:

   I. *Stadium melancholicum (incrementi)*
   II. *Stadium maniae (acmes)*
   III. *Stadium perturbationis (decrementi)*
   IV. *Stadium dementiae (defectus)*

Wir haben hier also unsere alte Einheitspsychose, wie sie Zeller beschrieben hat, wieder vor uns, mit der wesentlichen Einschränkung auf einen Verlauf unter anderen, allerdings einen besonders typischen Verlauf. Kahlbaum stellt neben die *Vesania typica* dann noch die *Vesania progressiva*, das ist die progressive Paralyse. Später hat Kahlbaum dann noch seine *Vesania catatonica* hinzugefügt. Hatte Neumann von allen Geisteskrankheiten des Menschen nur das Irresein gelten lassen und sowohl theoretisch als auch beschreibend die affektiven Psychosen gänzlich vernachlässigt, so konnte der gänzlich empirische und unvoreingenommene Kahlbaum ihm hier nicht folgen.

[¶] Er stellte der Klasse *Vesania* die Klasse *Vecordia* zur Seite und definiert sie als idiopathische Seelenstörung von begrenztem Umfang der psychischen Symptome, welche meist nach der Pubertät auftritt. Innerhalb der Gruppe Vecordia

---

286 Hermann Reimer was das 15. Kind des oben erwähnten Berliner Verlegers Georg Andreas Reimer, der Schwager Albert Zellers. Neben vielen Arbeiten zur Klima- und Balneotherapie ließ er 1894 seinen satirischen Roman *Zweierlei Hoheit* unter dem Pseudonym Juvenalis minor erscheinen. Reimers Roman und der natürlich viel höherstehende „Maler Nolten“ von Eduard Mörike sind, soweit wir sehen, die einzigen Darstellungen der Einheitspsychose in Romanform. Wir wissen ja auch, daß Albert Zeller Mörike bei der Abfassung dieses Romanes beraten hatte. Vgl. Hermann Reimer, Zweierlei Hoheit: Roman von Juvenalis minor (Zürich: n.p., 1894). [Auslassung (ca. 550 Worte): weitere biografische Details zu Karl Ludwig Kahlbaum (1828–1899) und Hermann Reimer (1825–1906)].

287 Kahlbaum, *Die Gruppierung*.

unterscheidet Kahlbaum eine *Vecordia dysthymia* mit vorzugsweiser und primärer Ausbildung von Störungen des Gemütslebens, die sich weiter aufspaltet in *Dysthymia meläna* mit Vorwalten trauriger Affekte und in *Dysthymia elata* mit Vorwalten freudiger Affekte. Neben die Familie *Vecordia dysthymia* tritt dann die Familie *Vecordia paranoia* mit besonderer Ausbildung der Störungen in der Sphäre der Intelligenz, die *Vecordia diastrephia* mit Störungen vor allem innerhalb der Sphäre des Willens. Die letzte Familie der *Vecordia*-Gruppe nennt Kahlbaum *Vecordia insania*. Er möchte darunter ein partielle Störung ohne Vorherrschen einer besonderen dynamischen Richtung, jedoch mit Vorwalten anderer psychischer Symptome verstehen. Eine recht unklare Sache.

Die ganze Gruppe *Vesania* zeichnet sich aus durch eine gewisse Konstanz der Erscheinungsformen während der ganzen Verlaufsdauer sowie durch eine günstige Prognose.

Zu den beiden Gruppen *Vesania* und *Vecordia* tritt dann noch die Gruppe *Dysphrenia*. Kahlbaum möchte hierunter eine sympathische und symptomatische Seelenstörung, im Anschluß an einen speziellen physiologischen oder pathologischen Körperzustand sich entwickelnd, mit dem Charakter der Totalerkrankung des psychischen Lebens verstehen. Er teilt die *Dysphrenien* ein 1. in die *Neophrenia*, das ist eine Seelenstörung, welche vor, mit oder nach der Geburt im ersten Lebensjahr erworben wurde und die den Charakter des Mangels an psychischem Gehalt trägt. Der *Neophrenia* wird die *Paraphrenia* zur Seite gestellt. Unter diesem Begriff sammelt Kahlbaum die Seelenstörungen, welche im Anschluß an eine Übergangsperiode der biologischen Entwicklung auftreten. In dieser Gruppe unterscheidet Kahlbaum die *Paraphrenia hebetica*, die *Paraphrenia senilis* und die *Paraphrenia hypnetica*. Unter *Paraphrenia hebetica* versteht er die Pubertätsstörungen. Er kennt hiervorn zunächst nur eine Gruppe, die Hebephrenia. Später kommt die verlaufsgünstigere Heboidophrenie, das Heboid, hinzu. *Paraphrenia senilis* meint die im Greisenalter auftretenden und *Paraphrenia hypnetica* die in Schlafzuständen vorkommenden Störungen, zum Beispiel den Somnambulismus.

Es wäre durchaus interessant und lohnend, sich weiter mit Kahlbaums Psychiatrie zu befassen, vor allem mit seiner Unterscheidung zwischen Krankheitsprozeß, Habitualformen und Elementarformen. An dieser Stelle ist es jedoch nicht erlaubt und wir müssen lediglich feststellen, daß Kahlbaum aus der einen Psychose mit typischen Verlaufsstadien eine Krankheitsklasse unter fünfen gemacht hat. Kahlbaum ist somit derjenige, welcher die Lehre von der einen Geisteskrankheit endgültig überwunden hat. Der Weg zu immer klarerer Unterscheidung von Krankheitseinheiten ist frei geworden. Diese Entwicklung ist keineswegs auf die Psychiatrie beschränkt. Auch in der übrigen Medizin wurden die Krankheiten immer schärfer voneinander getrennt, vor allem seitdem die sich rasch entwickelnde Bakteriologie die Spezifität bestimmter Krankheiten erweisen konnte. Man denke hierbei nur an Robert Koch (1843–1910) und dessen Postulate.

Man könnte meinen, daß die Einheitspsychose damit eines natürlichen Todes an dem wachsenden Beobachtungsmaterial gestorben sei. Sie war allerdings zunächst nur scheintot. Rudolf Gottfried Arndt (1835–1900), der Ordinarius für Psychiatrie in Greifswald, ließ sie in seinem Lehrbuch für Psychiatrie 1883[288] noch einmal zum Leben erwachen, und zwar im selben Jahr, in welchem Emil Kraepelin (1856–1926) die erste Auflage seines Compendiums der Psychiatrie erscheinen ließ.[289]

TEIL 3.6

Rudolf Arndt und das biologische Grundgesetz

Arndt stammt aus dem Kreis Marienwerder.[290] Er besucht in Ratibor das Gymnasium. Er studierte in Greifswald. 1866 bis 1867 war er Volontärarzt an der Provinzial-Irrenanstalt in Nietleben bei Halle. Am 18. Dezember 1867 habilitierte er sich in Greifswald für innere Medizin, in deren Bereich teilweise noch die Psychiatrie gehörte. 1873 wurde er außerordentlicher Professor. Als solcher vertrat er das Fach Psychiatrie bis zu seinem Tode. Arndt war ein merkwürdiger Mensch. Streng formell, oft schroff, eigenbrötlerisch und empfindlich, nur durch seine starken wissenschaftlichen Interessen mit seiner Umwelt verbunden. Sein Denken war das eines modernen Naturwissenschaftlers, allerdings mit starker Neigung, gefundene Gesetzmäßigkeiten zu verallgemeinern.

Bekannt bis auf den heutigen Tag wurde Arndt durch die Entdeckung und Formulierung der sogenannten Arndt-Schulzschen Regel. Diese lautet: „Schwache Reize fachen die Lebenstätigkeit an, stärkere und mittelstarke beschleunigen, fördern sie, starke hemmen und stärkste heben sie auf." Der Greifswalder Pharmakologe H. Schulz hatte in dieser Regel das Grundprinzip der Arzneimittelwirkung erkannt und exakte Beweise hierfür geliefert, zum Beispiel durch Experimente mit den sogenannten Hefegiften, welche in kleiner Dosis das Wachstum der Hefen beschleunigen. Für Arndt wurde diese Regel zum biologischen Grundgesetz, dessen Anwendungsmöglichkeit unbegrenzt war und das er so unbekümmert zur Erklärung der verschiedenartigsten Erscheinungen heranzog. Die Entstehung von Plattfuß und Klumpfuß, Riesen und Zwergen, Schwarz und Weiß bei Tier und Menschen, Körperwärme und Fieber erklärten sich ihm so auf eine einfache Weise. Daß bei einer so breiten Anwendung eines allgemeinen Gesetzes auch Treffer sein würden, versteht sich von selbst. Arndts Versuch, das Pflügersche Zuckungsgesetz mit Hilfe des biologischen Grundgesetzes zu erläutern, war ein

[288] Rudolf Arndt, *Lehrbuch der Psychiatrie für Aerzte und Studirende* (Wien und Leipzig: Urban und Schwarzenberg, 1883).

[289] Emil Kraepelin, *Compendium der Psychiatrie: Zum Gebrauche für Studirende und Aerzte* (Leipzig: Abel, 1883).

[290] Die Persönlichkeit und das Werk Arndts wurden eingehend gewürdigt von W[illy] Vorkastner und Pophal, „Rudolf Gottfried Arndt 1835–1900," in *Deutsche Irrenärzte*, hg. von Theodor Kirchhoff, vol. 2 (Berlin: J. Springer, 1924), 138–142.

solcher Treffer.[291] Arndt hat seither einen festen Platz in der Neurophysiologie. Johann Gottschick schreibt in seinem Buch *Die Leistungen des Nervensystems*: „Nicht nur durch den elektrischen Strom [...], sondern auch durch andere physikalische und chemische Faktoren [...] kann die Erregbarkeit des Neurons eine Änderung erfahren. Im allgemeinen kommt es zunächst zu einer Erregbarkeitssteigerung und später zu einer Erregungsverminderung. Wie lange diese einander entgegengesetzten Stadien der Erregungsänderung anhalten, hängt von der Einwirkungsintensität und -dauer ab. Es gilt auch an nervösen wie an allen lebenden Substanzen die Arndt-Schulzsche Regel, daß schwache Einwirkungen die Lebenstätigkeit anfachen, etwas stärkere sie beschleunigen und fördern, starke sie hemmen und stärkste sie ganz aufheben. Was allerdings dabei als schwache und starke Einwirkung anzusehen ist, hängt stets von den betreffenden physikalischen Gegebenheiten oder chemischen Konstitutionen ab; so kann ein Stoff bei einer bestimmten Konzentration noch erregungsfördernd wirken, bei der ein anderer Stoff schon hemmt. Auch diese Tatsachen beweisen aber, daß Reiz und Erregungssteigerung am Neuron mit Vorgängen übereinstimmen, die in einem stärkeren Grade der Ausprägung zu Neuron*schädigung* führen.“[292]

Hatte Arndt somit bei der Anwendung seines biologischen Grundgesetzes auf die Gesetze des ermüdeten und absterbenden Nerven Glück gehabt, so mußte es ihm naheliegen, dies auch bei Geisteskrankheiten zu versuchen, zudem ja schon Griesinger Geisteskrankheit und Neuralgie in Analogie gesetzte hatte. Er schreibt in seinem Lehrbuch: „Das alles legt nun den Gedanken nahe, daß, wie jede Psychose nichts Anderes als der Ausdruck, d. h. die Reaktionsweise des in seiner Ernährung beeinträchtigten Nervensystems, insbesondere des Gehirns ist, daß so auch diese letztere an sich wieder nichts Anderes als bloß ein Ausdruck des Zuckungsgesetzes des in seiner Ernährung geschädigten Nerven überhaupt ist, und daß somit jede Psychose in ihrem Verlaufe dem Zuckungsgesetze des ermüdeten oder absterbenden Nerven folgt. Und so ist es auch in der Tat! Nur muß man sich mit dem Gedanken vertraut machen, daß das Absterben unter Umständen sehr lange dauert, sich Jahre und Jahrzehnte hinzieht, wie das der Fall bei dem Vorgang ist, den wir Involution nennen. Die Involution ist ja nur der Gang zum Tode [....] Die *initiale Melancholie* entspricht der Reaktionsweise des einfach ermüdeten Nerven, ist die des ermüdeten, beziehungsweise leicht ermüdenden psychischen Organs. Die *Manie* entspricht dem ersten Stadium des absterbenden, beziehungsweise leicht erschöpfbaren psychischen Organs, und die *sekundäre Melancholie* dem mehr oder minder erschöpften und daher mehr oder minder auch gelähmten psychischen Organe. [....] Wie das Zuckungsgesetz des in seiner Ernährung geschädigten Nerven überhaupt eine große Mannigfaltigkeit in seiner Erscheinungsweise an den Tag zu legen vermag, so auch die Psychosen. Das wechselvolle, in jedem einzelnen Falle anders gestaltete Bild, das sie darbieten, hat hierin seinen Grund. Wenn die einzelnen Stadien einer

---

[291] [Eduard Pflüger (1829–1910) beschrieb 1859 die Auslösung von Muskelzuckungen bei bipolarer Reizung eines motorischen Nerven mit galvanischem Strom].

[292] [Johann Gottschick, *Die Leistungen des Nervensystems* (Jena: Fischer, 1955), 32].

Psychose, sowohl nach Dauer als auch nach Stärke, ziemlich gleichmäßig ausgebildet sind, sodaß die Manie mit derselben Deutlichkeit in die Erscheinung tritt wie die initiale und sekundäre Melancholie und auf diese Weise ein ganz bestimmter Typus in ihrem Ablauf zur Erscheinung kommt, so heißt man die Psychose nach dem Vorgange Kahlbaums eine *Vesania typica*. Andernfalls führt sie andere Namen: *Dysthymia* oder auch *Melancholia*, *Mania* schlechtweg, *Lypémanie*, *Chaeromanie*, *Tobsucht* usw.; oder sie wird auch, zumal wenn das bezügliche Stadium sich über lange Zeiträume erstreckt und so gewissermaßen habituell geworden erscheint, und Parästhesien, Parabulien, Paralogien, sowie Parergasien überhaupt sich daneben geltend machen, zu einer Psychose quasi sui generis, zur sogenannten Verrücktheit oder Narrheit, der *Paranoia, Moria, Dementia*."[293] An jeder ausgebildeten Psychose kann man sonach 3 Stadien unterscheiden, das Stadium der initialen oder primären Melancholie, das Stadium der Manie und das Stadium der sekundären Melancholie. Jede psychische Krankheit beginnt und endet mit einer Melancholie.

Wir sehen so, daß Arndt im Grunde Griesingers Weg, wie er ihn in seinen beiden Arbeiten „Über psychische Reflexaktionen" und „Neue Beiträge zur Physiologie und Pathologie des Gehirns" begonnen hatte, konsequent fortsetzte.[294] Darüberhinaus ist er mit Griesinger aber auch darüber einig, daß Geisteskrankheiten funktionelle Krankheiten seien, das heißt Störungen der Gehirnfunktion. Arndt steht aber dennoch auf dem Standpunkt Zellers, daß der ganze Körper Seelenorgan sei. Arndt schreibt: „Alle Vorgänge des gesammten Körpers werden Quellen des psychischen Lebens. Es kommt nur darauf an, daß diese Vorgänge in irgendeiner Form dem großen Gehirne übermittelt und in demselben zu Bestandteilen des Vorstellens, des Bewußtseins werden."[295]

Arndt ist somit tatsächlich der letzte Vertreter der Einheitspsychose im Sinne Zellers und Griesingers. Die einzelnen abgrenzbaren Bilder von Seelenstörungen sind lediglich Phasen im Verlaufe eines umfassenderen Geschehens. Alle Geisteskrankheiten verlaufen nach demselben Schema, auch die progressive Paralyse. Die Variation der Bilder kommt dadurch zustande, daß verschiedene Phasen verschiedenartig stark hervortreten und daß sie von der Eigenart der erkrankten Persönlichkeit gefärbt werden. So entstehen paranoische Bilder dadurch, daß sich die *Vesania typica* auf dem Boden einer paranoetischen Veranlagung entwickelt. So Veranlagte können auch primär an Paranoia erkranken.

Nachdem wir Zellers Einheitspsychose als romantische Einheitspsychose charakterisierten, müssen wir hier fragen, ob denn auch Arndt noch zu den Romantikern gehöre. Diese Frage ist leicht zu verneinen. Es besteht ein prinzipieller Unterschied zwischen dem Denken Arndts und dem der romantischen Ärzte. Im romantischen Denken steht alles mit jedem in Bezug, überall wird Verbindendes gesehen, Ganzes, das lebendig sich entwickelt. Bei Arndt wird Einheit erreicht durch Verallgemeinerung und Verabsolutierung eines an sich richtigen Grundgesetzes. Dies sind

[293] Arndt, *Lehrbuch*, 253 f.

[294] Griesinger, „Ueber psychische Reflexactionen"; ders., „Neue Beiträge".

[295] [Arndt, *Lehrbuch*, 4].

gegensätzliche Wege. Man könnte sagen, für die Romantiker ist das Besondere nur interessant als Bestandteil eines Ganzen. Für Arndt wird auch das Allgemeinste nur Beispiel einer besonderen Regel. Wenn dieser Ausdruck nicht zu respektlos wäre, könnte man bei Arndt von der monomanen Auffassung von der Einheit der Psychosen sprechen.

TEIL 3.7

Abschliessende Zusammenfassung

Wir haben nun das breite Band der Erscheinungen, in welchem der Gedanke von der einen einheitlichen Psychose, welche in typischen Stadien von Melancholie zur Manie und weiter zu Verrücktheit und Blödsinn prozesshaft fortschreitet, in der Zeit vor Emil Kraepelin aufmerksam durchgemustert.

Es haben sich dabei 3 Auffassungen deutlich gegen einander abgehoben:

eine romantische (Albert Zeller),
eine positivistisch-skeptische (Heinrich Neumann),
eine monomane (Rudolf Arndt).

Die Lehre von der Einheitspsychose endete mit Karl Ludwig Kahlbaum, für welchen die eine einheitliche Psychose zu einem, allerdings typischen Verlauf unter anderen wurde. Sie heisst seit Kahlbaum „*Vesania typica completa*".

Fassen wir die Entwicklung der Lehre von der Einheitspsychose rückblickend kurz zusammen:

Wir sehen, dass schon Sydenham, Reil und Autenrieth Geisteskrankheiten beschrieben hatten, deren Verlauf dem später aufgestellten Schema der Einheitspsychose entsprach.

Autenrieths Schüler Albert Zeller war dann der erste, welcher die Lehre in seinem 2. Bericht über die Wirksamkeit der Heilanstalt Winnenthal 1840 klar aussprach. Wir bemühten uns, den persönlichen und geistesgeschichtlichen Wurzeln dieser Lehre bei Albert Zeller im Detail nachzugehen. Dabei fanden wir das Einheitsstreben der Romantik als den eigentlichen Grund der Zeller'schen Einheitspsychose. Infolge seiner Erziehung, seines persönlichen Wesens und seiner Berührung mit dem Kreis um Georg Andreas Reimer in Berlin, insbesondere mit Schleiermacher, war Zeller der Romantik tief verbunden. Infolge seiner Wesensart und des Ergebnisses seiner Selbstbeobachtung wurde ihm das Problem des Gestimmtseins zum Ausgangspunkt seiner psychopathologischen Überlegungen. Joseph Guislains Lehre vom Seelenschmerz als Fundamentalstörung der Geisteskrankheiten musste klärend auf Zellers Gedanken wirken, welche, wie wir sahen, in dieselbe Richtung gingen. Man kann somit sagen: *die Geburtsstunde der Lehre von der Einheitspsychose schlug, als Zeller mit dem Gedanken Guislains bekannt wurde.*

Keiner ist der Vorgänger des anderen. Das Zusammentreffen mit dem ähnlich Denkenden befruchtete beide.

Zellers Schüler Griesinger brachte dann die Lehre von der Einheitspsychose zu fast allgemeiner Anerkennung. Er formulierte sie entschiedener, als Zeller dies getan hatte, er liess Ausnahmen nicht mehr zu und trennte scharf die primären, affektiven Zustände von den sekundären, nicht affektiven, welche für ihn den Charakter von Schwächezuständen trugen.

In dieser apodiktischen Form war die Lehre von der Einheitspsychose indes in hohem Masse angreifbar geworden. Der Angriff erfolgte dann auch durch Ludwig Snell auf der Naturforscherversammlung von Hannover im September 1865. Snell trug 8 Fälle vor, welche wir heute als paranoid-halluzinatorische Schizophrenien diagnostizieren würden, und legte dar, dass diese Zustände primär ohne vorhergehendes *stadium melancholicum* aufgetreten seien. Diese Einwendungen waren so überzeugend, dass Griesinger 1867 in seinem Vortrag anlässlich der Eröffnung der psychiatrischen Klinik in Berlin die Lehre von der Einheitspsychose gründlich verwarf. Er entwickelte ein neues Forschungsprogramm, in welchem die Erforschung der Initialstadien der von ihm so genannten Primordialdelirien einen breiten Raum einnehmen sollte. Dass er dennoch 1867 die alte Lehre von der Einheitspsychose erneut in der unveränderten 3. Auflage seiner *Pathologie und Therapie* propagierte, ist einer der wirklich tragischen Momente in Griesingers Leben, welchem der frühe Tod 1868 die Klärung dieses Zwiespaltes versagte.

Wir haben Griesinger als einen Mann des Übergangs an der Schwelle der grossen Wandlung in der 1. Hälfte des 19. Jahrhunderts dargestellt; halb noch Romantiker, halb schon positivistischer Naturforscher. Auch in der Geschichte der Einheitspsychose war Wilhelm Griesinger ein Mann der Wandlung; brachte er doch einerseits die Lehre zur breitesten Anerkennung, andererseits war er der erste, der sich von ihr abwandte.

Die skeptisch-positivistische Form der Einheitspsychose trat uns bei Heinrich Neumann klar und deutlich entgegen. Neumanns Denken fusste auf den Forschungen Griesingers; er brach aber in seinem Lehrbuch entschieden mit jedem Systematisierungsversuch. Lieber gar keine Systematik als eine falsche. Neumann war so eigentlich der Begründer nicht eines Einheitssystems, sondern, wie Kahlbaum mit Recht sagt, eines Non-Systems. Wenn er dennoch zu einer einheitlichen Auffassung der Geisteskrankheiten kam, so geschah dies auf eine recht gewaltsame Weise: er setzte Geisteskrankheit mit Irresein gleich und liess die ganzen affektiven Zustände, die Primärstadien der Zeller-Griesingerschen Lehre unter den Tisch fallen. Die Melancholie war für ihn lediglich ein Begleitsymptom, das in jeder Phase des Irreseins auftreten konnte und dem keine Selbstständigkeit zukam. Es konnte so erstmals geklärt werden, dass Zellers und Neumanns Einheitspsychose wesensmässig verschieden sind; man sollte die Namen der beiden Männer nicht mehr in einem Atemzuge nennen.

Die 3. Form, in welcher uns die Einheitspsychose vor Kraepelin begegnete, war die von Rudolf Arndt 1883 in seinem Lehrbuch der Psychiatrie niedergelegte. Arndt hatte die sogenannte Arndt-Schulz'sche Regel entdeckt und mit dem Pharmakologen Schulz zusammen experimentell erhärtet. Diese wichtige Regel wurde ihm zum biologischen Grundgesetz schlechthin, das zur Erklärung des Verschiedenartigsten dienen musste. Auch die Geisteskrankheit war ihm nur ein Beispiel für die Richtigkeit dieses Grundgesetzes. An den von Zeller und Griesinger aufgestellten Verlaufsstadien hielt er im wesentlichen fest; er brachte sie in Analogie zum Verhalten des absterbenden und ermüdeten Nerven und damit zum Pflüger'schen Zuckungsgesetz. Arndt ging den von Griesinger begonnenen Weg konsequent zu Ende. Das Wesentliche an seiner Auffassung ist aber dennoch, dass für ihn die Geisteskrankheit nur ein Spezialfall eines in seiner Anwendung überdehnten, an sich richtigen Grundgesetzes war. Wir sprachen von der monomanen Form der Einheitspsychose.

Kahlbaum hat dann die Lehre von der Einheitspsychose harmonisch in die nun aufbrechende Erforschung der Krankheitseinheiten hinübergenommen. Die Einheitspsychose wurde für ihn zu einem typischen Verlauf unter anderen, zur „*Vesania typica*".

Wir haben uns in der vorliegenden Arbeit in erster Linie bemüht, den geistesgeschichtlichen und biografischen Hintergrund aufzuhellen, auf welchem sich in der Zeit vor Kraepelin die Lehre von der Einheitspsychose in ihren verschiedenen Formen und Fassungen entwickelte. Damit sollte dieser Lehre keineswegs jeder Erfahrungsgrund abgesprochen werden. Wir sehen allerdings diese Verläufe heute doch recht selten und möchten daher ganz am Ende unserer Untersuchung die Frage aufwerfen, ob sie nicht zur Zeit Albert Zellers häufiger gewesen sein könnten. Albert Zeller wies immer wieder darauf hin, dass in seinem Erfahrungsgut die Dinge so liegen würden, wie er sie beschrieben habe. Er wunderte sich selbst darüber, dass anderwärts andere Formen überwogen. In seinem 1. Bericht über die Wirksamkeit der Heilanstalt Winnenthal schrieb er folgendes: „Merkwürdig bleibt es übrigens, wie selten die in Frankreich alle anderen Formen überwiegende Narrheit sich hier beobachten liess, und wie sehr die Form der Schwermut bei den Frauen, und die der partiellen Verrücktheit bei den Männern überwog."[296]

Im schwäbischen Volkscharakter herrscht auch heute noch, wie jeder Erfahrene weiss, eine subdepressive Grundstimmung vor, und wir dürfen diese in Zusammenhang bringen mit einer hohen prozentualen Beteiligung der pyknischen Konstitutionstypen an der schwäbischen Bevölkerung. Vor der industriellen Völkerwanderung mit ihrer zunehmenden Nivellierung der Stammescharaktere war der Anteil der Pykniker in Schwaben wahrscheinlich noch höher. Zeller und Griesinger mussten dann in ihrem schwäbischen Beobachtungsgut vorwiegend Depressionen oder stark gebremste Schizophrenien sehen. In Ludwig Snells Beobachtungsgut in Hildesheim war dies wohl nicht in diesem Masse der Fall. Ihm drängten sich mehr die Bilder der Kernschizophrenien auf. Sein Einwand könnte so gleichermassen auf Beobachtung gegründet gewesen sein wie die Lehre von der Einheitspsychose wenigstens in Schwaben.[297]

---

[296] [Albert Zeller, „[Erster] Bericht," 334].

[297] [In seinen späteren Veröffentlichungen hat sich Zeller über diese epidemiologische Deutung der Entstehung der Einheitspsychose relativiert und geistesgeschichtliche Momente stärker betont.

Die historische Untersuchung hat den ganzen Fragenkomplex der Einheitspsychose aufgeworfen. Angesichts der intensiven Bemühungen der älteren Ärzte um die einheitlich verlaufende eine Psychose sei der Wunsch ausgesprochen, dass mit den Mitteln der modernen Psychiatrie, insbesondere mit denen der Konstitutionslehre, der Gestaltpsychologie und der somatischen Psychosenforschung das Problem erneut auf breiter Basis aufgerollt werden möge.

Literaturverzeichnis[298]

Ackerknecht, Erwin Heinz. 1957b. *Kurze Geschichte der Psychiatrie*. Stuttgart: Enke.

Allgemeine Deutsche Biographie. Edited by Rochus von Liliencron and Franz Xaver von Wegele. Leipzig: Duncker & Humblot, 1875–1912. #|

Arndt, Rudolf. 1883. *Lehrbuch der Psychiatrie für Aerzte und Studirende*. Vienna and Leipzig: Urban und Schwarzenberg.

Artelt, Walter. 1949. *Einführung in die Medizinhistorik: Ihr Wesen, ihre Arbeitsweise und ihre Hilfsmittel*. Stuttgart: Enke.

Aschoff, Ludwig, and Paul Diepgen. 1945. *Kurze Übersichtstabelle zur Geschichte der Medizin*. 6th. ed. Berlin: Springer. #|

Autenrieth, J. H. F., and J. G. von Bohnenberger. 1815. Vorrede. *Tübinger Blätter für Naturwissenschaften und Arzneykunde* 1 (1): 1–10.

Bernd, Adam. 1738. *Eigene Lebens-Beschreibung Samt einer aufrichtigen Entdeckung, und deutlichen Beschreibung einer der grösten, obwohl großen Theils noch unbekannten Leibes- und Gemüths-Plagen, Welche Gott zuweilen über die Welt-Kinder, und auch wohl über seine eigene Kinder verhänget: Den Unwissenden zum Unterricht, Den Gelehrten zu weiterem Nachdencken, Den Sündern zum Schrecken, und Den Betrübten, und Angefochtenen zum Troste*. Leipzig: Johann Samuel Heinsius.

Birnbaum, Karl. 1928b. Geschichte der psychiatrischen Wissenschaft. In *Handbuch der Geisteskrankheiten*, ed. Oswald Bumke, vol. 1, 11–49. Berlin: Springer. #|

Bodamer, Joachim. 1944. *Wilhelm Griesinger und die Entwicklung der Psychiatrie im 19. Jahrhundert*. Medizinische Dissertation, Universität Heidelberg.

Bodamer, Joachim. 1948b. Zur Phänomenologie des geschichtlichen Geistes in der Psychiatrie. *Der Nervenarzt* 19:299–310. #|

Bodamer, Joachim. 1953b. Zur Entstehung der Psychiatrie als Wissenschaft im 19. Jahrhundert. *Fortschritte der Neurologie, Psychiatrie und ihrer Grenzgebiete* 21:511–535. #

de Boismont, Alexandre Jacques Francois Brierre. 1867. *Joseph Guislain: sa vie et ses écrits. Esquisses de médecin mentale*. Paris: B. Baillière. #

Broussais, François Joseph Victor. 1828. *De l'irritation et de la folie: ouvrages dans lequel les rapports du physique et du moral sont établis sur les bases de la médicine physiologique*. Brussels: Melle Delaunay.

Buder. 1934. Die Psychiatrie Albert Zellers. *Allgemeine Zeitschrift für Psychiatrie* 102:217–231. *#|

Cramer, Max. 1927. *Zellerbuch*. Stuttgart: Grüninger. #|

Vgl. G[erhart] Zeller, „Die Tübinger Psychiater-Schule," in *Wahn*, hg. von Walter Schulte und Rainer Tölle (Stuttgart: Georg Thieme, 1972), 102 f].

[298] Works cited in the introduction of the original typescript have been marked as (*), those later compiled in its bibliography as (#). Works cited, but not referenced by Zeller are unmarked, those added by the editors are marked as (†). Works that are otherwise not cited in the text body or have been abridged are marked as (|).

Damerow, Heinrich Philipp August. 1829. *Die Elemente der nächsten Zukunft der Medizin, entwickelt aus der Vergangenheit und Gegenwart*. Berlin: Reimer. #

Damerow, Heinrich. 1840. *Über die relative Verbindung der Irren-Heil- und Pflege-Anstalten in historisch-kritischer, so wie in moralischer, wissenschaftlicher und administrativer Beziehung. Eine staatsarzneiwissenschaftliche Abhandlung*. Leipzig: Otto Wigand.

de Boor, Wolfgang. 1954b. *Psychiatrische Systematik: Ihre Entwicklung in Deutschland seit Kahlbaum*. Berlin: Springer. #

Dessoir, Max. 1902. *Geschichte der neueren deutschen Psychologie*. Berlin: Duncker. #

Diepgen, Paul. 1959. *Geschichte der Medizin: die historische Entwicklung der Heilkunde und des ärztlichen Lebens. Vol. 2/1: Von der Medizin der Aufklärung bis zur Begründung der Zellularpathologie (etwa 1740 - etwa 1858)*. 2 vols, 2nd ed. Berlin: Walter de Gruyter. #

Eschenmayer, Carl A. 1830a. *Mysterien des innern Lebens: erläutert aus der Geschichte der Seherin von Prevorst*. Tübingen: Zu-Guttenberg. #

Eschenmayer, Carl A. 1830b. Das verschleierte Bild zu Sais. In *Mysterien des innern Lebens: erläutert aus der Geschichte der Seherin von Prevorst*, ed. Carl A. Eschenmayer. Tübingen: Zu-Guttenberg.

Esquirol, Jean-Étienne Dominique. 1838. *Des maladies mentales: considérées sous les rapports médical, hygiénique et médico-légal*. Paris: Baillière.

Fischer, Kuno. 1872. *Geschichte der neueren Philosophie*. Heidelberg: Winter. #

Flemming, Carl Friedrich. 1879. Zwei Nekrologe: A. v. Zeller und Chr. Roller. *Allgemeine Zeitschrift für Psychiatrie* 35:117–124. *#|

Fluegel, John Carl. 1947. *Probleme und Ergebnisse der Psychologie: Hundert Jahre psychologischer Forschung*. Stuttgart: Klett. #

Gaupp, Robert. 1921. Ferdinand Autenrieth (1772-1835). In *Deutsche Irrenärzte: Einzelbilder ihres Lebens und Wirkens*, ed. Theodor Kirchhoff, vol. 1, 55–58. Berlin: J. Springer.

Gaupp, Robert. 1939. Ein zyklothymer Psychiater über seine seelischen Krankheitszeiten. *Zeitschrift für die gesamte Neurologie und Psychiatrie* 166:705–710. *#

Gaupp, Robert. 1940. Albert Zeller. *Schwäbische Lebensbilder* 1:574–582. *#

Georget, Étienne Jean. 1821. *De la physiologie du système nerveux et spécialement du cerveau: Recherches sur les maladies nerveuses en général et en particulier sur le siège, la nature et le traitement de l'hystérie, de l'hypochondrie, de l'épilepsie et de l'asthme convulsif.* Paris: Baillière.

Goethe, Johann Wolfgang. 1917 [1817]. Der Verfasser teilt die Geschichte seiner botanischen Studien mit. In *Sämtliche Werke*, 252–272. Leipzig: Insel.

Gottschick, Johann. 1955. *Die Leistungen des Nervensystems*. Jena: Fischer. #|

Gregor, Adalbert. 1921. Johann Christian Reil (1759-1813). In *Deutsche Irrenärzte: Einzelbilder ihres Lebens und Wirkens*, ed. Theodor Kirchhoff, 28–42. Berlin: J. Springer.

Griesinger, Wilhelm. 1843. Ueber psychische Reflexactionen. Mit einem Blick auf das Wesen der psychischen Krankheiten. *Archiv für physiologische Heilkunde* 2:76–113.

Griesinger, Wilhelm. 1844a. Neue Beiträge zur Physiologie und Pathologie des Gehirns. *Archiv für physiologische Heilkunde* 3:69–98.

Griesinger, Wilhelm. 1844b. [Rezension von] M. Jacobi: *Die Hauptformen der Seelenstörungen, in ihren Beziehungen zur Heilkunde nach der Beobachtung geschildert*. Erster Band: Die Tobsucht. *Archiv für physiologische Heilkunde* 3:278–296.

Griesinger, Wilhelm. 1845. *Die Pathologie und Therapie der psychischen Krankheiten*. Stuttgart: A. Krabbe. #

Griesinger, Wilhelm. 1867. Vortrag zur Eröffnung der psychiatrischen Klinik zu Berlin am 2. Mai 1867. *Archiv für Psychiatrie und Nervenkrankheiten* 1:143–158.

Griesinger, Wilhelm. 1872. In *Gesammelte Abhandlungen*, ed. C. A. Wunderlich. Berlin: Hirschwald. #|

Griesinger, Wilhelm. 1876. *Die Pathologie und Therapie der psychischen Krankheiten für Ärzte und Studierende*. 4th ed. Braunschweig: Wreden. #|

Gruhle, Hans Walter. 1932. Geschichtliches. In *Handbuch der Geisteskrankheiten*, ed. Oswald Bumke, vol. 9, 1–30. Berlin: Springer. #

Guislain, Joseph. 1826. *Traité sur l'aliénation mentale et sur les hospices des aliénés*, 2 vols. Amsterdam: J. Van der Hey et Fils.

Guislain, Joseph. 1833. *Traité sur les phrénopathies, ou doctrine nouv. des maladies mentales, basée sur des observations pratiques et statistiques, et l'étude des causes, de la nature, des symptomes, du pronostic, du diagnostic et du traitement de ces affections*. Bruxelles: Établiss. encyclographique.
Guislain, Joseph. 1838. *Abhandlung ueber die Phrenopathien oder neues System der Seelenstörungen, gegründet auf praktische und statistische Beobachtungen und Untersuchung der Ursachen, der Natur, der Symptome, der Prognose, der Diagnose und der Behandlung dieser Krankheiten. Mit einem Vorwort und Zusätzen von Dr. Zeller*. Translated by Wunderlich. Stuttgart: Rieger. *#
Guislain, Joseph. 1852. *Leçons orales sur les phrénopathies, ou Traité théorique et pratique des maladies mentales*. Ghent: L. Hebbelynck.
Guislain, Joseph. 1854. *Joseph Guislain's Klinische Vorträge über Geistes-Krankheiten*. Translated by Heinrich Laehr. Berlin: Hirschwald. #l
Haeser, Heinrich. 1881. *Geschichte der Medicin in der neueren Zeit*. Vol. 2. 3rd ed. Jena: Fischer. #
Hagen, Friedrich Wilhelm. 1870. Der Werth und die Bedeutung der Psychologie für die Psychiatrie. In *Studien auf dem Gebiete der ärztlichen Seelenkunde: gemeinfassliche Vorträge*, ed. Friedrich Wilhelm Hagen, 3–38. Erlangen: Besold. #
Haller, Johannes. 1950. *Die Epochen der deutschen Geschichte*. Stuttgart: Port Verlag.
Hartmann, Nicolai. 1923. *Die Philosophie des deutschen Idealismus*. Berlin: de Gruyter. #l
Hayner, Christian August Fürchtegott. 1817. *Aufforderung an Regierungen, Obrigkeiten und Vorsteher der Irrenhäuser zur Abstellung einiger schweren Gebrechen in der Behandlung der Irren*. Leipzig: Göschen.
Herbart, Johann Friedrich. 1816. *Lehrbuch der Psychologie*. Königsberg.
Herbart, Johann Friedrich. 1824/1825. *Psychologie als Wissenschaft*. Königsberg.
Herting, Johannes. 1921. Maximilian Jacobi, 1775-1858. In *Theodor Kirchhoff*, ed. Deutsche Irrenärzte, 83–94. Berlin: Springer.
Herting, Johannes. 1925. Die erste rheinische Irrenanstalt Siegburg: Eine geschichtliche Studie, unter Benutzung amtlicher Quellen zur 100jährigen Wiederkehr ihres Eröffnungstages 1. Januar 1825. *Allgemeine Zeitschrift für Psychiatrie* 81:163–241. #
Herting, Johannes. 1930. *Carl Wigand Maximilian Jacobi: Ein deutsche Arzt (1775–1858)*. Görlitz: C. A. Starke. #
Hirsch, August, ed. 1884–1887. *Biographisches Lexicon der hervorragenden Ärzte aller Zeiten und Völker*. Vienna, Leipzig: Urban & Schwarzenberg. #l
Hoche, Alfred Erich. 1912. Die Bedeutung der Symptomenkomplexe in der Psychiatrie. *Zeitschrift für die gesamte Neurologie und Psychiatrie* 12:540–551.
Hoffbauer, Johann Christoph. 1802. *Untersuchungen über die Krankheiten der Seele und die verwandten Zustände*. Halle: Hahn.
Hoffbauer, Johann Christoph. 1807. *Psychologische Untersuchungen über den Wahnsinn, die übrigen Arten der Verrückung und die Behandlung derselben*. Halle: Hahn.
Hoffbauer, Johann Christoph, and Johann Christian Reil, eds. 1808–1812. *Beyträge zur Beförderung einer Kurmethode auf psychischem Wege*. Halle: Curt.
Huch, Ricarda. 1951. *Die Romantik: Ausbreitung, Blütezeit und Verfall*. Tübingen: Wunderlich. #l
Ideler, Carl Ludwig. 1895. Carl Wilhelm Ideler und seine Stellung in der Entwicklung der Psychiatrie. *Allgemeine Zeitschrift für Psychiatrie* 51:851–883. #
Jacobi, Maximilian, ed. 1825. *Sammlungen für die Heilkunde der Gemütskrankheiten*. Elberfeld: Schönian. #
Jacobi, Maximilian, ed. 1830. *Beobachtungen über die Pathologie und Therapie der mit Irreseyn verbundenen Krankheiten*. Elberfeld: Schönian. #l
Jacobi, Maximilian, ed. 1844. *Die Hauptformen der Seelenstörungen*. Leipzig: Weidmann. #
Jacobi, Maximilian, ed. 1856. *Auswahl geistlicher Lieder für Privaterbauung*. Bonn: Marcus. #l
Jaspers, Karl. 1948. *Allgemeine Psychopathologie*. 5th ed. Berlin: Springer. #
Kahlbaum, Karl. 1863. *Die Gruppierung der psychischen Krankheiten und die Einteilung der Seelenstörungen*. Danzig: A. W. Kafemann. #

Kant, Immanuel. 1956. *Kritik der reinen Vernunft*. Hamburg: Felix Meiner. †
Kerner, Justinus. 1830. Zur Geschichte des Geistersehens der Seherin von Prevorst. In *Mysterien des innern Lebens: erläutert aus der Geschichte der Seherin von Prevorst*, ed. Carl A. Eschenmayer, 84–97. Tübingen: Zu-Guttenberg.
Kerner, Justinus. 1957. *Das Bilderbuch aus meiner Knabenzeit*. Leipzig: Koehler & Amelang. #I
Kerner, Justinus. 1958. *Die Seherin von Prevorst*. Stuttgart: J. F. Steinkopf. #I
Kierkegaard, Søren. 1844. *Der Begriff Angst*. Leipzig: Fr. Richter.
Kirchhoff, Theodor. 1912. Geschichte der Psychiatrie. In *Handbuch der Psychiatrie, Allgemeiner Teil, 4. Abschnitt*, ed. Gustav Aschaffenburg. Leipzig and Vienna: Deuticke. #
Kirchhoff, Theodor. 1921a/1924. *Deutsche Irrenärzte: Einzelbilder ihres Lebens und Wirkens*. 2 vols. Berlin: J. Springer. #
Kirchhoff, Theodor. 1921b. Wilhelm Griesinger. In *Deutsche Irrenärzte: Einzelbilder ihres Lebens und Wirkens*, vol. 1, 1–14. Berlin: J. Springer.
Kluckhohn, Paul. 1953. *Das Ideengut der deutschen Romantik*. Tübingen: Niemeyer. #
Kolle, Kurt. 1956–1963. *Grosse Nervenärzte*. 3 vols. Stuttgart: Thieme. #I
Kornfeld, Sigmund. 1905. Geschichte der Psychiatrie. In *Handbuch der Geschichte der Medizin*, ed. Max Neuburger and Julius Pagel, vol. 3, 601–728. Jena: Fischer. #
Kraepelin, Emil. 1883. *Compendium der Psychiatrie: Zum Gebrauche für Studirende und Aerzte*. Leipzig: Abel.
Kraepelin, Emil. 1918. Hundert Jahre Psychiatrie: Ein Beitrag zur Geschichte menschlicher Gesittung. *Zeitschrift für die gesamte Neurologie und Psychiatrie* 38:161–275. #
Kretschmer, Ernst. 1919. Über psychogene Wahnbildungen bei traumatischer Hirnschwäche. *Zeitschrift für die gesamte Neurologie und Psychiatrie - Originalien* 45 (3/4): 272–300. #
Kretschmer, Ernst. 1936. *Körperbau und Charakter: Untersuchungen zum Konstitutions-Problem und zur Lehre von den Temperamenten*, 11th and 12th ed. Berlin: Springer. †
Kreuser, Heinrich. 1885. *Die Königliche Heil- und Pflegeanstalt Winnenthal. Fünfzigjähriger Anstaltsbericht*. Tübingen: Fuess. #I
Kreuser, Heinrich. 1904b. Zu Albert Zellers Gedächtnis. *Medicinisches Correspondenz-Blatt des Würtembergischen Ärztlichen Vereins* 74:935–939. *#
Kronfeld, Arthur. 1928. Einige Bemerkungen über die ersten psychotherapeutischen Veröffentlichungen insbesondere J. C. Reil. *Allgemeine Zeitschrift für Psychotherapie* 1:46–51. #
Kuhn, Roland. 1957. Griesingers Auffassung der psychischen Krankheiten und seine Bedeutung für die weitere Entwicklung der Psychiatrie. In *Beiträge zur Geschichte der Psychiatrie und Hirnanatomie*, ed. Alfred Glaus, vol. 100, 41–67. Basel: Karger. #
Laehr, Hans. 1921. Johann Gottfried Langermann, 1768-1832. In *Deutsche Irrenärzte*, ed. Theodor Kirchhoff, 42–51. Berlin: Springer.
Laehr, Heinrich. 1893. *Gedenktage der Psychiatrie und ihre Hilfswissenschaften in allen Ländern*. 4th ed. Berlin: G. Reimer. #
Laignel, M., and Jean Vinchon. 1930. *Les malades de l'esprit et leur médecins du 16e au 19e siècle*. Paris: Maloine. #
Lang. 1878. *Zur Todesfeier und zum Gedächtnis des Ober-Med. Rats Dr. A. v. Zeller*. Grabrede. #I
Leibbrand, Werner. 1937. *Romantische Medizin*. Hamburg: H. Goverts.
Leibbrand, Werner. 1956. *Die spekulative Medizin der Romantik*. Hamburg: Claassen. #I
Llopis, Bartolomé. 1960b. Das allen Psychosen gemeinsame Achsensyndrom. *Fortschritte der Neurologie und Psychiatrie* 28 (2): 106–129. #
Meuret, Gustav. 1879. *Dr. Albert Zeller: Blätter der Erinnerung*. Stuttgart: Steinkopf. #I
Müller, Ernst. 1960. Forschung, Erziehung und Lehre untersucht nach den Druckschriften der Carlsschule. In *Die Hohe Carlsschule [Ausstellungskatalog]*. Stuttgart: Turmhaus. #
Neuburger, Max. 1913. *Johann Christian Reil*. Stuttgart: Enke. #I
Neumann, Heinrich. 1847. *Der Arzt und die Blödsinnigkeits-Erklärung*. Breslau: Gosohorsky. I
Neumann, Heinrich. 1859. *Lehrbuch der Psychiatrie*. Erlangen: Enke. #
Paulus, H. E. G. 1830. Die Unterleibs-Kranke zu Weinsberg, vornehmer genannt: Die Seherin von Prevorst. *Sophronizon* 12 (2): 22–90. #I
Pelman, Carl. 1912. *Erinnerungen eines alten Irrenarztes*. Bonn: Friedrich Cohen. #I

Pflüger, Eduard Friedrich, and Wilhelm. 1853. *Die sensorischen Functionen des Rückenmarks der Wirbelthiere: Nebst einer neuen Lehre über die Leitungsgesetze der Reflexionen*. Berlin: Hirschwald.
Reil, Johann Christian. 1910 [1795]. *Von der Lebenskraft*. Leipzig: Johann Ambrosius Barth. #
Reil, Johann Christian. 1968. *Rhapsodieen über die Anwendung der psychischen Curmethode auf Geisteszerrüttungen*. Halle: Curt, 1803; reprint. Amsterdam: Bonset. #
Reil, Johann Christian. 1805. *Über die Erkenntnis und Kur der Fieber*. Vol. 4. 2nd ed. Halle: Curt. #
Reil, Johann Christian. 1807. Über die Eigenschaften des Ganglien-Systems und sein Verhältniss zum Cerebral-System. *Archiv für Physiologie* 7 (2): 189–254. #
Reil, Johann Christian. 1811. Anhang über die Organisation der Versorgungsanstalten für unheilbare Irrende. In *Joseph Mason Cox: Praktische Bemerkungen über Geisteszerrüttungen*. Halle: Renger. #
Reimer, Hermann. 1856. Zur Kompression der Karotiden bei Epilepsie. *Deutsche Klinik* 8 (24): 251–252. #I
Reimer, Hermann. 1878. Königin Johanna die Wahnsinnige und ihre Nachkommen. *Im Neuen Reich* 8 (1): 561–578. #I
Reimer, Hermann. 1889. *Handbuch der speciellen Klimatotherapie und Balneotherapie mit besonderer Rücksicht auf Mittel-Europa: zum Gebrauch für Aerzte*. Berlin: Reimer. #I
Reimer, Hermann. 1894. *Zweierlei Hoheit: Roman von Juvenalis minor*. Zürich: n.p. #
Reimer, Hermann. 1895. *Klimatische Winterkurorte: Leitfaden für Ärzte und Laien*. 4th ed. Berlin: G. Reimer. #I
Reimer, Hermann. 1897. *Klimatische Sommerkurorte: Leitfaden für Ärzte und Laien*. 3rd ed. Berlin: G. Reimer. #I
Reimer, Hermann. 1869. *Klimatische Winterkurorte mit besonderer Rücksicht auf die Winterstationen der Schweiz, Tirols, Oberitaliens und des südlichen Frankreichs: Ein Leitfaden für Aerzte u. Laien*. Berlin: Reimer. I
Reimersche Familienkalender. 1928. Berlin. #I
Roller, Christian Friedrich Wilhelm. 1845. Zeller's Aufsätze in Ersch und Gruber allgemeiner Encyclopädie. *Allgemeine Zeitschrift für Psychiatrie* 2 (4): 736–738.
Roller, Theodor. 1924. *Georg Andreas Reimer und sein Kreis: Zur Geschichte des politischen Denkens in Deutschland um die Zeit der Befreiungskriege*. Berlin: Weidmann. #I
Schiller, Friedrich. 1959a. *Medizinische Schriften: eine Buchgabe der Deutschen Hoffmann-LaRoche AG aus Anlaß des 200. Geburtstages des Dichters, 10. November 1959*. Berlin: Fischer. #
Schiller, Friedrich. 1959b [1779]. Philosophie der Physiologie. In *Friedrich Schiller: Medizinische Schriften. Eine Buchausgabe der Deutschen Hoffmann-La Roche AG aus Anlaß des 200. Geburtstages des Dichters*, 37–62. Miesbach: W. F. Mayr.
Schiller, Friedrich. 1959c [1780]. De discrimine febrium inflammatoriarum et putridarum. In *Friedrich Schiller: Medizinische Schriften. Eine Buchausgabe der Deutschen Hoffmann-La Roche AG aus Anlaß des 200. Geburtstages des Dichters*, 63–134. Miesbach: W. F. Mayr.
Schiller, Friedrich. 1959d [1780]. Versuch über den Zusammenhang der thierischen Natur des Menschen mit seiner geistigen. In *Friedrich Schiller: Medizinische Schriften. Eine Buchausgabe der Deutschen Hoffmann-La Roche AG aus Anlaß des 200. Geburtstages des Dichters*, 135–180. Miesbach: W. F. Mayr.
Schleich, Gustav. 1910. *Ein Stück aus der Geschichte der medizinischen Fakultät der Universität Tübingen*. Tübingen: University of Tübingen. #
Schleiermacher, Friedrich. 1834. *Über die Religion: Reden an die Gebildeten unter ihren Verächtern*. 4th ed. Stuttgart: Hausmann. #I
Schleiermacher, Friedrich. 1843. *Predigten*. Berlin: Reimer. #I
Schleiermacher, Friedrich. 1860. *Aus Schleiermachers Leben in Briefen*. 2nd ed. Berlin: Reimer. #I
Schleiermacher, Friedrich. 1869. *Monologen: Eine Neujahrsgabe*. Leipzig: Brockhaus. #I

Schopenhauer, Arthur. 1860 [1840]. Über die Freiheit des menschlichen Willens. In *Die beiden Grundprobleme der Ethik, behandelt in zwei akademischen Preisschriften*, 3–106. Leipzig: Brockhaus.
Sigerist, Henry E. 1932. *Grosse Ärzte: Eine Geschichte der Heilkunde in Lebensbilder*. Munich: Lehmann. #
Sioli, Franz. 1921. Friedrich Nasse, 1778-1851. In *Deutsche Irrenärzte: Einzelbilder ihres Lebens und Wirkens*, ed. Theodor Kirchhoff, 105–117. Berlin: Springer.
Snell, Ludwig Daniel, and Christian. 1865. Über Monomanie als primäre Form der Seelenstörung. *Allgemeine Zeitschrift für Psychiatrie und psychisch-gerichtliche Medizin* 22:368–381. #
Spurzheim, Johann Caspar. 1817. *Observations on the deranged manifestations of the mind, or insanity*. London: Baldwin, Cradock and Joy.
Stahl, Georgii Ernesti. 1708. *Theoria Medica Vera*. Hallae: Orphanotropheum.
Stahl, Georgii Ernesti. 1831–1832. *Georg Ernst Stahl's Theorie der Heilkunde*, translated by Carl Wilhelm Ideler, 3 vols. Berlin: Enslin.
Stickler, Georg. 1939/1940. Wunderlich, Roser, Griesinger: 'Die drei Schwäbischen Reformatoren der Medizin'. *Sudhoffs Archiv* 32: 217–274 and 33: 1–54. #
Stickler, Georg. 1941. Karl August Wunderlich. In *Schwäbische Lebensbilder*, vol. 2. Stuttgart: Kohlhammer. #l
Stübler, Eberhard. 1948. *Johann Heinrich Ferdinand v. Autenrieth (1772-1835)*. Stuttgart: Schröder. #
Sudhoff, Karl, and Julius Leopold Pagel. 1922. *Kurzes Handbuch der Geschichte der Medizin*. 4th ed. Berlin: Karger. #l
Verwey, Gerlof. 1985b. *Psychiatry in an anthropological and biomedical context: Philosophical presuppositions and implications of German psychiatry, 1820–1870*. Dordrecht: Reidel. †
Vorkastner, Willy, and Pophal. 1924. Rudolf Gottfried Arndt 1835-1900. In *Deutsche Irrenärzte*, ed. Theodor Kirchhoff, vol. 2, 138–142. Berlin: J. Springer.
von Aster, Ernst. 1932. *Geschichte der Philosophie*. Leipzig: Kröner. #
von Autenrieth, Johann Heinrich Ferdinand. 1801–1802. *Handbuch der empirischen menschlichen Physiologie*. 3 vols. Tübingen: Heerbrandt. #
von Autenrieth, Johann Heinrich Ferdinand. 1807. Bemerkungen über die Verschiedenheit beider Geschlechter und ihrer Zeugungsorgane, als Beytrag zu einer Theorie der Anatomie. *Archiv für die Physiologie* 7 (1): 1–139.
von Autenrieth, Johann Heinrich Ferdinand. 1834–1835. *Specielle Nosologie und Therapie. Nach dem Systeme eines berühmten deutschen Arztes und Professors*, ed. Carl Ludwig Reinhard, 2 vols. Würzburg: Etlinger. #
von Autenrieth, Johann Heinrich Ferdinand. 1836a. Verbindung der Seele mit dem organischen Körper: Entwicklung des Charakters der Persönlichkeit in der Reihe der Wesen. In *Ansichten über Natur- und Seelenleben*, ed. Johann Heinrich Ferdinand von Autenrieth, 345–396. Stuttgart: Cotta.
von Autenrieth, Johann Heinrich Ferdinand. 1836b. *Ansichten über Natur- und Seelenleben*. Stuttgart: Cotta. #
von Mohl, Robert. 1902. *Lebens-Erinnerungen von Robert von Mohl (1799-1875)*. Stuttgart: DVA. #
von Nostiz und Jänckendorf, G. A. E. 1829. *Beschreibung der königl. Sächsischen Heil- und Pflegeanstalt Sonnenstein mit Bemerkungen über Anstalten für Herstellung oder Verwahrung der Geisteskranken*. 3 vols. Dresden: Walther. #l
von Zeller, Johann Friedrich. 1831. *Freier Mann, freies Gut! Oder ein Vorschlag zu einem Vergleich, durch die Verwandlung der Zehenten, Grund- und Boden-Gefälle und überhaupt jeder sogenannten Feudal-Last, in ablösbare Geld-Renten, im Königreich Würtemberg*. Stuttgart: Munder. #l
Walther, Luise, Hanns Wolfgang Rath, and Friedrich Walther. 1923. *Aus Mörikes Kreis und Stuttgarter Zeit: 150 Charakterköpfe in bisher meist unveröff. Schattenbildern*. Ludwigsburg: Schulz. #l
Weller, Karl. 1957. *Württembergische Geschichte*. Stuttgart: Silberburg-Verlag. #l

Westphal, Carl. 1868. Nekrolog. Nach einer Rede gehalten zur Gedenkfeier für Griesinger. *Archiv für Psychiatrie und Nervenkrankheiten* 1:760–774. #

Wunderlich, Carl August. 1839. *Die Nosologie des Typhus: Eine Beleuchtung der wichtigsten Ansichten über dieselbe*. Stuttgart: Rieger.

Wunderlich, Carl August. 1859. *Geschichte der Medizin: Vorlesungen gehalten im Sommersemester 1858*. Stuttgart: Ebner & Seubert. #

Wunderlich, Carl August. 1869. Wilhelm Griesinger: Nekrolog. *Archiv für Heilkunde* 10:113–150. #

Zeller, Albert. *Versuch über den Consens der inneren Organe und Systeme, 1824*. Berlin: Albert Zeller Papers. *

Zeller, Albert. 1826. *Untersuchungen über die Einwirkung verschiedener Stoff des organischen und anorganischen Reiches auf das Leben der Pflanzen*. University of Tübingen. *#

Zeller, Albert. *Studientagebücher, 1824-1827*. Berlin: Albert Zeller Papers, Privatbesitz. *

Zeller, Albert. 1830. *Das verschleierte Bild zu Sais oder die Wunder des Magnetismus von einem Freunde der Wahrheit*. Leipzig: Weidmann. *#

Zeller, Albert. 1834. Mitteilungen über die neu errichtete Irrenheilanstalt Winnenthal. *Medicinisches Correspondenz-Blatt des Würtembergischen Ärztlichen Vereins* 3 (5/14): 34–36, 108. †

Zeller, Albert. 1837. [Erster] Bericht über die Heilanstalt Winnenthal von ihrer Eröffnung, den 1. März 1834 bis zum 28. Februar 1837. *Medicinisches Correspondenz-Blatt des Würtembergischen Ärztlichen Vereins* 7:321–335. *#

Zeller, Albert. 1838. Ueber einige Hauptpunkte in der Erforschung und Heilung der Seelenstörungen. *Zeitschrift für die Beurteilung und Heilung der krankhaften Seelenzustände* 1 (3): 515–569. |

Zeller, Albert. 1840. Zweiter Bericht über die Wirksamkeit Heilanstalt Winnenthal von ihrer Eröffnung, den 1. März 1837 bis zum 29. Februar 1840. *Medicinisches Correspondenz-Blatt des Würtembergischen Ärztlichen Vereins* 10:129–147. *#

Zeller, Albert. 1843. [Dritter] Dreijähriger Bericht über die Wirksamkeit der Heilanstalt Winnenthal vom 1. März 1840 bis zum 28. Februar 1843. *Medicinisches Correspondenz-Blatt des Würtembergischen Ärztlichen Vereins* 13 (38–39): 297–310. #

Zeller, Albert. 1844. [Dritter] Bericht über die Wirksamkeit Heilanstalt Winnenthal von ihrer Eröffnung, den 1. März 1840 bis zum 28. Februar 1843. *Allgemeine Zeitschrift für Psychiatrie* 1:1–79. *

Zeller, Albert. 1845a. Irre, Irren, Irrereden, Irrwahn. In *Allgemeine Encyklopädie der Wissenschaften und Künste, Sect. 2, Th. 24*, ed. J. S. Ersch and J. G. Gruber. Leipzig: Brockhaus. *#

Zeller, Albert. 1845b. Irrenanstalten, Irrenhäuser. In *Allgemeine Encyklopädie der Wissenschaften und Künste, Sect. 2, Th. 24*, ed. J. S. Ersch and J. G. Gruber. Leipzig: Brockhaus. *#

Zeller, Albert. 1847. *Lieder des Leids*. Berlin: Reimer. #|

Zeller, Albert. 1848a. [Vierter] Bericht über die Wirksamkeit Heilanstalt Winnenthal, vom 1. März 1843 bis 28. Februar 1846. *Allgemeine Zeitschrift für Psychiatrie* 5:163–209.

Zeller, Albert. 1848b. [Vierter] dreijähriger Bericht über die Wirksamkeit Heilanstalt Winnenthal von ihrer Eröffnung, den 1. März 1843 bis zum 28. Februar 1846. *Medicinisches Correspondenz-Blatt des Würtembergischen Ärztlichen Vereins* 18:9–20. *#

Zeller, Albert. 1850. *Sprüche und Lieder*. Heidelberg. #|

Zeller, Albert. 1854. [Fünfter] Bericht über die Wirksamkeit Heilanstalt Winnenthal von ihrer Eröffnung, den 1. März 1846 bis zum 28. Februar 1854. *Medicinisches Correspondenz-Blatt des Würtembergischen Ärztlichen Vereins* 24:297–318. *#

Zeller, Albert. 1855. [Fünfter] Bericht über die Wirksamkeit Heilanstalt Winnenthal vom 1. März 1846 bis 28. Februar 1854. *Allgemeine Zeitschrift für Psychiatrie* 12 (4): 693–700.

Zeller, Albert. 1887. *Lieder des Leids*. 7th ed. Berlin: Reimer. #|

Zeller, Albert. 1901. *Trost und Rat*. Basel: R. Reich. #|

Zeller, Gerhart. 1957. *Albert Zeller im Lichte der modernen Psychiatrie*. Ein Vortrag. #|

Zeller, Gerhart. 1968b. Welcher psychiatrischen Schule hat Wilhelm Griesinger angehört? *Deutsches Medizinisches Journal* 19:328–334. †

Zeller, Gerhart. 1969b. Bonhoeffers wissenschaftliches Werk. Entwicklung und Bedeutung. In *Karl Bonhoeffer: Zum hundertsten Geburtstag am 31. März 1968*, ed. Erwin Straus von Jürg Zutt and H. Scheller. Berlin: Springer. †

Zeller, Gerhart. 1972b. Die Tübinger Psychiater-Schule. In *Wahn*, ed. Schulte von Walter and Rainer Tölle, 95–104. Stuttgart: Georg Thieme. †

Zeller, Gerhart. 1981. Von der Heilanstalt zur Heil- und Pflegeanstalt: Ein Beitrag zur Geschichte des psychiatrischen Krankenhauswesens. *Fortschritte der Neurologie und Psychiatrie* 49:121–127. †

Zeller, Gerhart. 1998. Hat das psychiatrische Reformprogramm Wilhelm Griesingers aus dem Jahr 1868 heute noch eine Bedeutung? In *Rehabilitationspsychiatrie*, ed. Jürgen-Helmut Mauthe. Stuttgart: Enke. †

Zeller, Gerhart. 2007. *Albert Zellers medizinisches Tagebuch der psychiatrischen Reise durch Deutschland, England, Frankreich und nach Prag von 1832 bis 1833*. 2 vols. Zwiefalten: Psychiatrie und Geschichte. †

Zeller, Hermann. 1921. Ernst Albert Zeller. In *Deutsche Irrenärzte: Einzelbilder ihres Lebens und Wirkens*, ed. Theodor Kirchhoff, 208–218. Berlin: J. Springer. *#

Zilboorg, Gregory. 1941. *A history of medical psychology*. New York: Norton. #

Index

G. Zeller et al., *A History of Unitary Psychosis*, Theory and History in the Human and Social Sciences, https://doi.org/10.1007/978-3-031-90182-9

Z

The manufacturer's authorised representative in the EU is Springer Nature Customer Service Centre GmbH, Europaplatz 3, 69115 Heidelberg, Germany. If you have any concerns regarding our products, please contact ProductSafety@springernature.com

Printed and bound by CPI Group (UK) Ltd, Croydon, CR0 4YY

01/10/2026

02225849-0001